The Good Doctors

The Good Doctors

The Medical Committee for Human Rights
and the Struggle for Social Justice in Health Care

JOHN DITTMER

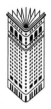

BLOOMSBURY PRESS

New York　Berlin　London

Published by Bloomsbury Press, New York

All papers used by Bloomsbury Press are natural, recyclable products made from
wood grown in well-managed forests. The manufacturing processes conform to the
environmental regulations of the country of origin.

LIBRARY OF CONGRESS CATALOGING-IN-PUBLICATION DATA

Dittmer, John, 1939–
The good doctors : the medical committee for human rights and the struggle for
social justice in health care / John Dittmer.—1st ed.
p. cm.
ISBN-13: 978-1-59691-567-1
ISBN-10: 1-59691-567-6
1. Social medicine—United States. 2. Right to health care—United States.
3. Civil rights movements—United States. 4. African American
physicians—Southern States. I. Title.

RA418.3.U6D58 2009
362.1097509'046—dc22
2008042878

First U.S. Edition 2009

1 3 5 7 9 10 8 6 4 2

Typeset by Westchester Book Group
Printed in the United States of America by Quebecor World Fairfield

For Craig and Caitlin, and Grace and Rose

Contents

Preface

Of all the forms of inequality, injustice in health
care is the most shocking and inhumane.

—Martin Luther King Jr.[1]

In the fall of 1979, veterans of the civil rights movement gathered on
the campus of historically black Tougaloo College for a conference
to celebrate the fifteenth anniversary of Mississippi's Freedom
Summer—a time when nearly a thousand volunteers, most of them
northern white college students, came down to work with local black activists in voter registration projects and freedom schools in communities
across the state. The opening assembly took place in Woodworth Chapel,
the scene of inspirational mass meetings in the 1960s. Outside, on the
chapel steps, the college physician, Robert Smith, was handing out leaflets
protesting the failure of the conference's organizers to include a session on
the Medical Committee for Human Rights (MCHR), an organization he
had helped found. I had been on the faculty at Tougaloo for a dozen years
and was only vaguely aware of the Medical Committee. Fifteen years
later, in the spring of 1994, I was invited to participate in the thirtieth anniversary commemoration. I had just completed a book on the black freedom struggle in Mississippi, whose solitary paragraph on the work of
MCHR contained two errors of fact. This time there was a session on the
Medical Committee—Dr. Smith had been persistent—and out of curios-
ity I joined the audience in the basement of the Tougaloo library. The

panel consisted of men and women who had played a key part in MCHR's work in the South, including Tom Levin, Alvin Poussaint, and Josephine Martin. Their stories were fascinating and opened my eyes to a whole new chapter of the civil rights movement. I realized then that I had given the Medical Committee short shrift. This book, I suppose, is in part an act of atonement.

Begun in the summer of 1964 as an ad hoc support group for the volunteers and veteran activists, the Medical Committee for Human Rights became a permanent organization of health care professionals with chapters in major cities across the country. MCHR provided medical care for civil rights workers in the South, desegregated area hospitals, and picketed at conventions of the American Medical Association to protest the AMA's refusal to require its southern affiliates to admit black physicians. In the late sixties and early seventies MCHR moved on to support causes associated with the New Left, including opposition to the war in Vietnam. Its local chapters developed task forces to deal with problems ranging from prison reform to occupational health and safety.

The history of MCHR provides insight into the internal dynamics of the social reform movements of that era. Most of the organization's founders were established Jewish physicians, the children of Eastern European immigrants. Born and raised in New York City, they were active in groups associated with what would later be called the Old Left. Several of them had been or still were members of the Communist Party. The second wave of health care activists became politically involved as medical and nursing students in the mid-1960s, influenced by the egalitarian platform of the Students for a Democratic Society (SDS). While there were periods of tension, the Medical Committee was unique in that Old and New Left radicals bridged generational and ideological gaps to march together under the banner "Health Care Is a Human Right."

Although its first three chairpersons were black, the Medical Committee was essentially a white organization. The successful efforts of these privileged, older white professionals to reach out to dedicated, angry young black militants adds a new dimension to our understanding of the struggle for civil rights in the South. And their attempts—most of them unsuccessful—to forge alliances with black physicians in the National Medical Association demonstrate the limits of interracial cooperation during a time of social upheaval.

There was something Zelig-like about the Medical Committee. Wherever there was a demonstration or confrontation, be it at the Edmund

Pettus Bridge outside Selma or on the Meredith March in the South, in Resurrection City with the Poor People's Campaign, at Columbia University during the student rebellion, in the streets of Chicago outside the Democratic National Convention in 1968, or at Wounded Knee with the American Indian Movement, men and women in white coats and Red Cross armbands were on the scene, providing "medical presence" and assistance to the people who were putting themselves at risk. Viewing these historic events from the perspective of health care professionals enhances our understanding of that turbulent era.

Throughout it all, Medical Committee activists were in agreement that health care in the United States was inadequate, unjust, racist, and in need of a major overhaul. MCHR members established free health clinics in inner cities and created the model for the comprehensive community health center. They also campaigned for a national health service that would provide quality care for everyone. Indeed, what is striking about the debates over national health insurance then and now is the degree to which the problems, the issues, and the arguments have remained unchanged. For more than four decades, MCHR alumni have been activists in the struggle to democratize the American health care system.

Finally, a word about the title. I do not mean for it to be taken ironically. Although this book records many examples of naïveté, wrongheadedness, and ego-tripping (among other shortcomings), I admire these "good" doctors for who they were and are, and for what they have done and are still doing. As for "doctors," think of the broader dictionary definition, that of "medical practitioner." Most MCHR members were physicians, but many were not, and their contributions, particularly those of the nurses working in the South, were significant, to say the least. And while the Medical Committee for Human Rights is at the center of this study, other organizations and individuals played an important role in the postwar movement to provide a health care system for all Americans based on egalitarian principles, free from discrimination by race or social class. These activists saw firsthand the debilitating impact of racism and poverty on the delivery of medical services, and they worked relentlessly to right these wrongs.

Two Roads to Atlantic City

O n June 17, 1963, Robert Smith boarded a Delta flight in Jackson wearing a borrowed blue suit and his brother's dress shoes. The twenty-six-year-old African American doctor was bound for Atlantic City to join a small group of health care professionals who were protesting the racially discriminatory practices of the American Medical Association. The AMA was holding its annual convention at the New Jersey resort, and to get there Smith had to fly down to New Orleans, change planes for Philadelphia, and then take a bus to Atlantic City. The Philadelphia flight was delayed, and he missed the last bus. Bob Smith spent the night curled up on a bench in the terminal, looking like a well-dressed hobo, and hoping the early morning bus would get him to the boardwalk on time.

That evening, New York physician Walter Lear and a half-dozen other health care activists were gathering at an Atlantic City hotel. Lear became concerned when the man from Mississippi did not appear. "We waited and we waited, and I was getting close to hysterical because my vision of this was that Bob Smith *had* to be on that picket line. He was not there. Well, finally about seven o'clock in the morning he arrived at the hotel and of course we were very delighted to see him."[1]

The ninth of twelve children, Bob Smith grew up on a cattle farm in Terry, Mississippi, twenty miles south of the capital in Jackson. His father, Joe, a livestock dealer and farmer, liked to say that he was "descended from a tramp." After the Civil War, Bob's grandfather, John Smith, was a sharecropper on a Delta plantation. At the end of one season, while set-tling up he saw he was being cheated, said so, and words led to blows. Once the reality set in that black men did not question white economics in the Delta—let alone fight for their rights—young Smith jumped on a slow-moving freight he assumed was headed north to the Promised Land. But the train was going south (shades of *Huckleberry Finn*), and after two hours he disembarked in Terry because he was getting hungry.[2]

Terry proved to be a good jumping-off place. The land, with its green, gently rolling hills, dense woods, and ponds full of fish, stands in sharp contrast to the piney woods of South Mississippi and the flat expanse of the Delta to the north. During Reconstruction, an interval between the horrors of slavery and the imposition of a rigid caste system, a few enter-prising blacks established themselves as independent farmers in the coun-tryside around the hamlet of Terry. Earning money by doing odd jobs, Smith soon began to acquire land, which he left to his son Joe, who be-came one of the most successful black farmers in the county, owning more than two hundred acres.

The Smith family lived in a big house on a self-contained farm, grow-ing vegetables and raising chickens, hogs, and cows. Bob's mother came from a family of devout Christians and was a student at Jackson State College when she married Joe Smith. By the time Bob was born, half his siblings had grown up and left home. One of his two sisters got married and moved to Minneapolis, where he would later spend his summers. Four brothers had served overseas in the armed forces during World War II, and all came back to live in Mississippi. If not idyllic, his early child-hood was filled with good times and adventure. With three older brothers at home, he did not need to plow behind a mule or perform other field chores. His mother taught the youngest three boys to do housework, and Bob helped her with the cooking. He had time to roam the fields, fish, play with his friends (several of whom were his nieces and nephews), and accompany his father on his rounds.

The Smith children attended the all-black public school in Terry, where four teachers taught all eight grades. They were strict disciplinari-ans. "Reading and doing arithmetic were requirements for not being hit." Although one of the teachers was his cousin and the other three were members of his church, Bob was not a model student. He always did well in his subjects and mastered them quickly, but then he grew bored. "I was always a nuisance in grade school," he recalls. "I was always picking on teachers and other students."

He flirted with the idea of becoming a musician, but gave up the piano at age fifteen because he could not play by ear. Bob then decided on a career in medicine, and after that he never seriously considered any other line of work. He received encouragement from a Jewish physician, a Dr. Kahn, who worked for the Veterans Administration and hunted birds with his father. When Kahn retired, he gave Bob his medical books. The Smith family physician was a good white doctor from Crystal Springs named Eubanks, whom Joe Smith took into rural areas to see black patients.

While in his teens Bob took up the family business raising prize beef cattle, winning the grand prize and a substantial cash award at a regional (segregated) 4-H Club competition. He joined the New Farmers of America (the black version of the Future Farmers of America) in high school and became a national officer his senior year. At the group's annual convention in Atlanta he introduced Mayor William B. Hartsfield to the assembled delegates. The following year in Washington he met President Dwight Eisenhower while touring the White House with an NFA delegation. Bob's travels and experiences outside the state set him apart from most Mississippi youths, black or white.

Smith came of age in Jim Crow America. At home, his father did everything he could to protect his children from the worst ravages of racism. He refused to let Bob do odd jobs for white people because "if you go down there and get into trouble, or if something comes up missing, I can't do a thing for you." Joe Smith did not allow his children to go to segregated movie theaters in Jackson or to patronize Jim Crow restaurants. "I can't ever remember as a child having something handed to me through a window," Bob recalls. As a result, the young farm boy did not get to know many white people, nor did he have white friends as playmates. Yet he knew about racism. "Everything was separate. White kids on the bus, throwing things at you, you couldn't help but be aware."

Upon his graduation from high school in 1953 it was a foregone conclusion that Bob would enroll at Tougaloo College. The small liberal arts institution, founded in the aftermath of the Civil War by the American Missionary Association on a cotton plantation north of Jackson, was the only black school in the state to offer a true premed program. A number of its faculty came from leading institutions of higher learning, including Bob's mentor, St. Elmo Brady, the first African American to receive a Ph.D. in chemistry. In keeping with its missionary tradition, Tougaloo had always had a white president, and a majority of its faculty members were white as well. Simply existing as an interracial college in a state best known as a bastion of white supremacy was no small achievement. Tougaloo's reputation as an open institution, however, would be severely tested in the 1950s.

On May 17, 1954, Chief Justice Earl Warren spoke for a unanimous U.S. Supreme Court when he wrote that "separate educational facilities are inherently unequal." Mississippi senator James O. Eastland spoke for the majority of his white constituents when he warned that "the South will not abide by nor obey this legislative decision of a political court . . . We will take whatever steps are necessary to retain segregation in education." The impact of *Brown v. Board of Education* extended far beyond the question of the future of the public schools. For Mississippi whites the Supreme Court decision had been a wake-up call, and preserving the "southern way of life" soon assumed all the trappings of a holy crusade. Black leaders, believing that the federal government had at long last come down firmly on the side of racial justice, pushed voter registration campaigns as well as school desegregation. Things were deceptively quiet for the rest of 1954, but when the court handed down its implementation decision in early 1955, the Citizens' Council, an organization of white business, political, and professional leaders that was, in the words of newspaper editor Hodding Carter II, an "uptown Ku Klux Klan," used economic intimidation and threats of violence to crush NAACP efforts to desegregate any public schools. (Not until the fall of 1964, ten years after *Brown*, would the first public elementary schools be integrated in Mississippi.) Using similar tactics, the Citizens' Council retaliated against all kinds of black leaders, including prominent health care professionals.[3]

In the post–World War II decade, physicians and dentists were at the forefront of black protest activity in Mississippi. Emmett J. Stringer, a Columbus dentist, is a case in point. A World War II veteran and graduate of Meharry Dental School, Stringer opened his practice in 1950 and organized the Columbus branch of the NAACP three years later. Under Stringer's leadership, in little over a year more than four hundred blacks had joined the local branch, making it the largest in the state. In 1953 the young activist was elected president of the NAACP State Conference of Branches, but after the *Brown* decision Stringer's life became a nightmare. Banks, once eager to extend credit, now refused to loan him money, and his automobile insurance was canceled. Stringer's dental practice declined. Former patients stopped him on the street to explain that their white employers were insisting they patronize another dentist. Stringer had a young family to support, and the economic pressures became unbearable. In late 1954 Stringer announced he would not accept a second term as state NAACP president.[4]

By keeping a lower profile, Stringer was able to maintain his practice in Mississippi. Others were not so fortunate. Clinton Battle, the young physician who had built Indianola's NAACP branch, learned that he could no longer ply his trade in the birthplace of the Citizens' Council and fled the state. Also driven out was Natchez physician Maurice Mackel, who founded the NAACP branch there in 1940 and then led the school petition drive fifteen years later. The most prominent figure forced into exile was T. R. M. Howard, who moved to the all-black town of Mound Bayou in the early 1940s to become the chief surgeon at the Knights and Daughters of Taber Hospital. A tall, powerful man in his early forties, Howard enjoyed life in the fast lane. He built a large plantation mansion, played the horses, and loved flashy cars. In 1951 Howard founded the Regional Council of Negro Leadership, a racial advancement organization that brought prominent black national figures like congressional representative William Dawson and NAACP attorney Thurgood Marshall to speak to thousands of blacks who gathered on Howard's estate in Mound Bayou. Howard's lifestyle and politics were anathema to the Citizens' Council, which ruined him financially and put a thousand-dollar price on his head. Reluctantly, Howard cut his losses and moved his practice to Chicago's South Side, believing that "I can do more alive in the battle for Negro rights in the North than dead in a weed-grown grave in Dixie." After Howard left, the only two black physicians publicly involved in civil rights work were A. B. Britton in Jackson and Gilbert Mason on the Gulf Coast.[5]

Life was difficult even for those African American physicians who stayed clear of politics. Indeed, the most striking fact about black doctors in Mississippi is that there were so few of them, only about fifty-five in 1960. Most of them practiced in urban areas; fifty-two of the state's eighty-two counties had no black physicians at all. With only about four thousand black doctors in the entire country in 1960, African Americans comprised less than 3 percent of all medical students in the United States. The two black medical schools, Howard and Meharry, remained "the almost exclusive source of the limited supply of black physicians." Fewer than two hundred blacks were graduating from medical school each year. Almost none of them would consider setting up shop in the Magnolia State.[6]

There are a number of reasons why the state with the largest percentage of black citizens had the fewest black health care professionals. Like their white counterparts, many black doctors placed a high priority on the acquisition of wealth and the prestige that went with it. While Mississippi's black physicians were not starving, it was hard for them to make much money in an area where most of their patients were either poor or indigent. Mississippi also lacked the cultural, educational, and entertainment amenities desired by many physicians and their families. Nor were most black doctors eager to confront Jim Crow. T. R. M. Howard told a national meeting of physicians in 1957 that "too many Negro doctors in this nation have not concerned themselves about this 'all-out fight for first class citizenship for our people,'" adding that "we are spending too much money on Cadillacs, yachts, and mansions in this grave hour."[7]

Most of all, black physicians stayed clear of Mississippi because of the difficulties inherent in practicing medicine in the nation's most segregated state. The problem was most evident in the paucity of hospital facilities for blacks. Many counties lacked hospitals that would accept black patients. In those that did, the facilities were both segregated and inferior, and blacks were routinely denied admission if they did not have cash in hand. University Hospital in Jackson, part of the medical school, received referrals from all over the state and often had long waiting lists for black patients because there were so few beds available for them.[8]

Jackson's Baptist Hospital admitted black patients but crammed them into the "Green Annex," a segregated area with fewer than forty beds where "everything took place . . . surgery, delivery, pediatrics, whatever." One physician recalled seeing "a kid about nine years old being treated. And in the bed next to him was an old guy with tubes running out of everything, with cancer." This situation was common throughout the state. When Gilbert Mason opened his practice in the racially "moderate" Gulf Coast city of Biloxi in 1955, the hospital annex consisted of two rooms, each containing a four-bed ward. Mason recalled that "regardless of their ailments or relative medical conditions, whether infectious or life threatening, men were confined in one room and women in the other. New mothers, if they were black, were confined in this exposed ward with their new babies."[9]

To make matters worse, most black physicians could not even see their hospitalized patients. In Mississippi—and throughout the South—hospital privileges were restricted to members of the all-white county medical societies. To gain membership in the American Medical Association, the politically powerful parent organization, one had to belong to the county and state associations. Blacks, then, fell victim to a medical version of catch-22. Appeals to the AMA to force the county societies to admit black physicians—and thereby award them hospital privileges—fell on deaf ears. In 1948 the organization adopted a resolution officially proclaiming that "the county medical society is the sole judge of whom it shall elect to membership." In subsequent years the AMA position, restated ad nauseam, was that while it opposed racial discrimination and encouraged its southern chapters to admit blacks, it was powerless to compel them to integrate.

Beginning in the 1950s, a few Mississippi county medical societies admitted selected black doctors as "scientific members" who could attend professional gatherings but not social functions. In Jackson, A. B. Britton was the only black "scientific" member of the local medical society before the early 1960s, and he did gain limited hospital privileges at Baptist. The most visible black physician in town, Britton was a Tougaloo graduate who had served in World War II and in the Korean conflict before taking his medical degree at Howard. Britton had became politically active in the 1960s, serving as a member (and later chairman) of the Mississippi State Advisory committee to the U.S. Commission on Civil Rights. He was Medgar Evers's personal physician.[10]

With a ratio of one black physician for every seventeen thousand black citizens in Mississippi, the majority of African Americans who saw a physician patronized white doctors, either by choice or necessity. A number of white physicians did treat destitute blacks; others followed the hospitals' policy of cash up front. Historian James C. Cobb writes of one Delta doctor who said, "If there is a nigger in my waiting room who doesn't have three dollars in cash, he can sit there and die. I don't treat niggers without money." For blacks who had the money up front and endured Jim Crow indignities—separate entrances and waiting rooms—there was still no guarantee of satisfactory treatment. According to one black Delta patient, "Most often I sits on one side of the office and he sits on the other asking questions. There ain't no listening or thumping or looking in the mouth like white folks get."[11]

Black physicians looked on while potential paying customers lined up in Jim Crow fashion to see white doctors who, very often, directed indigent African American patients to the black doctor's front door. When Douglas Connor opened his practice in Starkville in 1951, he found that most of his patients were from rural areas, while the blacks in town patronized white doctors. Connor observed that "to this day, among a segment of the black community, especially among the middle class, there is an attitude that if something is done by a white person it is done better."

In Vicksburg, Dr. Aaron Shirley knew "middle-class black patients were going to white doctors . . . and some of them would brag about it." Excluded from local and state medical societies, denied hospital privileges, and forced to compete with white physicians for the few black patients who could pay for their services, black doctors in Mississippi struggled to survive in a hostile environment. It is no wonder that the new graduates of Howard and Meharry decided to locate elsewhere.[12]

Bob Smith was the only one of several Tougaloo seniors applying to medical school who was admitted "on the first pass." Because the University of Mississippi Medical Center did not accept blacks, the state had implemented a program granting tuition and loans to black students to attend any accredited medical school outside the state. The five thousand dollars in loans would be forgivable at a rate of one thousand dollars a year for each year the returning physician practiced medicine in Mississippi. The subsidy presented Smith with a crisis of conscience, for in taking it he was profiting from the Jim Crow system. But as he later told a reporter from *Time* magazine, "If I hadn't taken it, I wouldn't be a doctor today."[13]

Smith applied to and was accepted at both Howard and Meharry. He chose Howard in part because he had visited there while in high school. Bob soon adapted to his new environment, despite his awareness that "most of my classmates were upper-class compared to me." Many, he noted, "were looking forward to getting Howard behind them, and moving on to Los Angeles or New York to be society doctors." But this "country boy from Mississippi" soon found his own circle of friends, developed an active social life, and "never spent a lonely day in Washington."[14]

At Howard, Bob stayed informed about the racial stirrings in the Deep South. It was there that he first met Martin Luther King Jr., who occasionally spoke at the Sunday chapel services. Other activists like Thurgood Marshall and theologian Howard Thurman were visible presences on the Howard campus. Completing his medical training at Howard in 1960, Smith did his internship in Chicago, which in many ways was his second home. Two of his brothers lived there, and for years he had spent his summers boarding with their families while working in the city. He continued this routine during medical school, holding down two summer jobs, working at Cook County Hospital during the day and as a short-order cook at night. For Bob, that hospital—"a big Greek temple"—was a powerful symbol, and he determined that he would return there for his internship.

What he found in Chicago was a health care system that in many ways mirrored that of Mississippi. While there were no racially discriminatory laws on the books, de facto segregation was pervasive in the city's hospitals. Until the mid-1950s only a handful of black doctors had privileges outside of Provident, the city's all-black hospital on the South Side. Chicago hospitals used various subterfuges to deny black patients admission. The interracial Committee to End Discrimination in Chicago Hospitals (CED) had formed in 1951, headed by Dr. Arthur Falls, one of the nation's eminent black physicians. Bob joined the CED, and he became friends with a politically active group of interns, many of whom would become civil rights activists in their home communities. His plans to continue his studies in Chicago were put on hold when, in the aftermath of the closing of the border with West Berlin in August 1961, his draft board ordered him back to Mississippi following completion of his internship to await a call-up for active military duty. He looked upon his return home as temporary. He would serve his time as an army physician and then return to Chicago, where he had been promised a residency in obstetrics-gynecology, one of only a few blacks nationally to have such an opportunity.

By the time Smith arrived back home in Terry in July of 1962, black Mississippians had begun their final assault on the Jim Crow system. Joining them were a dedicated cadre of newcomers, or "outside agitators," as the segregationists labeled them. In the spring of 1960 the sit-ins in the upper South had signaled a new militancy among black college students, and out of this movement came the Student Nonviolent Coordinating Committee (SNCC), which began its Mississippi operation in McComb in the summer of 1961. That spring the Congress of Racial Equality (CORE), an interracial organization formed in the early 1940s, staged a freedom ride through the Deep South to test a U.S. Supreme Court decision banning racial discrimination in bus and train terminals. The NAACP had been active locally on a number of fronts. Nine members of the Tougaloo College NAACP youth council made headlines when they sat in at the Jackson Public Library, a tax-supported facility that refused to admit blacks. Gulfport NAACP president Dr. Gilbert Mason led a "wade-in" along Gulf Coast beaches that was broken up by white men wielding pipes, chains, and baseball bats. In the Delta, state NAACP president Aaron Henry, a Clarksdale pharmacist, was laying the groundwork for a full-scale assault on segregation in Coahoma County, and state field secretary Medgar Evers was working with local people in the Jackson area who were staging a boycott of downtown merchants. To coordinate the burgeoning protest movement, in early 1962 leaders of SNCC, CORE, SCLC (Southern Christian Leadership Conference), and the state NAACP, together with local groups, formed the Council of Federated Organizations— COFO—the umbrella agency that directed the Mississippi movement during the period of its ascendancy.[15]

Drawn into the movement, Bob Smith became a devoted ally of Medgar Evers and attended movement gatherings in Jackson, where he met SNCC people like Bob Moses and Lawrence Guyot. "I learned so many things by attending those mass meetings," he recalled. "Between July and December of 1962 was my real education, my great awakening."

For Walter Lear, the decision to picket the AMA was predictable, if not inevitable, for the forty-year-old physician had been fighting against racism in the medical profession since his days as an intern. Born in the Bronx in 1923, he grew up in a nonreligious Jewish family. Lear's father had belonged to a revolutionary group in Russia as a teenager, but when he came to the United States shortly after the turn of the century he gave up politics. Determined to become a successful professional, he worked hard to assimilate and learned to speak English without an accent. Living on the Lower East Side of Manhattan, he attended medical school in Brooklyn, and then became a general practitioner in the Bronx before going to Europe to study ophthalmology. Rheumatoid arthritis cut short his practice, and for reasons of health he moved the family to Miami Beach when Walter was seven. Arriving in America's leading resort city at the onset of the Great Depression, the Lears soon adapted to their new surroundings. Walter's mother, an educator, started a private school, and her income helped the family make ends meet.[16]

A good student, Walter graduated first in his class from Miami Beach High School and from there went to Harvard, where he became politically involved and joined a group of students favoring the entry of the United States into World War II. Harvard student Joseph Lash led this organization, and he arranged for Walter and other pro-war students to have tea with his friend Eleanor Roosevelt in the White House. During his senior year, Lear became chairman of the Harvard premedical society. For him, becoming a physician had always been a given. His father "felt very strongly" that Walter should enter the medical profession, and his dutiful son was glad to oblige. The problem was that it was difficult for Jewish applicants to gain admission to medical schools, for most of them had a rigid quota for Jews as well as for blacks. Eventually Lear won admittance to the Long Island School of Medicine—during the middle of World War II—under a government program that enabled him to defer his military obligation until he finished his medical training.

A debate on the merits of a national health insurance program proved a turning point in his career. "I was just overwhelmed, and pretty well convinced that this area that was being debated was the area on which I had to concentrate," he recalls. "The issue of the organization, financing, etc., of medical care was really going to be my specialty." It did not take long for Lear to get connected with the Association of Internes and Medical Students (AIMS), an organization concerned mainly with medical students' rights, but which also embraced ideas—such as national health insurance—considered anathema by the AMA. AIMS identified with leftist student movements during the war, and afterward it lobbied aggressively for racial equality in the medical profession. Lear served as the national director of AIMS for two years; then he became chair of the AIMS Committee Against Discrimination in Medicine. In 1948 he spoke at the final general session of the National Health Assembly, a conference that met in Washington to discuss the nation's health problems. Lear took issue with the assembly's final report, which lacked "a forceful reaffirmation of the principle of equal educational opportunity for all regardless of race, and a condemnation of the shameful and undemocratic practices of segregation and discrimination in the education and training of health personnel." The young doctor's demand that the assembly endorse the health-related recommendations of President Truman's Commission on Civil Rights—and oppose federal funding for medical institutions that practiced discrimination and segregation—was met with stony silence.[17]

Lear interned at Kaiser Hospital in Oakland, California. A pioneer in providing a group practice, prepayment health insurance plan during World War II for its shipyard workers, Kaiser was now expanding its coverage to other groups. In 1948 Lear returned to New York and enrolled in the School of Public Health at Columbia University, where he received his M.S. in hospital administration. To fulfill his obligation to the military, he worked from 1948 to 1951 in the Industrial Hygiene Division of the U.S. Public Health Service, and then he served as associate medical director of the Health Insurance Plan of Greater New York from 1952 to 1961. He was also the New York chair of the antinuclear organization SANE.

The sit-ins and freedom rides had inspired Lear, and he continued to work for racial equality in the medical profession. From 1961 to 1963 he was a consultant for the National Urban League, doing research and writing that led to the publication of *Health Care and the Negro Population*. He also attended the annual meetings of the IMHOTEP Conference on Hospital Integration, the organization begun in 1956 by Howard University's W. Montague Cobb. Named after the ancient African-Egyptian physician Imhotep ("he who cometh in peace"), this largely black but interracial group of health care professionals met annually to discuss legal and political strategies to open up hospitals to African American patients and physicians. The American Medical Association was the major stumbling block to progress in this area, and Lear came away from the 1963 IMHOTEP meeting convinced that "we had to do something about the AMA." He then hit upon the idea of a picket line at the AMA convention in Atlantic City.

Lear's plan received support from the Physicians Forum (PF). Organized in 1941, this New York–based group of doctors embraced the radical notion that "medical care is a right for all" and advocated a program of national health insurance. Many of its members had a history of political activity dating back to the Communist Party in the 1930s. A few had participated as medical volunteers on the side of the Loyalists during the Spanish civil war. An independent socialist himself, Lear joined the group when he moved to New York in the late 1940s and became a board member in 1954. His colleagues in the Physicians Forum would be of assistance to Lear as he planned his offensive against the AMA. Still, PF was an overwhelmingly white organization, and Lear knew that without support from southern black physicians—the group directly affected by AMA policy—the Atlantic City protest would lack credibility. He turned to the National Medical Association (NMA) for assistance.

Formed in Atlanta in 1895, the NMA was the Negro alternative to the AMA. A month later, in the same city, Booker T. Washington gave his famous "Atlanta Compromise" speech. The NMA charter reflected much of Washington's message of racial solidarity and self-help, and most of its members embraced the Tuskegean's conservative philosophy of racial accommodation. The NMA published its own medical journal, held annual meetings, and, as the years passed, tried to open a dialogue with the AMA. A "good-will" committee created in 1938 lobbied the AMA to accept NMA membership as sufficient qualification for AMA affiliation and to support admission of black physicians to staff positions at tax-supported hospitals. The AMA ignored both requests.[18]

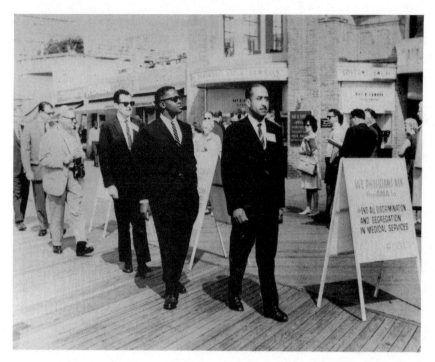

Physicians picketing the American Medical Association at its annual convention in Atlantic City, 1963. Physicians in the dark suits are (right to left) John L. S. "Mike" Holloman, Robert Smith, and Walter Lear. (Institute of Social Medicine and Community Health)

Stung by the rebuff, the NMA waited nearly two decades before approaching the AMA again. In the meantime, younger physicians like Montague Cobb became impatient over the organization's apparent lack of purpose. In a scathing critique of the NMA's 1947 convention, Cobb denounced the assembly for failing to "combat discriminatory practices in medicine" and labeled the gathering itself as "a painful example of generalized inadequacy as tragic as it was unconvincing." A year later Cobb became editor of the *Journal of the National Medical Association*, and for the next two decades his column, "The Integration Battle Front," focused on the issue of racism in the profession. The NMA as a whole, however, continued its cautious approach, particularly in its reluctance to confront the AMA.[19]

Although Lear knew Cobb from the IMHOTEP conferences, he turned to another prominent NMA member, John L. S. Holloman, a general practitioner in Harlem, for support. "Mike" Holloman was born in Washington in 1919, graduated from the prestigious Dunbar High

School and Virginia Union University (where he later served as president), and earned his medical degree from the University of Michigan. A captain in the army during World War II, Holloman served as a medical officer in the unit headed by Benjamin O. Davis, the first black general. After he returned from the war, he established his practice in Harlem, joined the Physicians Forum, and became a board member of the NMA, working with Cobb and other black physicians to push that organization to take a more aggressive stance on civil rights issues. With Lear as catalyst and general coordinator and Holloman as temporary chairman, the Medical Committee for Civil Rights (MCCR) was organized just two weeks before the AMA convention.[20]

In the fall of 1962, Bob Smith was growing restless waiting for his draft board to decide whether to call him up for active duty. When he learned that the state hospital for the mentally ill, located outside of Jackson in Whitfield, had once employed a Negro physician, he arranged for an interview with Cecil Jaquith, the hospital's director, who hired him at an eight-to-five job. Smith's civil rights activities took him out to Tougaloo for mass meetings, where he learned that college physician A. B. Britton would no longer be able to provide medical services. Tougaloo president Daniel Beittel asked Smith to take on that responsibility—for free. Smith told his boss that he would be seeing students in his off hours, and Jaquith, although aware of the college's reputation as a civil rights bastion, replied that as long as nobody complained he would look the other way.

A month after Smith started seeing patients at Tougaloo, a Mississippi highway patrolman stopped him at the campus gates. At that time the school was under heavy police surveillance. Its civil rights commitment had won it the sobriquet "Cancer College," and the state legislature was looking for ways to lift its accreditation and shut it down. Now that the segregationists were onto Dr. Smith, Jaquith advised him to stop going to Tougaloo. Ignoring the warning, Smith continued to provide medical care for the students. In addition, he began to treat civil rights workers for a range of ailments, from minor infections to acute stress. Now a police target himself, Smith was stopped on a trumped-up speeding charge while driving from Tougaloo to the state hospital. Instead of issuing a ticket, the officer briefly jailed the young physician, the first of several such arrests.

As Lear was organizing his AMA protest, Tougaloo student members of an NAACP Youth Council were initiating a boycott of downtown merchants in Jackson, charging them with a broad pattern of discrimination against black workers and consumers. Their demands included equality in hiring and promotion, the use of courtesy titles, and an end to Jim Crow practices. John Salter, a Tougaloo professor, was the faculty adviser to the youth council, and NAACP state field secretary Medgar Evers was also supportive. The "Jackson movement" hit full stride in late May of 1963 after a sit-in at the downtown Woolworth drugstore led to a riot (and one of the most famous photographs to come out of the civil rights movement). The Woolworth sit-in transformed the boycott into a mass movement. Scenes of enraged whites attacking peaceful protesters appeared on television screens across the country, and that night nearly one thousand enthusiastic blacks at the Pearl Street AME Church sang freedom songs and greeted the sit-in participants with a standing ovation. Over the next few days, events moved at a frantic pace. Police assaulted black high school students demonstrating during their lunch hour. National NAACP head Roy Wilkins came to town, and he and Evers were arrested on a picket line on Capitol Street in downtown Jackson. Soon Wilkins would move to apply the brakes to the demonstrations, but his actions would be overshadowed by what transpired on the night of June 11.

Earlier that evening, President John F. Kennedy made a historic television address, endorsing for the first time a comprehensive civil rights bill. Evers had missed the speech, for he was speaking at a church rally in Jackson. At 12:20 A.M. he pulled into his driveway and got out of his car carrying a bundle of NAACP T-shirts. As his wife, Myrlie, and their children jumped up to meet him, a Citizens' Council member named Byron De La Beckwith, crouching 150 feet away in a honeysuckle thicket, fired one shot from a high-powered rifle, dropped the gun into a patch of weeds, and fled. The slug hit Evers's back just below the shoulder blade, knocking him to the ground. He staggered to his feet, groped toward the kitchen door, and collapsed in a pool of blood. He died in an ambulance taking him to the hospital.

More than four thousand black men, women, and children packed the Masonic Temple for Evers's funeral. During the service Bob Smith sat silently, grieving for his friend and mentor. Smith's idyllic childhood in Terry, the good years at Tougaloo and Howard, the successful internship in Chicago, and the vibrant movement he discovered on his return to Mississippi—all that just weighed on him now. He remembers the murder of Evers as a turning point. "I was devastated and wanted to do something." Two days later he received a call from Dr. Britton, who passed on

Lear's request for a southern black presence at the AMA protest. Britton asked whether Smith would be interested in making a hurried trip to Atlantic City. The young doctor jumped at the chance. "Yes, yes, please," he told Britton.[21]

In Atlantic City the physicians waiting for Smith's arrival were becoming nervous about the protest itself. Mike Holloman admitted that he had "reservations about my role and what we in the committee were planning. I had reservations because doctors had never picketed doctors before. How would the public react? What would be the reaction of my colleagues? I was uneasy, but Birmingham was boiling then. If it meant only a handful of us on that line, I would be one of them." The day before the picketing Holloman and Lear met with the Atlantic City police chief. "We wanted everything to be understood and approved," Lear recalls. "We did not want to get arrested." There was a legal issue to be resolved. Atlantic City had an ordinance prohibiting placing stationary objects on the boardwalk. The physicians had prepared signs on sandwich boards and wanted to display them on the boardwalk. The chief asked the two men why they just didn't carry their signs as they walked. "Because," Lear informed him, "doctors do not carry picket signs." It was, Lear later reflected, "an interesting cultural comment on the medical profession. It just didn't seem the right thing to do, to carry a sign. If we were to have doctors participating in this event we could not demand that they shed this other professional image." After hearing Lear's argument, the chief agreed. "Yes, I understand. Doctors don't carry signs." At a press conference later that day Holloman assured reporters that "we will not behave like a labor union."[22]

The picketing itself went peacefully. A small group of fewer than twenty physicians and other health care workers, most of them white, marched for three hours under a hot sun around six signs set in a line about forty feet long in front of the convention hotel. A few AMA delegates passing by joined the line for a short time. The Medical Committee for Civil Rights had earlier written to the AMA demanding that it take a stand against discrimination and segregation in "all phases of medicine and health services," only to be rebuffed. So after the picketing ended, Holloman, an AMA member, walked the length of the hall to the dais to present AMA president Edward R. Annis with a similar letter calling on the AMA to expel any state or local affiliate that refused to accept black physicians as full members.[23]

AMA officials responded condescendingly. Later that day, the chairman of its board of trustees issued a statement calling it "unfortunate that this incident has tended to obscure the achievements in medical science being reported at this meeting, which will improve the health of all people regardless of race." President Annis told the delegates at a later session that the protesters were "typical . . . of those who are trying to force their ideas on the masses of the American people," concluding that "in the American Medical Association anybody of any race or creed who wants to work, is recognized. The profession recognizes men by their achievement, and not the color of their skin." Annis had nothing to say about skin color and AMA membership. The AMA president-elect, Norman A. Welch, did address that issue, telling reporters that while he favored the admission of "qualified Negroes" to local societies, the AMA would "not interfere in those constituent groups that bar Negroes."[24]

The dissident doctors were satisfied with their demonstration. It had gone off without a hitch, forcing the AMA leadership to deal with the fact, if not the substance, of their protest, which had received good press coverage, including stories and photographs in major city newspapers. The *New York Times* also published a photograph of doctors Holloman, Smith, and Lear walking the line. After long sessions with newspaper and television interviewers, in which he told his story about race and health care in Mississippi, a bone-tired Bob Smith boarded a bus to retrace his route back to Jackson. The Atlantic City protest had transformed the young doctor. Returning home, he "realized for the first time that from then on things would never be the same. I saw that I was serving a purpose, that there was a higher calling, and that this thing needed the kind of leadership and pushing that we were bringing, and that we would never give up until we had achieved some of these goals."[25]

CHAPTER I

The Good Doctors

During the summer of 1963 civil rights activity intensified throughout the South. Direct action protests rocked Birmingham, Greensboro, Atlanta, and more than a hundred other cities in eleven southern states. The unleashing of police dogs on demonstrators in Birmingham helped persuade President Kennedy to submit a civil rights bill to Congress, which debated its controversial provisions throughout the summer and into the fall. Although the section desegregating public accommodations such as restaurants and hotels was the most prominent feature of the bill, the provision calling for an end to discrimination in federally assisted programs was of special interest to advocates of equal treatment in medical facilities.

In 1946 Congress had passed the Hospital Survey and Construction Act, more commonly called the Hill-Burton Act, after its principal sponsors. The law, providing millions of dollars of federal funds annually for hospital construction and expansion, stated that the facilities be available to "all persons . . . without discrimination on account of race, creed, or color." Senator Lister Hill of Alabama then added the following wording: "But an exception shall be made in cases where separate hospital facilities are provided for separate population groups, if the plan makes equitable provision on the basis of need for facilities and services of like quality for each such group." This separate-but-equal clause was, in the words of political scientist David Barton Smith, "the only one in federal legislation of this century that explicitly permitted the use of federal funds to provide racially exclusionary services."[1]

The Hill-Burton Act in practice did not provide equal hospital facilities for blacks. Ninety hospitals that had received federal construction grants from Hill-Burton refused to accept black patients, and as we have seen, throughout the South hospitals that did admit blacks subjected them to inferior and unhealthy accommodations. The National Medical Association had long opposed Hill-Burton, and in 1963 congressmen Adam Clayton Powell Jr. and John Dingell vowed to fight the discriminatory clause when the act came up for renewal. At the same time, the NAACP Legal Defense Fund had filed suit in federal court, maintaining that Hill-Burton as written and interpreted was unconstitutional.[2]

On July 17 Walter Lear, representing the Medical Committee for Civil Rights, testified before the House Judiciary Committee, then holding hearings on the Kennedy civil rights bill. Lear supported the measure, noting that it would "clearly invalidate the 'separate but equal' clause of the Hill-Burton Act." But the point of his testimony was to expand the public accommodations section of the measure to include "non-profit, non-governmental hospitals, nursing homes, clinics, and other health facilities which provide an essential public service that would otherwise be provided by government agencies." "It seems anomalous," he told Congressman Powell, "that commercial enterprises serving the general public should be covered by this legislation but that non-profit hospitals serving the general public are not." This provision for expanded coverage was added to the final bill.[3]

Lear's congressional testimony is evidence of the credibility the Medical Committee had acquired in a short time. That summer its first newsletter went out to ten thousand health care personnel, including the entire membership of the NMA. Fund-raising letters resulted in enough money to pay Lear's business expenses, and the American Friends Service Committee provided space in its New York office. A national advisory board included such luminaries as Paul Dudley White, who had been President Eisenhower's personal physician. MCCR meetings attracted nurses, dentists, and other health care workers in addition to physicians. The group stepped up its attack on the AMA, which had refused to "use its well-known and greatly respected strength to help desegregate hospitals, medical societies, and all other aspects of medicine and health services." Unwilling to come out against the Jim Crow provisions of Hill-Burton, the AMA stood by its pallid 1950 resolution that "constituent and component societies having restrictive membership provisions based on race, study this question, with a view to taking such steps as they may elect to eliminate such restrictive provisions." As earlier, AMA leaders consistently maintained that they could not force state and local societies to admit black members.[4]

On July 31, 1963, Lear and Mike Holloman submitted a list of questions to AMA president Edward R. Annis. They asked if Dr. Annis opposed racial segregation in general, and in particular the racially exclusive policies of medical societies and the segregation of patients in hospitals. Annis did not respond, but the issue would not go away. The AMA adopted a strategy to ignore MCCR and start talking to the less confrontational National Medical Association.[5]

The MCCR Atlantic City protest had an impact on the NMA, for here a predominantly white group of physicians had taken the lead in attacking racial segregation in medicine while the major black medical society sat on the sidelines. "We're friendly with the AMA," explained John T. Givens, the NMA's executive secretary. "I wouldn't do anything to embarrass them." But shortly after the MCCR demonstration, NMA president John A. Kenney Jr. asked AMA officials for a meeting "to discuss racial problems in organized medicine," and the AMA agreed, suggesting its headquarters in Chicago as the site. That session, and its immediate aftermath, symbolized the changes taking place in the NMA leadership. On Tuesday, July 2, President Kenney and a delegation of black physicians met with AMA officials and agreed to hold further discussions, in which NMA representatives would lay out "specific charges of injustices against Negro physicians." The next day NMA president-elect, Kenneth Clement, was part of an NAACP-sponsored demonstration outside the AMA headquarters. Marching with Clement were Montague Cobb and two other members of the NMA board. When asked about the apparent rift in the NMA, Kenney replied that Clement had been invited to the meeting with the AMA, but he had refused to attend. "He'd rather picket," observed Kenney, concluding that "there is a new militancy in our organization."[6]

The AMA reached out, briefly, to members of the black medical association. In August its president-elect, Norman A. Welch, addressed a plenary session of the NMA convention. Assuring delegates that the AMA opposed racial discrimination, he conceded that some county medical societies still refused to admit black physicians. "You are impatient and I don't blame you," he said, but he could only point to the earlier meeting between representatives of the two groups as a sign of progress. And Welch reaffirmed his earlier statement that he would not interfere with those southern medical societies that barred black doctors from membership.[7]

By the end of the summer of 1963, the Medical Committee for Civil Rights had more than two hundred active members, most but not all from the New York City area. To demonstrate their visibility, and to show support for the civil rights movement, MCCR made plans for medical people to participate as a group in the March on Washington. More than two hundred health care workers assembled in Washington on the morning of August 28. The MCCR contingent lobbied members of Congress and had lunch at a local restaurant before assembling for the march itself. Lear recalls that day as "a very moving experience. What was very special was the range of support we had for the medical contingent, much broader than for the picketing of the AMA. The NMA turned out, marching under the MCCR banner, as did the American Nurses Association."[8]

MCCR assisted civil rights workers in an unheralded program that began during the summer of 1963. While attending the IMHOTEP conference in Atlanta that spring, Lear stopped by the Student Nonviolent Coordinating Committee office to talk with executive secretary James Forman, who agreed to lend SNCC support to the MCCR program. During the course of their conversation, Forman mentioned that a number of SNCC veterans were "getting very burned out, and they really needed to get away and rest up." Lear immediately thought of "the lovely summer

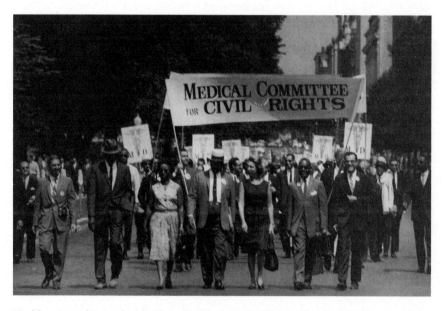

Health care workers at the March on Washington. Dr. Walter Lear is in the front row, right. (Institute of Social Medicine and Community Health)

homes in Westchester County and on Long Island of a number of the physicians I knew," and when he got back to New York he asked Trudy Orris to take on this project.[9]

Born Gertrude Weissman, Trudy came from a poor family in New York. A full-time factory worker at age fourteen, she was active in the labor movement and at an early age became involved in the Communist Party. During World War II she was elected union steward at the clothing store where she worked. By that time she had met and married a young physician named Leo Orris. Brought up in a conservative, orthodox Jewish home, Leo became interested in socialism while in college. "In the thirties and forties if you were not a young leftist who were you? If you had any progressive ideas you were a leftist." Orris served as a military doctor during World War II. During the 1950s the Orrises supported accused atomic spies Julius and Ethel Rosenberg and became involved in the civil rights movement. Leo belonged to the Physicians Forum, and he was in that small group of physicians who picketed the AMA in Atlantic City. Trudy was the more politically involved of the two. An official in the Women's International League for Peace and Freedom, she also became committed to the black protest movement. In early 1963 she took their sixteen-year-old son Peter with her on a freedom ride to Maryland, and responded enthusiastically when Lear told her of his plans for a rest-and-recreation retreat for civil rights workers.[10]

During the summer of 1963, Trudy Orris made weekly trips to New York bus and train stations to meet arriving black SNCC activists. She showed them the city, gave them some orientation about the upper-middle-class families they would be staying with, and then sent them off to Westchester, Fire Island, and Martha's Vineyard vacation homes to enjoy a week of beach time, movies, good food, and conversation. At the end of the week, each host family held a fund-raising party, which raised twenty-five thousand dollars for SNCC that summer. SNCC made all the decisions about who would participate in the program, with Forman taking an active role and spending some time in New York himself. He and other SNCC leaders selected people suffering from burnout (or "battle fatigue," as it would later be called). Most never suspected they had been singled out for any reason except to raise money for SNCC. The summer R & R program was a great success, and it was repeated the following year. Trudy Orris and the white women who supported her worked hard so that the young black activists they admired so much could enjoy a carefree week

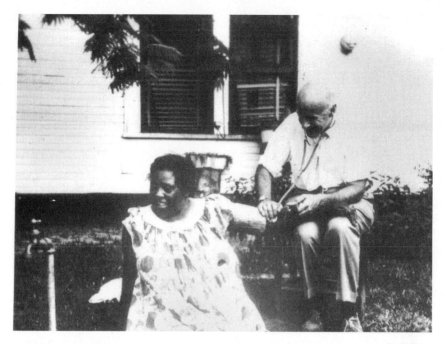

Dr. Leo Orris examining Mrs. Fannie Lou Hamer, Ruleville, Mississippi, summer 1964. (Institute of Social Medicine and Community Health)

before returning to the dangerous life of a SNCC field secretary in the Deep South.[11]

After his eventful trip to Atlantic City, Dr. Robert Smith returned to Jackson and his job at the state mental hospital. He had met a number of progressive northern physicians at the AMA protest, who told him to call on them if he ever needed assistance, a promise he would remember. Smith did not return home a conquering hero, however, at least not in the eyes of the local medical establishment. To have one's picture prominently displayed in the *New York Times*—the symbol of the left-wing, integrationist press—was not the kind of visibility a young black physician desired if he wanted to continue to ply his trade in Mississippi. Smith resumed his work as the Tougaloo physician, attended movement meetings in the evenings, and recruited people for the March on Washington, although he did not go himself. He soon gained a reputation as the "doctor to the movement," as civil rights activists came to him with a variety of minor complaints as well as more serious physical and emotional problems. Often he would be called out of the city to treat victims of police abuse. With only a handful of black physicians in Jackson, most of whom were nearing retirement age, Smith saw most of the COFO workers himself.[12]

Although Smith had managed to stay out of trouble, his visibility as a civil rights activist and physician proved to be too much for his boss at the state mental hospital, who fired him in October of 1963. By then he knew he was not going to be drafted and was free to return to Chicago, where a residency in ob/gyn had been held open for him. Such a move would have benefited him professionally. But by now he was firmly committed to the black freedom struggle in his native state, and with the support of people like Dr. Britton, Bob Smith opened his own practice in the heart of the black community, near Jackson State College.[13]

In the spring and summer of 1963, the movement was at high tide, with massive demonstrations in cities like Birmingham and Greensboro, the March on Washington Martin Luther King Jr.'s "I have a dream" speech, and President Kennedy's civil rights bill, which promised to end the Jim Crow system in the South. But then came the September church bombing in Birmingham with the death of four young black girls, followed by the assassination of John Kennedy on November 22. While movement activists did not regard Kennedy as a civil rights champion, his death came as a blow, especially since his successor, Lyndon Johnson, was a southerner with few civil rights credentials. And as the congressional debate over the civil rights bill dragged on month after month, supporters in the North became discouraged as well.

Walter Lear did not need to read the newspapers to know that the civil rights movement had lost some of its momentum. In the late spring he had put together the Medical Committee for Civil Rights. Within a short time nearly everyone in the medical profession knew of its existence, and it had gained credibility with the major civil rights organizations and their leaders. By late summer MCCR made plans to conduct health surveys in hospitals in ten southern cities, to increase its pressure on the AMA, and to expand its base by recruiting nurses, dentists, and other health workers. As with the movement as a whole, however, MCCR experienced a decline during the fall of 1963. It did not survive into the new year.[14]

One major problem was lack of funding. According to Lear, he was "putting full time into MCCR work," and "could not afford to do that without being paid." At a steering committee meeting in late June, the question of putting him on salary was "deferred until the future activity and strength and finances [were] clarified." Attempts to raise money through mass mailings to physicians were unsuccessful, and by the fall the organization had contracted debts it could not pay. According to Lear, "We did not have the skill or energy to raise a lot of money." But to say that MCCR folded because it went broke is to beg the question. Civil rights for African Americans was not fashionable that fall. Without dramatic headlines of racial confrontations in the South, many white liberals, including physicians, turned their attention elsewhere.[15]

As for Walter Lear, he accepted a position as deputy commissioner for the Department of Health in the city of Philadelphia, and "after a month or so I closed the Medical Committee for Civil Rights." The unpaid MCCR bills followed him to Philadelphia, where he was hounded by creditors representing the Occidental Restaurant, where the medical group had dined before the March on Washington. It seems that some of the doctors had not paid for their meals, and as the coordinator he was held responsible. After sympathizing with the restaurant management about "the organization [MCCR] that took advantage of you and me [and is] now defunct," Lear paid the bill out of his own pocket. He would not be among the founding members of the Medical Committee for Human Rights.[16]

Mississippians, both black and white, faced the new year with foreboding. In early 1964 Jim Crow still held sway in the Magnolia State, with black Mississippians relegated to inferior jobs, schools, and health care. Many black physicians had either retired or left the state. Almost no younger doctors were choosing to follow Dr. Smith's example and live and work in "The Closed Society." Two who did, Aaron Shirley and James Anderson, would have a major impact on both health care and on race relations in the months and years to come.

The youngest of eight children, Aaron Shirley never knew his father, who died when Aaron was an infant. His mother, a nurse's aide, moved the family to Jackson from the Madison County hamlet of Gluckstadt, where they owned a farm and other property. Aaron spent his summers on the farm, planting, chopping, and picking cotton, hauling water and cutting wood. He had two brothers. One died in childhood; the other, a soldier, was killed in the D-Day invasion. Aaron's oldest sister, a nurse, influenced him to become a doctor. He preceded Bob Smith at Tougaloo. Shirley belonged to the college NAACP chapter, but was not politically active as a student. Upon graduation he enrolled at Meharry Medical School, and after completing his internship he came back to Mississippi to

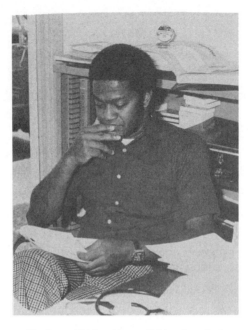

Dr. Aaron Shirley. (Aaron Shirley donation)

work off his tuition obligation. In 1960 he and his wife Ollye settled in Vicksburg because the only black physician there, who was retiring, encouraged Aaron to take over his practice.[17]

A Mississippi River town, Vicksburg is best known to students of the Civil War for its surrender after a long siege on July 4, 1863. The Confederate spirit lived on there (for generations local whites refused to celebrate Independence Day), but Vicksburg was known for its racial moderation. The Shirleys found out quickly, however, that they had not moved to a "New South" city. Just after he opened his practice Aaron applied for staff privileges at the hospital, the first time a black doctor had done so. This "upset everybody. I was about to disrupt the tranquility of peaceful relationships that the races had always enjoyed." He was denied hospital privileges for five years, although Cuban refugee physicians who moved to Vicksburg in 1963 gained them immediately. "They welcomed these doctors with open arms, because they were fleeing the Communists. But their native son . . ."

The new doctor again angered local whites when he stood up to a white motorist who backed into his car. When a police officer arrived, Shirley asked if he was going to give the guilty party a ticket. Instead, the officer demanded that Shirley move his car, and then turned to apologize to the white man for the inconvenience. Shirley recalls what happened next:

> Well, this was after the hospital had turned me down, and my wife had had a couple of incidents in one of the stores, so I just handed the officer the keys and I said, "You can do what you want to, I'm gonna leave." I walked home, about five miles, and came to find out that the guy who backed into me owned the lumber company, and he was *the* man in town! I wasn't any wild-eyed radical . . . but to have this guy yelling and screaming and calling me "boy" and "get out of the way . . ." They called me the next day from the Ford dealership and told me they were working on the car, and I could pick it up several days later. I don't know who paid for it.

Shirley survived these early battles with Jim Crow in Vicksburg and soon had a huge practice, with patients from as far as Port Gibson, forty miles away, coming to his office on the second floor of a downtown building. Without hospital privileges, he set up "a little birthing room" in his office. Like most doctors he made house calls. "I'd get home at ten or eleven o'clock at night. My wife would have patients sitting in the living room." He established a good relationship with a couple of the white doctors because "I made quality referrals. I had a reputation of sorts." (In 1965 Shirley would be the first black admitted to the residency program at the University of Mississippi Medical Center.)

His medical reputation notwithstanding, Shirley continued to be targeted for abuse, this time because of his increasing political activity. The murder of Medgar Evers had angered and radicalized him ("I kept thinking about my brother who was lost on a segregated ship, and what was he fighting for?"), and he became active in the Warren County Improvement League, which had an ongoing voter registration program. The Shirleys were forced out of their rented house after it became a gathering place for local activists, and bought an "old, old house, sitting on a hill. And we renovated it, with the potential of having to defend it in mind." (Such precautions were necessary. The Ku Klux Klan was now active in western Mississippi, and later in the summer it bombed the COFO headquarters in Vicksburg.) The Shirley home became a center of civil rights activity, as their commitment to the struggle intensified.

As Dr. Shirley was getting established in Vicksburg, James Anderson found himself thrust into the middle of the movement in McComb, a city that did not enjoy a reputation for moderation in racial matters. "Andy" Anderson, the tenth of twelve children, grew up in Jackson. His father, a mechanic at a local fertilizer factory, was a union man who managed to send all his children to college. At the end of his sophomore year in high school, Anderson won a scholarship to Morehouse, the most prestigious of the Negro colleges, and there he developed an interest in medicine. He then went on to Meharry, where he received his M.D. degree in June of 1961. Anderson volunteered for service in the Air Force during the Berlin Wall crisis, but he was not due to report until December. With some time on his hands, he went down to McComb to help out the town's black doctor, who had to be away for several months.[18]

Anderson arrived in McComb shortly after Bob Moses came to town to lead SNCC's first Mississippi voter registration campaign. The SNCC headquarters was just down the street from Anderson's office, and Moses and Anderson quickly became friends. As more SNCC workers arrived in the area, white opposition to civil rights activities turned violent. When Billy Jack Caston, a cousin of the sheriff, attacked Moses, Dr. Anderson was there to "sew his head up." When Moses returned to have the stitches removed, the McComb police chief called Anderson and demanded to know why he was associating with these "agitators." From then on Anderson was active in the McComb movement. He took care of the SNCC workers' medical needs, and bailed them out of jail with funds sent to him by northern activists like Harry Belafonte. He and local leaders negotiated with the mayor for the release of the more than a hundred black high school students arrested after a march protesting the expulsion from school of two student leaders. Later, when a white mob attacked a group of Congress of Racial Equality freedom riders integrating the bus terminal, Anderson treated the badly beaten demonstrators at his office. When he arrived in McComb in the summer of 1961, James Anderson "didn't know nuthin about that racial stuff. I just went down to practice medicine." By the time he left six months later a white government official had identified him (incorrectly) as the leader of the McComb movement.

In January of 1962, Anderson received his draft notice, with only three days to report for duty at Fort Sam Houston in Texas. His wife had to close down his office. (Anderson believes that his political activity led to his being drafted.) He served as an army doctor for two years, and then returned to Mississippi to work out his tuition obligation to the state. He had plans to open a practice in Clarksdale in the Delta, but he decided to set up shop in Jackson after he learned that a black doctor named James Vines was fleeing the state for the more comfortable climate of California. Bob Smith welcomed Anderson with open arms.

Shirley, Anderson, and Smith were all contemporaries. They grew up within a few miles of each other, attended good black liberal arts colleges, and received their medical education at Howard and Meharry. They came from large families, where parents and older siblings made sure they excelled in their schoolwork. Poor performance in any arena was not tolerated. With much encouragement from their families, all three boys decided on careers in medicine early on, although they had few black role models to follow. Although they returned to Mississippi ostensibly to work out their tuition obligations, they could have made more money faster in northern cities and retired their debts quickly. The three young physicians chose to work in Mississippi communities because they had seen firsthand the paucity of health care services available to black citizens, and they knew that the problem was political as well as medical. Men of great personal courage, they embraced the opportunity to be both professional health care givers and civil rights agitators.

On the evening of January 31, 1964, Louis Allen was gunned down outside his home in Amite County, not far from McComb. Married and the father of four children, the forty-five-year-old independent logger was hit in the face with two loads of buckshot, dying almost instantly. His "crime" was witnessing the murder, three years earlier, of black activist Herbert Lee by a Mississippi state legislator, and since that time Allen had been a marked man. Allen's murder coincided with the rebirth of the Ku Klux Klan in Mississippi. Throughout the winter and spring of 1964, night riders roamed unchecked across the state. Cross burnings announced the Klan presence in the area—on one night in May crosses burned in sixty-four counties—followed by bullets and bombs. Black churches, businesses, and homes were the targets, and local people began to stand guard at night with their own shotguns and rifles.[19]

All this took its toll on SNCC, CORE, and NAACP activists working under the COFO banner. Bob Moses recalled that by the beginning of 1964 the staff was exhausted. "They were butting up against a stone wall, with no breakthroughs." Veteran organizers "were already burnt out. They had been out there for a couple of years, and that's a long time in that situation." Moreover, so long as white hoodlums and police could attack black people with impunity, it would be extremely difficult for the civil rights forces to make substantive gains without some degree of protection from retaliation. All previous efforts to persuade the Kennedy administration to safeguard human rights in Mississippi had failed. Now key movement strategists grudgingly conceded that they must set aside for a time their program of patient low-key, long-term community organizing and instead reach out to the largely indifferent national public and shock it into demanding federal intervention. To do so meant attracting the media to Mississippi and providing television cameras with action footage. The Mississippi movement was about to enter a new phase.[20]

Discussions had begun in the fall of 1963 about the possibility of having a "Summer Project" in 1964. This ambitious program called for continuing voter registration efforts, the opening of community centers, establishment of "freedom schools" for black children, and organization of a new Freedom Democratic Party (FDP) to challenge the legitimacy of the regular segregationist delegation at the national party convention in Atlantic City. Most controversial was the proposal, supported by COFO leaders like Bob Moses and Dave Dennis, to bring in hundreds of outside volunteers—most of them white—to help staff the project. Veteran Mississippi SNCC activists opposed the idea. They believed that the movement should stick to what it did best: community organizing. They saw white volunteers as a hindrance to building black consciousness and developing indigenous, independent local leadership. Some feared that the presence of whites in black neighborhoods would attract attention and threaten the security of the community, or that white college students, confident of their superior technical skills, would attempt to take over leadership positions.[21]

The major argument favoring the volunteer presence was tactical. Unless America was awakened to what was going down in Mississippi, local whites would destroy the movement through brute force and terror. Moses recalls that he decided to weigh in with his considerable influence after learning of Louis Allen's murder. "There was no real reason to kill Louis, and they gunned him down on his front lawn . . . We were just defenseless, there was no way of bringing national attention . . . People were just going to be wiped out." So long as it was black people being brutalized, white Americans would pay little heed. But "they would respond to a thousand young white college students," CORE's Dave Dennis believed. White volunteers would bring visibility and publicity and might force a reluctant federal government to intervene directly to protect organizers working in the state. That argument eventually carried the day, and throughout the spring SNCC recruiters and supporters visited northern university campuses in search of summer volunteers.[22]

When Smith first learned about a summer project that could involve at least a thousand outside volunteers, he called up Anderson and said, "My God, Andy, what can we do? How are we going to manage?" He and Anderson were already spending much of their office time dealing with the medical problems of civil rights workers in the Jackson area. Smith also went out of town to demonstrations in Canton and Greenwood in the spring of 1964, carrying his black bag, taking care of victims of police and mob brutality. The influx of a thousand new workers was bound to increase the level of violence across the state. The volunteers would also need medical attention for problems resulting from stress as well as for the normal ailments afflicting people moving into a new and strange environment. Smith assumed, correctly, that with few exceptions white Mississippi physicians would have nothing to do with these outside agitators. That left health care problems in the hands of the small number of black doctors—barely fifty of them—practicing in the state. Some of them would not treat civil rights workers—and certainly not white ones—for fear of retribution from whites in the community. Others would see activists, but only if they had cash on hand, always a problem for the SNCC organizers working for a wage of ten dollars a week. Only a handful of black physicians, including Smith, Anderson, Shirley, Britton, Matthew Page in Starkville, Cyril Walwyn in Yazoo City, and Gilbert Mason on the Gulf Coast had publicly identified with the movement and would treat movement workers for free. And Smith and Anderson were carrying the bulk of the caseload.[23]

Early in June, Anderson and Smith met with Moses, the director of the Summer Project, to discuss what might be done. At the meeting, Smith recalled that a year earlier in Atlantic City he had marched with a number of health care activists from New York, including psychologist Tom Levin. Perhaps this New York group could be of assistance. Moses agreed, and on June 18—only a few days before the Summer Project was to begin—Levin received a letter written by Carol Rogoff of the New York SNCC staff containing a detailed proposal for action during the summer.[24]

The letter stated that "northern physicians and those involved in auxiliary professions are sorely needed in the state, especially in light of our summer program," noting that blacks in Mississippi "have inadequate medical services available to them." COFO was asking for doctors to volunteer to work in the state on a rotating basis throughout the summer. The physicians could set up five medical centers, "perhaps in conjunction with the Community Centers," and work at the centers in teams for a minimum period of two weeks. After reading the letter Levin could hardly contain his enthusiasm. "I saw us as the Abraham Lincoln Brigade of the civil rights movement," he recalled. "I had such a romantic notion!"[25]

A short, solidly built bullet of a man, Levin looked like he would be at home organizing a group of longshoremen, and he did in fact come from working-class origins. Both his parents emigrated from Russia when they were two or three years old. In effect they were first-generation Americans. His father was a hat blocker who could barely read or write and who turned to drink when he could not find work during the Depression. During Tom's childhood the family lived in fourteen different homes. His mother eventually became a clerk in the city system, and it was from her that Tom developed his passion for learning. His parents "were good people who suffered a lot because they never thought they mattered." Tom was not a motivated student, and "was bounced out" of three high schools. One afternoon, aimlessly walking around Brighton Beach, Levin came across a lively scene. "There was a bunch of people dancing folk dances on the beach—kids my age, boys and girls, all together. The music sounded Russian and I prized my Russian heritage, and I learned that they all lived in a commune run by a very left-wing Zionist organization. So at age fifteen I left home and joined the commune." He also became a member of the Young Communist League. From there he went to work in a factory because "the Socialist Workers Party's stance was 'You don't go to school, you join the working class.'" During World War II he was drafted into the navy and later stationed on Okinawa. After the war he took advantage of the GI Bill to complete his high school education and enroll at Long Island University, where he was president of the college NAACP branch. He received his B.A. in only two years. Inspired by *Mine Own Executioner*, a Hollywood movie about the struggles of a lay analyst (played by Burgess Meredith), Levin decided to become a psychoanalyst. After receiving his Ph.D., he became a child analyst, opening a practice in New York.

Always politically involved, Levin was a romantic revolutionary—"To me, life began with the Spanish civil war"—who differed from many fellow Marxists in that he favored direct action over ideological analysis. Moved by Martin Luther King's Birmingham campaign in 1963, Levin contacted SCLC's Wyatt T. Walker, suggesting that he start an organization of academics to come south for demonstrations, to put their bodies on the line. Levin created the Committee of Conscience, spent time in Mississippi and Alabama in 1963, and "recruited some people. They went down to demonstrations, but then the organization disappeared" during the winter of 1963–64. COFO's call for health care professionals to come to Mississippi, then, was in line with the recruiting Levin had already been doing.

With the Summer Project getting under way, Levin moved quickly to put a group of doctors into Mississippi. First he touched base with civil rights activists to make sure they would welcome a medical presence for the summer. On June 20, the day after he received the COFO request, Levin spoke by phone with Charles Evers, the state NAACP field secretary, who was an independent actor in Mississippi's movement politics. Next Levin phoned COFO leaders Aaron Henry and Bob Moses, who were then in Oxford, Ohio, training the second wave of summer volunteers. Levin also contacted A. B. Britton and Bob Smith. On June 23 Levin told Evers that "everyone I spoke to, though cognizant of the dangers, felt the need for such a project very strongly." Moses told Levin to make this a COFO project and urged him to start it right away. Support also came from SNCC's Jim Forman, who wrote to Levin that "there is a desperate need for the kind of services that your committee is planning to offer," assuring him that COFO would make available "any assistance we can offer you to insure the success of the program."[26]

Levin invited area physicians who were interested in civil rights to a meeting at his home on the evening of June 24. Of the twelve people who showed up, most, like Levin, were Jewish. American Jews had been active supporters of black protest movements since the founding of the NAACP early in the twentieth century. As victims of discrimination and persecution themselves, they could empathize with another oppressed group. Moreover, as historian Debra L. Schultz has observed, "Antiracist activism is one expression of a universalist concern with justice that has roots in Jewish history, ethics, and political radicalism." Left-wing, secular Jewish physicians would play a significant role in health care activist organizations in the 1960s and 1970s.[27]

Levin's guests were New Yorkers with histories of involvement in progressive causes. They belonged to the Physicians Forum. But the problem with PF, according to a former member, was that it was little more than "a Sunday afternoon discussion club . . . that took positions on health care issues of the day, but it did not have a strategy of where to go with its views except to pass resolutions and mail them out." Levin believed, then, that he would need to push hard for a direct presence in Mississippi, and he also worried that ideological differences might hold sway at the meeting. A number of Physicians Forum members had been or were currently active in the American Communist Party. Levin, at one time a follower of the program of Leon Trotsky, was "aversive to Stalinists. I felt they wouldn't work, that they would stay theoretical, political, pure but ineffectual." Others involved in the discussion were independent socialists, along with one or two New Deal Democrats. Levin saw his task as putting together what "the Spanish Loyalists never achieved: a good United Front."[28]

His fears proved unwarranted. Earlier that week three civil rights workers had disappeared in Neshoba County, Mississippi, and had not been heard from since. Movement leaders assumed they were dead. Two of the three, Michael Schwerner and Andrew Goodman, were from Jewish families in New York and known to the physicians assembled in Levin's home. The doctors were not there to discuss Marxist theory. They wanted to take action. After the meeting an ebullient Tom Levin sent a telegram to Aaron Henry in Mississippi boasting of "ten commitments for medical service in Mississippi out of twelve participants. Funds and medical supplies pledged. Possibility of manning five full aid stations has unexpectedly developed due to enthusiastic support."[29]

The following day Levin joined a larger group at the 135th Street office of Mike Holloman. A number of those present were on the staff at Einstein and Jacobi, hospitals engaged in "social justice matters." Most were established physicians in their thirties and early forties. Martin Gittelman, a young psychotherapist working at Jacobi, remembers that when Holloman asked, " 'Who will go to the South?' every person in the room raised their hand." They chose a name for their organization—the Committee for Emergency Aid in Mississippi—and elected an executive board that included Edward Barsky, the legendary radical who had been the medical director of the Abraham Lincoln Brigade.[30]

On July 1, Holloman issued a press release on behalf of the board, announcing the formation of the new organization and calling for volunteer "physicians, surgeons, dentists, nurses, medical technicians, drivers, and other first aid personnel" to staff five medical aid stations in Mississippi. Four days later a delegation that included Levin, Leslie Falk, and Elliott Hurwitt, the chief of surgery at Montefiore Hospital, flew to Jackson

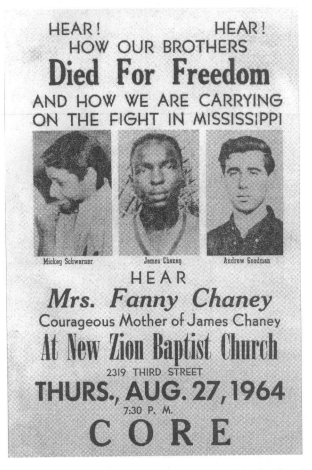

Poster of three missing civil rights workers. (Institute of Social Medicine and Community Health)

for a meeting at Smith's office on Lynch Street. There they spoke with local black doctors, COFO leaders, and representatives from the Delta Ministry, a new civil rights organization sponsored by the National Council of Churches that would figure prominently in movement activity in Mississippi over the next decade.[31]

The group met for five hours that hot Sunday afternoon and agreed on a four-point program for the summer: to recruit health care professionals to come to Mississippi for short periods to "visit and counsel with civil rights workers," to perform the "Good Samaritan function" (that is, to administer first aid to workers injured during demonstrations, or otherwise in need of immediate medical care), to gather and disseminate information on how movement workers could obtain care from Mississippi doctors and access to local hospitals, and to assist "Negro and white health care personnel" in their work. Originally, the northern doctors assumed they would come into the state, get licensed, and practice. But the Mississippi Department of Health, under the leadership of Archie Gray, a vehement segregationist, made it clear these outsiders would not get licenses. Administering first aid, however, was not prohibited, and that summer some doctors stretched the definition to fit the occasion. Still, doctors ran the risk of arrest for practicing without a license, a felony, and a number of the volunteer physicians decided to leave their black bags at home.

The second point of agreement was that the Committee for Emergency Aid would arrange and pay for medical care for the civil rights workers, summer volunteers, and COFO staff. The committee would also lend its expertise to write "grant requests to foundations and Federal agencies" for health projects in Mississippi. Finally, those present pledged to work to "help solve discriminatory and segregationist patterns in health services." They would rent an office on Farish Street in the heart of the black business district in Jackson. Bob Smith agreed to be the supervisor in charge of all medical personnel coming into the state during the course of the summer.[32]

The night following that meeting a large crowd gathered in Levin's office to hear from the delegation just back from Jackson. Attending were a number of people who would play prominent roles in the work of the committee, including Desmond Callan, Aaron Wells, and Leslie Falk. The group agreed that Levin should be the committee coordinator in New York, and that Falk would take the first shift as medical administrator in the new Jackson office. Finally, the question of a new name for the organization came up. This matter had been the subject of considerable discussion the day before in Jackson. Smith recalls that he suggested they continue with the name of the original group, the Medical Committee for Civil Rights, but "somehow that didn't seem acceptable." (Perhaps this was because the physicians did not want to be working under the banner of an organization they had so recently failed to support in its time of need?) At the Monday meeting the group agreed that the present name, the Emergency Committee, was too bland, and decided to call their organization the Medical Committee for Human Rights (Mississippi Project). Levin then sent a telegram to A. B. Britton in Jackson to spread the word that the "meeting last night brought complete and enthusiastic confirmation of the four-point program outlined in Jackson on Sunday afternoon." A week later he wrote to Art Thomas of the Delta Ministry that "at present we have more than enough physicians to staff the full five projected medical aid offices throughout the summer."[33]

CHAPTER 2

Freedom Summer in Mississippi

On Sunday, July 12, Bob Moses took time out from his busy schedule to pick up Leslie Falk at the Jackson airport. As the first medical care field adviser for the Medical Committee for Human Rights (MCHR), Falk had come down from his home in Pittsburgh to prepare for the visits of a dozen or more health care volunteers each week and to establish working relationships with COFO, the National Council of Churches' Delta Ministry, and black physicians across the state. He also hoped to meet with representatives of the white medical establishment. Falk did not have much time to touch base with his daughter Gail, a Freedom Summer volunteer.

At age forty-eight, Les Falk had already enjoyed a remarkable career. Born in St. Louis and raised in an affluent household—his father owned a clothing factory—Falk was a brilliant student who became a Rhodes Scholar in 1935. While studying in Oxford, he was a junior member of the medical research team that developed penicillin. He joined the Oxford Labour Club (where one of his drinking companions was Iris Murdoch, then an aspiring novelist). Falk became a Marxist and briefly flirted with the idea of joining the Abraham Lincoln Brigade in Spain, but instead stayed at Oxford to earn his doctoral degree in microbiology. Once war broke out in Europe, he returned to the United States and enrolled at Johns Hopkins medical school so he could study with Henry Sigerist, the internationally known medical historian and social activist. After getting his M.D. from Hopkins, Falk took a job with the Public Health Service (PHS). His support for the Progressive Party candidate for president, Henry Wallace, in 1948, for the Chinese Revolution, and for a comprehensive national health insurance program made him an inviting target, for by now the "red scare" was at high tide. Falk fell victim to the Truman loyalty campaign, created in 1947 to investigate government employees for Communist allegiances. Rather than "name names," he resigned from the PHS.

Fortunately, Falk found a challenging position in Pittsburgh as medical administrator of the United Mine Workers Health Program Fund, where he made dramatic innovations in health care delivery in the coalfields, particularly in the treatment of black lung disease. He also joined the faculty of the new School of Public Health at the University of Pittsburgh. A dedicated socialist, Falk could be rigid in his thinking (Tom Levin called him "one of the most doctrinaire men I have ever met"), but his vast experience and his commanding presence made him the ideal person to get the Medical Committee off the ground in Mississippi.[1]

After arriving in Jackson on Sunday, Falk met with three white ministers, Art Thomas, Warren McKenna, and Bruce Hanson—who represented the Delta Ministry, an organization that would prove invaluable to MCHR in Mississippi. The next day he met with Moses, COFO's medical liaison Lois Chafee, and Claire Bradley, the MCHR secretary and office manager in Jackson. He discussed logistics with doctors Smith, Britton, and Anderson, and then proceeded on to the State Health Department to meet its director, Archie Gray. Although he received Falk politely, Dr. Gray was a white supremacist who would oppose MCHR's every move in Mississippi. Finally, on that busy Monday, Dr. Falk examined Dennis Sweeney, a COFO summer volunteer from Berkeley, who had suffered a concussion from a bomb explosion the previous night at the Freedom House in McComb. During that first week Falk also met with attorneys for the NAACP Legal Defense Fund and with George Crockett from the National Lawyers Guild, a left-wing organization known for its defense of activists accused of being Communists. He also talked with the president of the white Mississippi State Medical Society and representatives of the black National Medical Association.[2]

By now the first wave of MCHR volunteers—doctors, nurses, and other health care workers—had arrived. Most had taken a week's leave (or used vacation time) and had left families behind. After checking in at the Sun-n-Sand (the only desegregated hotel in Jackson), they went to the COFO office on Farish Street, where Smith saw to their medical orientation. Then Moses or another COFO leader described the goals of the Summer Project and the difficulties the MCHR volunteers might encounter. Falk and his associate, David Miller, a physician from New Haven, stressed the need for the volunteers to insure their personal safety by keeping in contact with the Jackson office, calling in when they left one community project and arrived at another. The warnings were specific. "No one should go *anywhere* alone, but certainly not in an automobile, and certainly not at night. Travel at night should be avoided unless absolutely necessary . . . At night, people should not sit in their room without drawn shades. Remove all unnecessary objects from your cars which could be construed as weapons . . . When getting out of a car at night, make sure the car's inside light is out." While these precautions may appear extravagant, less than a month earlier the three civil rights workers had disappeared, and nobody knew what to expect next.[3]

All of the first volunteers were white, but with the arrival of black physicians from the North such as Aaron Wells, Henry Paul, and Vernal Cave (who had been the medical officer for the famous Tuskegee Airmen during World War II), the question arose as to whether black and white volunteers should travel to their projects together. At an MCHR executive committee meeting Falk argued that it would be too dangerous to have teams "traveling in Mississippi on an integrated basis." David Miller agreed that "we must have segregated teams for security reasons." Others, including Aaron Wells, vehemently objected, claiming that since integration was their goal it would be unthinkable for teams to work on a segregated basis. Their argument carried the day. There would be no segregation of MCHR people in Mississippi.[4]

The health care activists came to Mississippi with a common purpose, yet they arrived with different agendas. Although not mutually exclusive, the fledgling organization had a civil rights faction and a public health faction. Tom Levin, the driving force behind MCHR, was firmly in the civil rights camp and had little patience with "that group of orthodox, left-wing systems change people." For Levin, MCHR was in Mississippi to provide a medical presence: protection for civil rights workers. "I wanted the doctors to put their bodies on the line for both physical and legal danger," he recalled. "I couldn't care less about the health care system." Falk and Jack Geiger (of the Harvard School of Public Health), on the other hand, represented a group of activists who wanted to eliminate Mississippi's segregated, two-class health system, through negotiation and persuasion if possible, through litigation if necessary.[5]

Any dialogue with local white physicians and hospital administrators proved difficult, however, in part because of a remarkable letter written by two prominent white health care professionals. Harvard psychologist

Robert Coles and MIT's Joseph Brenner had signed on to work in Mississippi during the summer. Both had attended the first orientation program for the Freedom Summer volunteers, held in Oxford, Ohio, during the third week in June. At this point the Medical Committee was just forming, and there were no provisions for health care for the volunteers once they reached Mississippi. Acting on their own, the two physicians hit upon the idea of contacting all the white doctors in Mississippi, imploring them to overcome their prejudices and provide treatment for civil rights workers. Coles drafted a letter, Brenner signed it, and they sent it out on June 30, two weeks before the first MCHR team landed in Mississippi.

The "Dear Doctors" letter began by calling attention to the hundreds of volunteers who would soon be descending on the Magnolia State, and acknowledged that "the activities of these students . . . may be strongly resisted by many people of the state." Then Coles and Brenner, without mincing words, called upon their Mississippi colleagues, "whatever their social or political views," to obey the Hippocratic oath, helpfully quoting the relevant passage for their southern brethren, and ending the letter with the "sincere hope that a clear separation between social upheaval and medical need will be maintained."

Only some two hundred words long, the "Brenner-Coles Letter," as it came to be called, sent shock waves through the white Mississippi medical community. Whatever its intent, the letter was so obviously patronizing that it alienated even those physicians who might have been cooperative. Every time an MCHR volunteer met a white physician that summer, the letter would be topic number one. Two days after the first team arrived in the state, Miller warned that "nothing should be said to impugn the integrity of Mississippi physicians." MCHR acting director Elliott Hurwitt wrote that "at no time has this committee ever assumed the attitude or alleged that Mississippi physicians would not discharge their ethical and moral responsibilities to the practice of medicine." But the damage had already been done.[6]

It was a "primary policy" that summer to make contact with local white physicians. Some encounters were hostile (MCHR representatives who dropped in on a Batesville physician were "ordered off the premises with instructions not to return"), but most white doctors responded to MCHR overtures with civility, if not cordiality. Their offices were segregated and would remain so for years. Still, practically all the doctors interviewed said they would treat civil rights workers, provided they could pay. Information on the availability of medical services in the white community

JOSEPH H. BRENNER, M.D.
41 TENNYSON ROAD
WELLESLEY HILLS 81, MASSACHUSETTS

June 30, 1964

Dear Doctors:

For the past two weeks we have been caring for several
hundred American college students preparing themselves in
Ohio for a summer's work in Mississippi. We have treated
a variety of medical complaints ranging from lacerations,
sprains, infections and allergies, to an acute surgical
abdomen warranting emergency hospitalization.

We fully understand that the activities of these students
working for civil rights in Mississippi may be strongly
resisted by many people of the state. As physicians we
are concerned that they continue to receive adequate medical
care.

We are hopeful that the doctors of this nation, wherever
they live, whatever their social or political views, will
respond fully and without reservation to the words of the
Hippocratic oath: "The regimen I adopt shall be for the
benefit of my patients according to my ability and judgment,
and not for their hurt or for any wrong..."

We are sending this short letter to our fellow physicians
of Mississippi and to the county medical societies, in the
sincere hope that a clear separation between social upheaval
and medical need will be maintained.

Sincerely,

Joseph H. Brenner, M. D.
Medical Department
Massachusetts Institute of Technology

Robert Coles

Robert Coles, M. D.
Health Services
Harvard University

JHB:N

Copy of Joseph Brenner–Robert Coles letter to Mississippi physicians. (Institute of Social Medicine and Community Health)

was then passed on to the local COFO office, along with the promise that MCHR would foot the medical bills for civil rights workers in the project. This information was particularly useful in counties where there were no black physicians.[7]

Several white doctors who practiced in Jackson or taught at the Ole Miss medical school identified with the civil rights movement, including James Hendrick, who later played a prominent role in the effort to provide better health care for black children. Smith's major ally during the summer was Oscar Hubbard, a psychiatrist at the medical school. A transplanted northerner, Hubbard befriended the MCHR workers who came through Jackson, and in the fall during the presidential campaign he and Smith formed a physicians' committee for Johnson and Humphrey.[8]

There were, however, Mississippi health care people whose opposition to the movement—and to black people—was apparent. In Canton, a mean little town twenty miles north of Jackson, a local doctor refused to provide further treatment to a black woman when he learned that she worked with COFO. (MCHR volunteers sent her to a sympathetic doctor at the University Medical Center.) After a white pharmacist told a black man working with COFO that "it would be very easy to put something in these drugs that would kill you," Canton blacks became reluctant to have prescriptions filled locally. MCHR doctors fell under the eye of "one highly placed Canton physician" who warned that he was going to "monitor the MCHR carefully and that if he finds any evidence that in his opinion the law has been violated he will give the circumstance wide publicity and will seek to have the physician's license suspended in his home state."[9]

Unfortunately for the Medical Committee, the most hostile physician was also the most powerful man in Mississippi medicine, Archie Gray, the executive director of the Mississippi State Board of Health. Early in the summer, Dr. Alfred Kogon scheduled an interview with Gray to talk about MCHR's work. The conversation did not go well. When Kogon suggested that the State Board of Health initiate a statewide oral polio preventive program, Gray icily replied that he "did not care to help Dr. Sabin sell his vaccine." As the person in charge of issuing medical licenses, he made it clear to Kogon that none of the MCHR doctors would get one. Gray not only declined to give Kogon a letter of introduction to county health officers, he refused to provide a list of said officers. When asked if he would accept funds for use by his department, he replied, "Not if it came from Communist organizations like the National Council of Churches." Gray's attitudes toward African Americans were widely known. He treated Bob Smith with condescension and threatened to pull his license. Tom Levin also had his encounters with Gray. Always given to understatement, Levin observed that "Archie Gray is the most racist motherfucker I have ever met."[10]

MCHR volunteers who visited clinics and hospitals usually encountered chilly receptions, and when they were permitted to tour the facilities they found black patients and doctors Jim-Crowed at every turn. Virginia Wells, an African American registered nurse and a member of the first MCHR team sent to Mississippi, made an appointment to visit a white physician's clinic in the Delta hamlet of Como. "We arrived ten minutes early, and were immediately hustled out of the air-conditioned waiting room, having entered by the front door." They were then directed to the hot, poorly equipped Negro waiting room. And the doctor never showed up.[11]

Most visits were to public hospitals built with Hill-Burton funds. The Supreme Court had declared the "separate but equal" provision of the act unconstitutional in 1963, and Title VI of the new civil rights act forbade federal funding for any segregated institution. A team of MCHR physicians in Canton visited Kings Daughters Hospital, built in 1951 with Hill-Burton money. Hospital director S. L. Whittington answered "no comment" to all questions concerning racial segregation. When asked about hospital fees, Whittington replied that "information regarding charges for hospitalization or emergency care were none of our business," but the printed notices on the walls stated that a fifty-dollar deposit was required for admittance, a fee that would eliminate most black patients. Even the emergency room had a dollar-fifty admission charge. There was a waiting room for whites at the front of the hospital and a smaller one for blacks at the back. Interviews with local blacks confirmed that only the rooms for white patients were air-conditioned, and that although blacks comprised 70 percent of the county population, only twenty-two of the sixty beds were reserved for them. There were six African American nurses employed at the hospital. The two black doctors in town did not have hospital privileges. When visiting physician Desmond Callan asked whether a "Negro physician with high qualifications" would be accepted on staff, Whittington refused to answer. As they were leaving, staff physician C. H. Heywood told the visitors that "we consider this an intrusion on your part just as you would feel if someone were to check on your hospital." The experience at Kings Daughters was typical of MCHR hospital visits across the state, with one partial exception.[12]

The newly built St. Joseph's Hospital in Meridian, operated by an order of Catholic nuns, had opened as a completely integrated facility for its patients. MCHR physician Hyman Gold reported that "the hospital is magnificently equipped and beautiful." But shortly after its opening some white doctors and most of the white patients boycotted the desegregated facility. Faced with large deficits, St. Joseph's administrators reinstituted segregation, but the hospital still operated at only one-quarter capacity. Gold and other volunteers tried to persuade Meridian blacks to use the new hospital (they were reluctant to patronize a medical facility steeped in racial controversy) while lobbying hospital administrators to bring the town's black doctor on staff. It would be two years, however, before Mississippi hospitals began to desegregate, and then only after MCHR had gathered incriminating evidence on dozens of state health care facilities.[13]

While Medical Committee doctors regarded their "mission work" in the white medical community as a priority, they also tried to establish ties with black physicians practicing in the state. Shortly after the first wave of MCHR volunteers moved in, acting chairman Jerome Tobis wrote to each black doctor expressing "the admiration we feel for the outstanding job the Negro physicians of Mississippi have performed" in providing care for the "indigent sick" and for "those who have participated in the freedom movement during those turbulent days." Tobis asked for "advice and guidance . . . in seeking ways in which we may share the burden with you." Establishing a good working relationship with the majority of Mississippi's black physicians proved a formidable task for the Medical Committee, during Freedom Summer and beyond. Many of these doctors were middle-aged or near retirement. They were conservatives who did not want to risk their standing in the larger community by participating in the civil rights movement. Fewer than a dozen local black doctors would even treat civil rights workers during the early sixties.[14]

As they moved into their assigned communities, some MCHR doctors made it a point to contact local black physicians, but others ignored them. Summer coordinator Jack Geiger knew of several volunteers "who would never go to see the black doctors . . . and here's a black doctor, who had been serving the black community and the only health care resource for them, and a white doctor from Buffalo comes down and, in effect, says 'I'm going to rescue all you people.'" That the great majority of MCHR doctors were white alumni of the nation's best medical schools and had lucrative practices or prestigious academic appointments in the North only made things worse. Most MCHR volunteers had no prior experience with the southern movement, and thus came with the same baggage that many of the young white college students brought with them to Mississippi. They did not know black people or white Mississippi. Smith laughingly recalled the time early in the summer when the wife of MCHR medical director Elliott Hurwitt "put her arm around me as if we were lovers and walked me right into the Sun-n-Sand motel. You talk about different kinds of stress. This was another kind of stress I didn't need!"[15]

Even doing the right thing could create problems between a medical volunteer and a local black physician. Early in the summer the Medical

Committee responded to a COFO request that a doctor visit a civil rights worker beaten and jailed in Greenwood. Aaron Jackson, the only black doctor in town, was furious. It seems that in Greenwood a physician was to visit a prisoner only if the sheriff requested it. By violating this unwritten rule the MCHR physician angered the sheriff, who took out his wrath on Dr. Jackson.[16]

From the outset, MCHR leaders had sought support from the National Medical Association. NMA activist Montague Cobb, as we have seen, had been the leading opponent of Jim Crow medicine, and his IMHOTEP conferences constituted the only national forum for discussion of racial discrimination in the medical profession. Both he and his distinguished Howard colleague Paul Cornely became MCHR sponsors. But rank-and-file NMA members were much more conservative, and many stood aloof from civil rights struggles in their communities. When it came to medical activism, MCHR was the new kid on the block, garnering favorable media coverage for its Mississippi project. The typical NMA physician, then, had a difficult time warming up to these "Park Avenue doctors" who thought socialized medicine was a good idea.

Still, the Medical Committee wanted the black organization's endorsement for its civil rights work, a task that fell to Bob Smith. As an officer in the Mississippi NMA, Smith invited national leaders, including president Kenneth Clement, to come to the state on a fact-finding mission, hoping that they would issue a strong report at the annual convention stating that civil rights workers in Mississippi—and elsewhere—needed help. Smith had planned to take the delegation to the Delta, the center of black poverty and civil rights activism. But they never made it, getting only as far as Yazoo City before the impatient NMA president said, "I've seen enough. Take us back." With that "they were able to write up their report and hand it to the convention."[17]

When the delegates to the NMA convention assembled in early August, they were presented with a resolution introduced by the Illinois delegation that began with an NMA endorsement of the civil rights movement followed by a pledge to "participate to the best of our ability in the program outlined by the Medical Committee for Human Rights." The resolution also affirmed that "all members of the NMA will provide such medical care as they are capable themselves of rendering to those casualties of the struggle with no cost to the patient." The resolution failed, in large part because of "opposition by Mississippi delegates." During the discussion several Mississippi doctors took the floor to say that they could not afford to treat civil rights workers for free, then wryly suggested that "the idea is good if it would apply to M.D.s out of the South." They unfairly identified MCHR with the Brenner-Coles letter, which had "hurt their relations with local white Mississippi doctors." The convention did pass a compromise resolution appropriating five thousand dollars "for a medical project in the South but not just Mississippi." Shortly after the convention, Montague Cobb, who had grown increasingly unhappy with the largely white medical contingent in Mississippi, withdrew his name from the list of MCHR sponsors. Disappointed by the failure of earlier overtures, MCHR leaders hoped to attract more NMA support as the summer wore on.[18]

The Medical Committee was but a small part of the contingent of a thousand outsiders who flocked to Mississippi in the summer of 1964 to work in existing COFO projects, which were to be the staging area for expansion into new territory. A major goal of Freedom Summer was to create a truly statewide movement. Not surprisingly, most intense activity occurred in the Delta, where SNCC had been active since the spring of 1962. The volunteers assisted the veteran activists in a variety of ways. They helped staff community centers, where games and books were available, as were arts and crafts. Some of the males did traditional voter registration work, walking the streets and dusty roads to persuade blacks to take the test to try to register to vote. This activity increasingly gave way to registering local people for the new Mississippi Freedom Democratic Party, which would challenge the state's white segregationist delegation at the national party convention later in the summer. Most of the women volunteers (and some of the men) taught in the "freedom schools."

While the Summer Project expanded and extended existing COFO programs, the freedom schools were something new to the Mississippi movement, a creative response to the woeful education afforded blacks in the state's public schools. The curriculum encouraged maximum student participation, and was based on the assumption that "the teacher is not to be an omnipotent, aristocratic dictator." The key to the freedom schools was the awareness that the students brought with them valuable knowledge and experiences. The assumption was that the culture of black Mississippians was important and must be preserved. The curriculum reflected this emphasis. Children (and some adults) studied traditional subjects like reading, writing, and math, but each school devoted part of the day to black history and its relationship to the civil rights movement. Several of the medical volunteers took advantage of the freedom schools to talk with the students about health care issues.[19]

COFO projects differed in size and personality, but each had a "freedom house" that served as the staff residence, central office, and community center. Always filled with typewriters, mimeograph machines, books, staff members, Freedom Summer volunteers, and local black kids just hanging out, it had a chaotic yet friendly atmosphere. There was nothing fancy about doing civil rights work in Mississippi. Imagine the impact, then, when a new chauffeur-driven Oldsmobile pulled up in front of a freedom house and out stepped a white physician in coat and tie carrying his black bag.

In addition to Jackson, the Medical Committee sent teams to Clarksdale and Greenwood in the Delta, to Meridian and Canton in the central part of the state, and to Hattiesburg and McComb in the south. Health care workers fanned out from these bases to visit other COFO projects. After their orientation in Jackson, the physician and driver (and sometimes a registered nurse) set out to find the COFO headquarters in their assigned community and begin their duties. Exactly what constituted their "duties" was unclear. Originally, the idea was that these physicians would come to Mississippi and do what they did best, practice medicine. But thanks to Archie Gray that became impossible. The first MCHR volunteers were pretty much left on their own to see where they fit in, and they received little guidance once they arrived at their destinations. "Not only might you not be welcomed with open arms," their guidebook informed them, "it is entirely possible that no one will be expecting you, have ever heard of you or know why you are here . . . It becomes immediately apparent that flexibility is *the* required skill if you are to survive and if you are going to be truly helpful to the project."

An obvious way to help was to befriend the COFO staff and summer volunteers, treat their minor medical ailments (which MCHR doctors could do without violating the law), refer them to local physicians for more serious medical problems, and see to it that the Medical Committee paid the bills. The doctors treated gastrointestinal and upper respiratory ailments, and infections from cuts, abrasions, and mosquito bites. They believed that many medical problems stemmed from poor diet and unsanitary conditions in the freedom houses and COFO offices. In an early memorandum to "all COFO personnel," MCHR stressed "most emphatically your practice of the best level of hygiene possible. Teach by example better habits of personal, family, and community cleanliness. This requires that you keep yourselves, your homes, and your office as clean and tidy as possible."[20]

Such admonitions did not always sit well with the young activists. Here they were living as a family, enjoying the freedom of being away from home and on their own, when in walks someone in a suit telling everybody to shape up. The physician was, after all, an authority figure, accustomed to giving orders and seeing them carried out. Sally Belfrage, a journalist and volunteer who wrote of her experiences in Greenwood in her poignant memoir, *Freedom Summer*, recalls that

> the first few doctors who came to help us lurked around the library using up some of their endless good will by sprinkling the books with Borax, which was supposed to be lethal to cockroaches but only made the bindings soapy; assigning a variety of vitamin, iron, and salt pills to staff stomachs; directing "Now we will wash our hands" to those seen petting the resident kittens, Freedom and Now; and asking me to make posters reading PLEASE FLUSH THE TOILET. I tried to explain that those who didn't flush the toilet couldn't read, being for the most part under seven, but that didn't make any headway either.[21]

Other COFO complaints concerned the "sex lectures" delivered by doctors urging the young people to observe high moral standards and to practice celibacy, and criticisms directed at their personal appearance in general. One volunteer physician in Greenwood wrote that the "dress of the COFO workers is out of harmony with the community and needlessly careless. A beard can hide a peck of dirt." Such sanctimonious behavior could create animosity toward the next medical team. Nurse Mary Holman and physician Marvin Belsky visited Batesville, where they learned that "the COFO people joke bitterly about the preachy attitude of medical committee personnel about diet, morals, neatness." And in Clarksdale "the COFO people are angry about a lecture from medical personnel on morals." After learning what was going on, Aaron Henry let the MCHR know that its representatives "should not lecture or preach or patronize COFO or the local people." For the most part MCHR learned from its mistakes, and as a rule the volunteers who came later in the summer were less directive and more low key. Belsky and Holman repaired the damage done by the earlier team in Clarksdale—"We apologized and they forgave us"—and did good work in the Delta. Belfrage reported that after the initial debacle, "an effective new team, headed by Martin Gittelman, a psychologist, and June Finer, a physician, arrived to show what could be done."[22]

June Finer was born in London in 1935, and had vivid memories of spending nights in shelters during the Nazi air raids during World War II before being evacuated to the countryside with other children. The daughter of Jewish immigrants, she was educated in London and, after graduating from medical school in 1960, she moved to Chicago because she "wanted to travel for a while" and had relatives there. She did her internship at Michael Reese, a large, inner-city hospital. There for the first time she "saw the living conditions of the blacks, and I was stunned." June became a confidant of a local activist named Quentin Young, and through him became involved with the Committee to End Discrimination in Chicago Medical Institutions (CED). She joined the Chicago CED contingent that went to Mississippi. British, female, and fearless—a free spirit with tons of sex appeal—Finer did not fit the MCHR stereotype. Over the next fifteen months she would spend more time in the South than any other northern MCHR physician, working in hot spots like Jackson, Bogalusa, and Selma.[23]

Like Finer and Gittelman, most MCHR volunteers pitched in to do what was necessary in the projects. They used their rented automobiles to run errands and transport people to and from political meetings. (It soon became apparent that the MCHR "drivers" were unnecessary, and the later teams of physicians and nurses drove their own rented cars.) Those doctors who were also handy made necessary repairs on the COFO buildings, including the freedom schools. Excerpts from a report filed by physician Lee Hoffman during his week in Clarksdale are indicative of the range of activities an enthusiastic MCHR volunteer could perform:

> Attended a COFO worker who was beaten over the head . . . gave first aid . . . accompanied him to the hospital . . . Played football with local high school boys . . . Visited several sick local people, with nurse . . . Was arrested for being out after curfew . . . Visited citizen of Marks in jail at request of COFO to give her reassurance (I COULD NOT HAVE GOTTEN IN WITHOUT POSITIVE IDENTIFICATION AS AN MD) . . . Repaired a dangerous electrical connection in a local home . . . put a lock on a window in Freedom House . . . Attended funeral at request of family of a terminal patient I had seen earlier.[24]

Dr. Hoffman's visit to "several sick local people" was not part of the original MCHR mission. All the discussions in New York and in Jackson had focused on treating civil rights workers. Except for encouraging the white medical establishment to adopt a color-blind policy, taking on the health care problems of hundreds of thousands of poor black Mississippians was not on their agenda. But in each project, as word got out that there was a new doctor in town, indigent blacks heretofore denied health care asked for treatment. A few visiting physicians refused to see any patient who was not a civil rights worker, either because such work was not part of their assignment or because they feared for their licenses, but in most cases MCHR doctors and nurses helped as much as they could. In Clarksdale, for example, nurse Carolyn Lane "visited homes, taught infant care, dressed wounds, helped prepare meals and gave freely of her own money for things she felt people needed but couldn't get otherwise." She bought thermometers and taught mothers how to use them and supplied their children with toothbrushes. It was of course impossible for an MCHR volunteer in town for only a week to deal with the massive health problems facing hundreds of blacks in a particular community. One doctor described his work in the black community as "like touching the surface of a wave."[25]

In each area, MCHR representatives investigated the public health agencies charged with providing preventive care for the indigent and provided local people with information concerning these services. In many cases they found public health officials indifferent to the medical problems of blacks. Arthur Dunn reported from Holly Springs that "even the most casual survey reveals the extent of a grossly inadequate medical service for the Negro community . . . A conspiracy of silence existed among local white officials, making it difficult to find out exactly what the nature of the medical services 'theoretically' provided to the community really was." Some health officials were hostile, as when the public health nurse in Hattiesburg threatened to have a COFO nurse's license revoked for holding prenatal and personal hygiene classes for black women.[26]

Throughout the summer, MCHR volunteers put together a public health program of their own. They gave lectures at freedom schools and local churches on a range of topics, including prenatal and child care, nutrition, hygiene, family planning, and venereal disease. They immunized children and conducted door-to-door health surveys, gathering information on family health and living conditions. Poor sanitation was a universal problem. Richard Brenner reported that "many people living in the rural areas have privies at no specified distance from their wells." In Greenwood, Gittel-man and Finer organized the young people who had been hanging around the freedom house to build an outdoor shower and construct a system that would pipe fresh water into the community. Important as these projects were, they only called attention to the massive problems that remained.[27]

Most COFO staff members and summer volunteers were physically healthy, especially when compared with the black community as a whole, but across the state MCHR doctors and nurses encountered many cases of what psychologist Robert Coles labeled "battle fatigue." Coles spent time in Mississippi that summer, and later wrote that "in many ways these young civil rights workers are in a war and exposed to the stresses of war-fare." The symptoms, Coles reported, included fear, anxiety, and "anger no longer 'controlled' or 'managed.' Depressions occur. The youth af-fected may take to heavy drinking or become sullen, silent, and uncooper-ative." MCHR volunteer Des Callan agreed that "battle fatigue was in many ways the most serious health problem." He observed workers suffer-ing from insomnia, nightmares, "and some acting out and being crazed—really crazed." Callan also noted that the college students recruited for the summer were "energetic and often very half-formed young adults, who were already on the edge before they even set foot in the state." The main reason civil rights workers experienced psychological distress was, of course, the harassment and violence of Mississippi whites. Early in the summer, a SNCC organizer who had been shot in the head in 1963 be-came upset after a bloodied COFO worker he knew was taken to Baptist Hospital in Jackson. Fearing the young man would not get proper medical attention, the SNCC worker "provoked medical personnel, and spoke in a ranting, declamatory way . . . eyes bloodshot and staring . . . talking about people getting shot, including himself." He eventually left the hos-pital in a rage, accompanied by Tom Levin.[28]

Sam Block, the courageous young SNCC activist most responsible for launching the Greenwood movement, had paid the price with repeated jailings, beatings, and threats on his life. He talked with MCHR physi-cian Leon Redler, who reported that the activist "has had increasing anorexia, insomnia, anxiety, loneliness, bouts of depression and thoughts that perhaps death would be a solution to his problems." Plagued with ringing in his ears and hallucinations, Block told Redler, "I got to get out of here." The doctor observed that "he knows if he stays in or near Mis-sissippi he will not be able to resist running back to SNCC." Block left Mississippi that fall.[29]

Conditions inside the projects also contributed to worker stress. In a report written at the end of the summer, physician Emanuel Schreiber stated that "personal antagonisms, complexly related to many personal variables—color, education, region of orientation, sex—are abundant within the movement." Specifically, Schreiber found that "white COFO workers are not entirely excluded from the stored hate which the Negro holds for the white man, [and] in turn, the white workers are not free of a host of images of the Negro—the sensuous one, the incompetent one, and so on, which precludes free social relations." Add to this the problems created by sexual relations between workers, particularly interracial sex, and you have a mix COFO staff members found increasingly difficult to handle.[30]

That said, one should not exaggerate the incidence of battle fatigue. Most civil rights workers in Mississippi stayed physically and mentally healthy, even in the face of external threats and internal discord. From the outset of the summer, however, MCHR doctors, nurses, and psychiatrists saw that they had a role to play in alleviating the conditions produced by stress. One of the most ambitious projects took place in Greenwood under the direction of Martin Gittelman.

The son of immigrant parents, Marty Gittelman was brought up in a Jewish neighborhood in New York. He attended City College, did his graduate work in psychotherapy, and was a clinical psychologist on the staff at Jacobi Hospital in the spring of 1964 when he learned about the plans to send health care workers to Mississippi. An early and enthusiastic volunteer, Gittelman spent time in Canton before going on up to Greenwood, SNCC's major project and the organization's national headquarters for the summer. Shortly after he arrived in the Delta he recognized "what would become known as post-traumatic stress disorder, people who had been traumatized by a whole host of things." Here Gittelman began to experiment with group therapy, a discipline that would become his life's work. Each night at the freedom house the young psychologist would "get people to sit down and talk about the events of the day, and how they felt about it . . . particularly the folks who had been in jail and traumatized and abused." Most people welcomed these sessions, although "a few kids walked around, angry, irritable." Gittelman found race no obstacle, as black movement activists were happy to have an outside professional to talk with. He remembers several conversations with project director Stokely Carmichael (the two had attended the same high school). Disillusioned with his current role in the movement, Carmichael spoke of his desire to leave Mississippi and enroll in medical school. Others talked frankly about their own fears and aspirations. Once MCHR volunteers gained the confidence of civil rights activists they played an important role simply by listening.[31]

Sometimes, however, movement workers posed a threat to themselves or to others in the project. Normally these cases were referred to Bob Smith, who saw "people who actually suffered full breakdowns." He would arrange for them to have medical care available immediately in New York, with therapists such as Tom Levin, Josephine Martin, June Christmas, and Israel Zwerling.[32] MCHR came up with the idea of establishing a "rest and rehabilitation center" in Mississippi. Activists suffering from battle fatigue could get away for several days to "a place secluded both from unfriendly Mississippians and from the freedom fight." Here they would have the opportunity to "sleep well, to eat well, to listen to music, to read for pleasure, and to indulge in unpressured play." Formal and informal group discussions led by a mental health professional could be part of the retreat, but people with serious psychological problems would not be invited to the center. Near the end of the summer ten people participated in a trial two-day retreat at Tougaloo. The Medical Committee had rented two houses in Jackson during the summer, which for a time also served as a rest and recreation center. In the months that followed, MCHR found ways to provide activists with other opportunities to get away from the pressures that were preventing them from functioning effectively in the movement.[33]

Another important service provided by MCHR during Freedom Summer was that of "medical presence." Whether it was a demonstration or a march to the courthouse, MCHR volunteers were on the scene, easily identifiable by the Red Cross emblem on their sleeves and their professional appearance. ("We always wore a suit," one doctor recalled, "no matter how hot it was.") Their presence seemed to diminish the level of violence during a confrontation. "The police got nervous when they saw medical people or a car with a Red Cross band," observed one medical volunteer. "It was a bit of a deterrent to their brutality." This was also true when MCHR doctors went into the jails to examine civil rights workers who had been arrested. After such a visit, an activist was less likely to be beaten by the jailers, who knew the physician could testify to the previous condition of the inmate. MCHR doctors were also present when their professional status could provide reassurance, as when, at the end of the summer, they accompanied small children attempting to desegregate schools in Canton and Clarksdale.[34]

Medical presence also meant that any civil rights demonstrator beaten by a mob or by the police would get first aid from a physician or nurse, who would also arrange for hospital care, if needed. The summer of 1964 in Mississippi was the most violent since the last days of Reconstruction. There were thirty-five shooting incidents and sixty-five homes and other buildings burned or bombed, including thirty-five churches. One thousand movement people were arrested, and eighty activists suffered beatings. There were at least six murders. Violent racial confrontations were most prevalent in and around Greenwood. After a voter registration rally in mid-July, police arrested 110 people—including two women in advanced stages of pregnancy. MCHR physician Joel Bates reported that one of the women had received "a nasty head wound" that had not been treated. Bates went to the jail, saw six of the women who had been arrested, and arranged for the release of one woman who was nine months pregnant.[35]

Near the end of the Summer Project, COFO worker Silas McGhee had just driven volunteers to Lula's Café in Greenwood for a farewell party. As he sat alone in his car outside the café, someone drove by and shot him just below the temple. The bullet lodged in his throat. The celebrating summer workers and COFO staff members poured out of the café, saw McGhee bleeding, and rushed him to the hospital. June Finer arrived shortly thereafter, and as she offered her assistance she overheard one hospital worker say, "I hope they got one of them." Finer was soon ordered off the premises. McGhee was later transferred to Jackson for surgery, where he recovered from the gunshot wound. No one was arrested in the shooting.[36]

The Medical Committee also became involved in one of the most bizarre cases of violence that summer, one that occurred in a doctor's office in rural Leake County. On July 30, a Harvard student volunteer named John Polacheck sought treatment for a fungus infection at the clinic of Dr. A. L. Thaggard. When a staff member directed the white civil rights worker to the "Negro waiting room" Polacheck left, unwilling to patronize a segregated establishment. Learning of this, Ed Heininger, a National Council of Churches volunteer working in Leake County, called Thaggard and made an appointment for Polacheck at eleven A.M. the next day. They went together. Thaggard met them in the waiting room and began berating Reverend Heininger over his civil rights work. While they were talking, the two activists were ambushed from behind by at least a half-dozen men, who beat them to a pulp. Heininger, who later reported that Thaggard had pushed him into the arms of his attackers, was knocked unconscious. Police arrived and arrested the two volunteers—for disturbing the peace. Medical Committee leaders in Jackson helped arrange bail, and later doctors Herbert Cave, Robert Sager, and Charles Goodrich examined Heininger, who had suffered a severe injury to his left eye, lacerations of the scalp and face, and a swelling of the mouth and lips. MCHR leaders unsuccessfully petitioned the AMA to censure Thaggard for "a most flagrant case of unethical behavior." The Central Medical Society of Mississippi also refused to take action because "the testimony concerning the facts was equally opposing." Dr. Thaggard was a vice president of the Central Medical Society.[37]

The Medical Committee earned national recognition for its investigation into the case of the three civil rights workers murdered in Neshoba County. The tragic journey of black activist James Chaney, CORE worker Michael Schwerner, and summer volunteer Andrew Goodman into the heart of Klan country on Sunday, June 21, 1964, is the most depressingly familiar story of the Mississippi movement: their arrest by deputy sheriff Cecil Price on the outskirts of Philadelphia shortly after three P.M.; the incarceration in Sheriff Lawrence Rainey's jail; their release at about ten thirty that night. They were never seen alive again. For the next six weeks Mississippi officials claimed that their "disappearance" was a hoax, arranged by COFO as a publicity stunt, and that the young men were alive and well in Chicago, or Havana, or someplace. But then a paid informant told the FBI that the bodies were buried under an earthen dam at a Neshoba County farm. A bulldozer was hauled out to the dam on the morning of August 4, and by late afternoon the three bodies had been recovered.[38]

The disappearance of the three young men in late June had deeply shaken the New Yorkers who were organizing the Medical Committee for Human Rights. The doctors were familiar with the families of two of the victims. Carolyn Goodman, Andrew's mother, belonged to a family volunteer support group organized by Trudy Orris. Children of several of the physicians had preceded them as volunteers in Mississippi. Once the bodies had been found, MCHR wanted to do whatever it could to bring the killers to justice. The autopsies seemed a natural place to begin. William Kunstler and Arthur Kinoy, attorneys for the victims' families, requested that MCHR doctors be present. Both the FBI representative and the director of the University of Mississippi Medical Center (where the autopsies were to be held) agreed. However, when physicians Charles Goodrich and Alfred Kogon arrived at University Hospital at twelve thirty A.M. on August 5, the head of the Mississippi State Highway Patrol, flanked by police officers, turned them away. Goodrich's pleas that they were present on a purely personal "medical courtesy" mission representing the families of the victims were of no avail.[39]

The official autopsy, conducted by Jackson pathologist William Featherston, was not released, but the next day newspapers reported that examination of the badly decomposed bodies showed that all three young men had been shot, Schwerner and Goodman once and Chaney three times, with no evidence of mutilation or bodily injury. Medical Committee representatives in Jackson were suspicious. If the bodies were badly decomposed, then how could an official determination be made that there were no bodily injuries? Goodrich called his friend David Spain, a leading New York pathologist then vacationing on Martha's Vineyard, and asked him to come down at once.[40]

By coincidence, Spain flew down to Mississippi with Aaron Wells, who was on his way to Jackson for a two-week stint as MCHR field coordinator. Wells taught at Cornell Medical School and had a lucrative practice in Harlem. The two men checked into the Sun-n-Sands motel and were met with "hostile glances [and] angry epithets." (The Sovereignty Commission—the state spy agency charged with preserving the Mississippi way of life—was on the job and reported that on August 6, Dr. Spain shared a motel room "with a negro doctor from New York.") The following day the two men awaited word on whether Spain would be permitted to examine the bodies of Schwerner and Chaney. The remains of Andrew Goodman had been sent back to New York. Schwerner's body was still in Jackson because his parents wanted to have him buried next to his friend James Chaney. (That would prove impossible in Jim Crow Mississippi.) State officials went to great lengths to prevent the second autopsy. They required that the two families claim the bodies personally and then provide written permission before Spain could perform his examination. The Schwerners' call from New York authorizing Spain's autopsy was not good enough for Mississippi officials. Fannie Lee Chaney, James's mother, met with Goodrich and signed the consent forms. "I want everyone to know everything possible about what has happened," she said. "God must forgive them; it is very difficult for me to do so." Spain later wrote that "the pressure on Mrs. Chaney to refuse permission was tremendous . . . Without her, we would never see the body." Three weeks after she signed the form, Mrs. Chaney escaped injury after her home was bombed.[41]

When David Spain finally got in to examine James Chaney's body he was not prepared for what he saw. Reports of the official autopsy showed no bodily injury to any of the victims. Dr. Spain first noticed Chaney's face. "The lower jaw was completely shattered, split vertically, from some tremendous force." On the torso he found "the bones in the right shoulder were crushed—again, from some strong and direct blow." Spain's conclusion was quoted in newspapers around the world. "I could barely believe the destruction to these frail young bones. In my twenty-five years as a pathologist and medical examiner, I have never seen bones so severely shattered, except in tremendously high speed accidents or airplane crashes. It was obvious to any first-year medical student that this boy had been beaten to a pulp."

That the white Mississippians who conducted the official autopsy and the FBI agents who had observed it had either missed or had not seen fit to report the damage done to Chaney's body was proof to many of a conspiracy of silence. That James Chaney had been physically brutalized, while his white companions were not, was indicative of the depth and perversity of Mississippi racism. The story does not end there. While not disputing Dr. Spain's findings, the FBI later revealed that two Klansmen who confessed to the crime, interviewed separately, testified that the three men were shot. Neither said anything about beatings. Both the FBI and Justice Department prosecutors concluded that James Chaney's battered body was the result of contact with either the bulldozer that buried the three men in the dam or the dragline used by the FBI to exhume them.[42]

What happened or did not happen to James Chaney before he was killed has been the subject of controversy for more than four decades. In 2002, Jerry Mitchell of the Jackson *Clarion-Ledger* (whose investigative reporting has resulted in bringing to justice a score of men guilty of civil rights murders, beginning with Byron De La Beckwith, the man who shot Medgar Evers) wrote a series of articles revisiting the Neshoba case, for none of the assailants had ever been charged with murder. Mitchell had access to the full autopsy report, made available for the first time, and the files of the Mississippi State Sovereignty Commission. His investigation reopened the question of whether Chaney was beaten before he was shot. When the full autopsy was released for the first time, Mitchell contacted two prominent pathologists who said that the injuries to Chaney's body were inconsistent with damage from the bulldozer that buried them. An FBI agent on the scene when the bodies were uncovered said that they were not touched by the FBI's heavy equipment. State Sovereignty Commission investigator Andy Hopkins filed a secret report in January of 1965 that offers a plausible explanation for what happened to James Chaney that night. "He broke away from the group of men that were holding him captive. Shortly after he made the break, he was shot at several times by several different people, but was struck by only three bullets, each of which was alleged to have been fired from a different firearm." The autopsy report shows that Chaney was shot once in the back, an indication he was trying to escape. One of the Klan informants, James Jordan, had testified that Chaney was killed about forty feet from where Schwerner and Chaney had been shot. Anyone familiar with the psychology of a lynch mob knows that a victim attempting to escape is likely to suffer unspeakable brutality once apprehended. Although the controversy continues, Jerry Mitchell's conclusion that the Klansmen "just didn't kill the black activist, they tortured him before he died," appears to be the sad truth.[43]

David Spain's findings were a source of great pride to the medical volunteers. Without his efforts—and theirs—an important piece of the history of the murders of the three activists would have been lost. Just a few weeks earlier a handful of professionals had formed a group to assist civil rights workers in Mississippi. For the fifty-seven physicians, eighteen nurses, and thirty-five other health care professionals who came to Mississippi, the summer had been chaotic, exciting, humbling, and rewarding. They made mistakes. Few were prepared for their foray into the nation's most racially charged state. Still, the Medical Committee volunteers did good work in Mississippi during Freedom Summer. They reached out into the larger community and addressed the health needs of the civil rights workers. But more important was the simple fact that they were there, an adult professional presence providing a small sense of security to a besieged group of freedom fighters.

As for the COFO veterans, Freedom Summer had been a bittersweet experience. They had successfully brought off the most ambitious and extensive event in the history of the civil rights movement. The attention of the world had focused on the Magnolia State, and the Summer Project marked the beginning of the end of "massive resistance": White Mississippi no longer spoke with a single voice. But the activists were exhausted, and many turned bitter when the Freedom Democratic Party was not seated at Atlantic City, having been abandoned by their white northern liberal allies who feared that seating the FDP would deliver the South to Republican presidential candidate Barry Goldwater in November. "For many people," observed SNCC's Joyce Ladner, "Atlantic City was the end of innocence."

At the end of the summer the Medical Committee pledged to "continue its work in Mississippi as long as COFO exists." During the latter months of 1964, having resumed their professional lives in the cities of the North, the good doctors discussed the implications of this commitment, and how they would respond to an increasingly militant mood among civil rights activists.[44]

CHAPTER 3

The Medical Arm of the Civil Rights Movement

D uring the fall of 1964, the Medical Committee for Human Rights became a permanent organization, founded chapters in major cities, and made good on its promise to maintain a medical presence in Mississippi. The Medical Committee employed a full-time staff member to run its Jackson office and recruited nurses to work in African American communities. Several northern physicians, strongly influenced by their participation in the Summer Project, worked with Bob Smith and a new civil rights organization called the Delta Ministry to establish programs providing medical care for destitute Mississippi blacks. All this occurred at a time when civil rights activists in Mississippi and across the South were reassessing their commitment to the nonviolent movement and to working within existing institutions to effect social change.

On September 12, seventeen veterans of the Summer Project met in the New York home of Sidney Greenberg to chart MCHR's course. Most were from the immediate area; Jack Geiger and Count Gibson came down from Boston and Bob Smith flew in from Mississippi. Much of the meeting involved the mechanics of setting up an organizational structure, complete with constitution, bylaws, and committees. Aaron Wells was elected national chairman. Jerome Tobis, a celebrity in the medical profession, was chosen national vice-chairman, while Alfred Moldovan, who had coordinated the fund-raising campaign that had raised nearly forty thousand dollars over the summer, became treasurer. Jack Geiger and Count Gibson were in charge of program, Bob Smith was the liaison to the National

Medical Association, and Tom Levin chaired the recruitment and membership committee. Constance Friess, the only woman physician on the board, took charge of public relations. The group agreed that it should add more prominent sponsors, a list that already included medical luminaries like Benjamin Spock and Paul Dudley White.[1]

The organization's statement of purpose was simple and direct. "We are deeply concerned with the health needs of the socially deprived. It is our purpose to initiate activities to improve their health status and to provide professional support and assistance to organizations concerned with human rights." The group also agreed to "work on a national scope instead of just Mississippi—North, as well as South."

Fresh from their summer experience in Mississippi, doctors and other health care activists in several cities began forming MCHR chapters of their own. The eight affiliates included chapters in New York, Boston, Washington, D.C., Pittsburgh, Los Angeles, and Chicago. All wanted to become part of the national organization, but with authority to launch their own programs. Those attending the September meeting agreed on a broad statement advocating "the principles of federation with maximum local autonomy consistent with a functioning national body." Details of the relationship between the chapters and the national office in New York were to be worked out at an MCHR convention, scheduled for the spring of 1965 in Washington.[2]

The most contentious issue at the September meeting was whether to limit membership to medical professionals. Some believed that opening MCHR to the general public could lead to a "complete change in policies and direction" and thus sacrifice "its medical committee image." But the argument that "the majority will always be physicians, so let us act in magnanimity and not limit ourselves," carried the day. MCHR would be open to "all health care personnel and others who concur with our stated purposes." This was too much for Elliott Hurwitt, chief of surgery at Montefiore Hospital and one of the high-profile physicians who had gone to Mississippi. Two days after the meeting he wrote the following terse note: "The decisions reached at the meeting on September 12 are so totally at variance with my concepts of a *Medical* committee that I have no alternative but to withdraw. I should like this resignation to be effective as of this date." Hurwitt's wife, Claire, who had also volunteered in Mississippi, also quit the organization, icily stating that "I prefer to spend my time on other matters."[3]

After dispensing with the time-consuming details of establishing a national organization, the activists turned to what brought them together in the first place: support for the civil rights movement. Bob Smith reported on his current activities; others spoke of their own experiences as volunteers. Discussion quickly centered on a lengthy memorandum written by SNCC's Jesse Morris, addressed to "Medical Committee Personnel." A black activist from California who had come to Mississippi in 1963, Morris was now running the Jackson COFO office and the liaison between SNCC and MCHR. His report criticized MCHR's work in the summer and called for the committee to develop a health care program to address the needs of Mississippi's black poor.[4]

Morris did not mince words. "Can the medical committee develop a program which has the same goals and purposes as other programs administered and carried out by COFO—given the limitations in the form of state laws and regulations preventing the medical committee's personnel from completely utilizing their skills? . . . What can be undertaken by medical committee persons who cannot legally practice in the state, and who will only be in the state an extremely short period of time?" Morris acknowledged the positive contributions of MCHR volunteers during Freedom Summer, for "the mere presence of the doctors . . . gave the project an image within the state it wouldn't have otherwise had." The civil rights workers were also grateful for the physical exams. "But," he concluded, "none of this refutes the COFO staff's basic contention that the medical committee could have contributed more, if it had concentrated solely on serving the needs of local people . . . There is an overwhelming need for some type of health program to begin, and relatively soon." There was general agreement that participating in Freedom Summer was a good idea. But now in the fall changes were occurring inside the movement, and Morris, at least, was questioning COFO's future relations with MCHR. To learn more about the situation, the committee sent Jack Geiger to Mississippi.[5]

Of all the northern physicians who worked in black communities in Mississippi, Geiger would have the greatest impact. He returned time and again over the next four decades, and in the Delta he helped create the model for the comprehensive community health center. Jack Geiger was born in New York City in 1926. His father was a physician, and both his parents were German Jewish immigrants. A precocious student, Jack skipped grades and graduated from high school at age fourteen. During his senior year, as editor of the school paper he attended the stage production of Richard Wright's *Native Son*. After the play Geiger went backstage to interview the star of the show, African American actor Canada Lee. Lee befriended Geiger, and Jack subsequently visited the actor at his home on Sugar Hill in Harlem.[6]

Geiger needed this outlet, because at the time he was in the middle of "nonstop conflicts" with his parents. One Sunday he packed a bag, headed uptown and knocked on Lee's door, explained his problems at home, and asked if he could stay with the actor for a while. Later that evening Lee called the elder Geiger to say that he would send his son home in the morning, but since he would probably run away again, why not let him move in with Lee? Jack's parents agreed, and he "spent the rest of that year and much time subsequently at Canada's, which afforded me a kind of experience that I think that never ordinarily would have occurred." At Lee's home, Geiger got to meet Langston Hughes and Richard Wright. Duke Ellington "stopped by on occasion," as did actors, playwrights, athletes, and intellectuals. Politically progressive, Lee (who would later be blacklisted for his views) surrounded himself with "black and white liberal and radical folks." It was Lee who provided Geiger with the money for his first year of college at the University of Wisconsin.

At Wisconsin, Jack became politically involved. He picketed a factory that discriminated against blacks, and, after meeting with James Farmer in Chicago, Geiger and others founded the second CORE chapter, in Madison. At the end of 1943, Jack left school to enlist in the merchant marine, and for a good bit of the war sailed on the SS *Booker T. Washington*, "the only ship with a black captain." After the war Geiger enrolled at the University of Chicago and became civil liberties chairman of the left-wing American Veterans Committee. There he helped launch a two-year campaign to end discriminatory practices at the university hospital and to persuade the medical school to admit black applicants. Geiger's academic interests were biology and journalism, and for a time after he graduated he was the science editor of the International News Service. In 1954 he enrolled at Case Western Medical School.

As he began his second year Geiger had an epiphany. "One day standing on the steps of the medical school it occurred to me that out there in Cleveland, who got sick and who didn't and what they were sick with and their subsequent interaction with the health care system were all not just biological phenomena. They were *social phenomena*, and suddenly all the experiences from my earlier life clicked in. I got very excited and thought I had invented social medicine. I ran to the library and discovered they'd already done that for a hundred years."

A five-month fellowship from the Rockefeller Foundation, "which had funded something called community health centers in, of all places, South Africa," gave Geiger the opportunity to study there. He got a first-hand look at apartheid and made contact with members of the African National Congress. After getting his medical degree, Geiger did his internship in internal medicine at Boston City Hospital, and he went on to get a degree in epidemiology at the Harvard School of Public Health, where he joined the faculty in 1964. Through it all, his experiences with community health centers in South Africa stuck in his mind, and "it was clear to me what I was going to do was international health." But then Mississippi came along and his career took a different turn.

In 1961, Geiger was a founder of Physicians for Social Responsibility, a group dedicated to the elimination of nuclear weapons. Two years later he joined Walter Lear's Medical Committee for Civil Rights, and a year later was in the first wave of MCHR activists. Geiger spent a month in Mississippi as field director during Freedom Summer, and there he became aware of "the appalling problems of the black population and the nature of their health care." Now, in early October, he returned to the Magnolia State to meet with Morris and other COFO officials. Geiger also checked in with Claire Bradley, the MCHR staff member who ran the Jackson office. Bradley had tried to persuade Morris that MCHR would do right by COFO, and that he should not form another medical committee, as he once threatened to do. She argued that MCHR was interested in developing a health program for the larger black community, and that after a period of reorganization it would again work in tandem with COFO. Geiger reiterated these points in his meeting with Morris who, according to Bradley, came away "quite pleased with what we were doing and understanding a great deal more of the difficulties we faced."[7]

For Geiger it soon became clear that the Medical Committee's problems with COFO were minor compared to the struggles going on within the Mississippi civil rights movement. After the debacle in Atlantic City, where the national Democratic Party refused to seat the Freedom Democratic Party delegation's convention, many SNCC and CORE veterans turned their backs on the northern liberals who they believed had sold them out. Back home, the FDP supported the Johnson-Humphrey ticket and ran candidates of its own, but internally the movement was in disarray.[8]

COFO was also experiencing growing pains. Its leaders had assumed that the volunteers would go home at the end of the summer, but nearly two hundred of the students, most of them white, chose to remain and work in Mississippi. Racial tensions—kept under control during the summer—now surfaced, along with a breakdown in discipline and a loss of leadership. Both Bob Moses and Dave Dennis, the key people in COFO, had become disillusioned with the slow pace of change and no longer made their presence felt. The Jackson office, which only weeks before had been the state COFO headquarters and a haven for volunteers, was in turmoil. No one wanted to manage the office, so Morris reluctantly took the job. SNCC worker Hunter Morey wrote that "the state headquarters in Jackson is almost completely dysfunctional . . . Staff and volunteer discipline has broken down so far that the state headquarters has had several race riots, white workers are often subject to severe racial abuse, and even violence from Negro workers . . . juvenile delinquency appears to have taken over several offices." Although perhaps exaggerated, Morey's description of conditions was not far off the mark. Jackson staff member Charlie Horwitz observed that "there's a small-scale siege in the office every day." Things got so bad that Morris shut down the office for a week.[9]

The turmoil in COFO mirrored that of its parent organization, SNCC. At its September executive committee meeting, Jim Forman unveiled a plan to expand the Summer Project in 1965 to encompass the entire southern black belt. Enthusiastically received, the "black belt project" was the major agenda item at the October meeting of the SNCC staff, a much larger group. Here the project drew bitter opposition from a couple of Mississippi field secretaries, who may have been concerned that COFO would no longer be a SNCC priority. By the time the meeting ended a sharp division over SNCC's direction and leadership was apparent. The black belt project collapsed for lack of support, leaving SNCC without a program for the following summer. The Medical Committee was caught off guard, as its recruitment committee had already informed prospective volunteers that "next summer, in five states, two to three times the number of Medical Committee personnel will be required to support 'Black Belt' program." With another Freedom Summer now unlikely, what program should the MCHR pursue?[10]

Physician Robert Axelrod's earlier pledge that "as long as there is COFO, there will be doctors" was taking on unintended irony. Claire Bradley passed on COFO's request that no more doctors be sent to Mississippi unless a project specifically asked for them. She reiterated Morris's point that, with the Summer Project ended, short-term people "are of no use in the community" and just wasted the time of the movement people who had to entertain them. Still, several doctors did come down in the fall, mostly as observers.[11]

In addition to uncertainty over the direction of the civil rights movement, MCHR program planners were operating under financial strictures. Although the organization had raised forty thousand dollars during the summer, it spent more, leaving many unpaid bills in Mississippi. Treasurer Al Moldovan sent out an urgent appeal in late October to the volunteers, reminding them that many had said that "they would be willing to pay all or part of the cost of their Mississippi stay," but had failed to do so. (Plane fares to Mississippi and car rentals had accounted for nearly half of the MCHR budget.) By early September, MCHR had a stack of outstanding bills. "We need money, desperately," wrote Bradley from Jackson. "There are several sizeable hospital bills, rent due for the house and office due immediately, and automobile bills beyond belief." Until the organization could get on a solid financial footing, the more ambitious plans, like having a full-time medical director and staff working in Mississippi, would be put on hold.[12]

Fortunately, the Delta Ministry came to the rescue. With an energetic staff led by two northern white ministers, Art Thomas and Warren McKenna, and with significant financing from the parent National Council of Churches, the Delta Ministry opened an office in Greenville in the fall of 1964 and began looking for ways to have a long-term impact on poor blacks in the region. Health care was an obvious area of concern, and Thomas approached Geiger with an offer to support MCHR's Mississippi operation for the immediate future. Not only would it pay rent for the MCHR office and a house in Jackson, the Delta Ministry also promised to fund nurses to work in black communities. The first three MCHR nurses, Kathy Dahl, Phyllis Cunningham, and Josephine Disparti, had come down as summer volunteers with COFO and had stayed on into the fall. Dahl worked for MCHR in north Mississippi. Cunningham and Disparti signed on in early October and began community health projects in Hattiesburg and in the Delta.[13]

The oldest of six children, Phyllis Cunningham grew up in a working-class Catholic family in northern Minnesota. Her father owned a taxicab business and later bought a pool hall. Her mother, a homemaker, had gone to college for a year. Phyllis attended parochial schools and stayed in her hometown to enroll at the College of St. Teresa in 1957. Her political awakening occurred as an indirect consequence of her devout upbringing. "While at St. Teresa I had this terrible fear that I was going to lose my soul and go to hell, so I joined all the religious organizations I could possibly join to save my soul. It turned out that one of the groups

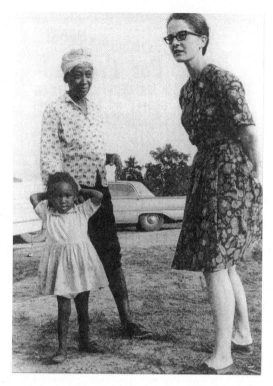

Phyllis Cunningham making a house call. (Charmian Redding)

was the Young Christian Students [YCS], which was the left-wing radical organization of the Catholic Church." Active in YCS, she organized a workshop on race relations, which brought leaders of the Minneapolis and St. Paul branches of the NAACP to campus. That meeting was "really an eye-opener" for the young nursing student, who had grown up in a town with few black residents. After graduation, with a degree in nursing, Cunningham took a job in Chicago organizing nursing students through the national office of the Young Christian Students, and worked full-time at local hospitals. After two years she moved to the Visiting Nurse Association, where she gained experience as a public health nurse. During her three years in Chicago, Cunningham got to know Quentin Young and June Finer through her participation in the Committee to End Discrimination. After meeting SNCC activists Tim Jenkins and Chuck McDew, she raised money for the movement through the Chicago Friends of SNCC. When Phyllis heard about the Summer Project she knew she had to be part of it. Denied a leave of absence, she did not hesitate before quitting her job and heading for Mississippi.[14]

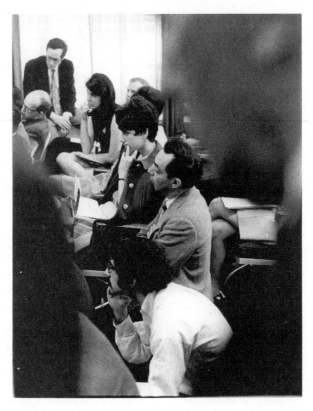

H. Jack Geiger (center, in sports jacket) and Josephine Disparti at an MCHR meeting. (Charmian Redding)

COFO assigned her to Hattiesburg. The only nurse in the project, she soon concluded that "it wasn't the volunteers who needed medical help; it was the need for health care in the black community." Dedicated, confident, yet unassuming, Cunningham started up neighborhood "health and welfare groups," and there led discussions on the politics of health care as well as health education. When MCHR physicians came to town they all wanted to talk to the resident nurse. A no-nonsense health care activist who did not suffer fools gladly, Cunningham resented this intrusion into her community work. Serving as a "tour agent" for a different group of doctors every week was frustrating, especially since many of them "would just get in our way." Eventually she wrote up a report of her activities that she presented to the visitors upon arrival "because I couldn't waste any more time educating these people, who had come down for one week and who would then go home thinking they had done something heroic." Cunningham does recall doctors who made a difference, like the pediatrician who gave local children comprehensive examinations. Still, years later she could not remember what most of the medical volunteers did, "except maybe take us out to dinner."

At the end of the summer, Sandy Leigh, the Hattiesburg project director, asked Cunningham to join the SNCC staff. When, a month later, MCHR offered her a job she put aside her earlier experiences with the visiting doctors. Aware that MCHR could provide medical and health support (as well as a salary), she signed on as the Medical Committee's first full-time nurse, with the provision that she could remain in Hattiesburg and continue her community work. Cunningham was the only MCHR employee directly connected to a movement organization. At times these dual roles led to conflicts, but "my first allegiance was always to SNCC." She never wore a nurse's uniform, and most of the local people saw her as a civil rights worker rather than an MCHR staff member.

Throughout the fall Cunningham expanded the work she initiated during the summer. The COFO office in Hattiesburg was responsible for the fifth congressional district, which covered the southeastern part of the state and extended to the Gulf Coast. Cunningham met with the project directors in the district and persuaded each to appoint a health officer. This staff member would organize a health committee comprised of local people, who would be responsible for disseminating information concerning health classes, lectures, and the nurse's "semi-clinic hours." As she had done in Hattiesburg, Cunningham encouraged health committee members to talk about discrimination in health care and the absence of medical facilities and services, with the ultimate goal of organizing people to act politically on these problems.[15]

After an MCHR supporter gave her a car, Cunningham spent much of her time on the road doing the work of nurse, teacher, and community organizer. She made house calls throughout the district, showing family members how to take care of a loved one suffering from a chronic disability like diabetes, asthma, or a stroke. She set regular times and places for her clinics, where, in addition to dispensing nonprescription medicines, she was available for consultation. Local people were reluctant to go to a physician—in part because of the expense—but they would talk to a nurse. Sometimes Cunningham would supply the encouragement needed to make an appointment with a doctor or to go to the hospital. And she also made contact with the community "healers," people who were highly respected and whose "home remedies really work in many cases."[16]

Nurses served an important role as teacher. Many poor blacks in Mississippi treated illnesses with herbs and other home remedies, but had little basic knowledge of hygiene and modern medicine. For Cunningham, a typical health-education class involved teaching young mothers to read thermometers and to treat worms and other common childhood illnesses. She also explained the need to take preventive measures like screening windows, moving and disinfecting privies, and properly disposing of garbage. Sometimes she was called in to deal with specific problems. Black parents in Gulfport asked her to offer pregnancy-prevention classes. A number of young girls were getting pregnant, which meant permanent expulsion from school. Officials would pressure a girl to name the father of her child, and if she did he too would be expelled. Teaching about birth control, including the use of contraceptives, was a delicate matter in the South. Many Protestant ministers, white and black, opposed sex education, believing that simply talking about ways to avoid pregnancy would encourage sexual promiscuity. The white teacher faced a particular problem, because by the 1960s some black militants were claiming that any effort to limit the size of black families was a racist plot tantamount to genocide. Still, the problem was apparent. Too many young black women were having too many children they could not afford to care for.[17]

Cunningham decided to talk about the hygiene aspect of birth control "with the morality left out." She recalls that "I probably did not talk about condoms . . . I wasn't comfortable." The program ended after three sessions. It seems that local white ministers got wind of these classes and threatened to cut off contributions to black churches if their ministers did not take action. Local public health officials went after Cunningham, accusing her of practicing medicine without a license. Nothing came of this, but the contretemps demonstrated once again that in Mississippi, health care advocacy and political activism were two sides of the same coin.

As a SNCC staff person, Cunningham used her MCHR work to recruit local people into the civil rights movement, where they could organize to demand better sanitation facilities in their neighborhoods, regular garbage pickup, and inoculation against disease. She encouraged the members of the community health committees to talk about discrimination in the local hospitals and in white doctors' offices. At the same time, she was telling COFO leaders to take more of an interest in the physical well-being of the black community and to incorporate health care advocacy into their program. While her main focus was on the needs of poor blacks in the Hattiesburg region, she became increasingly concerned over the problems movement activists were experiencing from stress and exhaustion.

In November of 1964, Cunningham attended the week-long SNCC retreat at Waveland, on the Mississippi Gulf Coast, called to discuss SNCC's goals, programs, and structure. In the aftermath of Freedom Summer, tensions were increasing between black and white staff members. Cunningham recalls that "there were a lot of SNCC people at Waveland who had problems. And I saw them, and recommended what should be done." She sent about ten people to local doctors that week, two of them suffering from bleeding ulcers. Most of all, she saw activists suffering from battle fatigue, a condition she had noticed in Hattiesburg and in the Jackson COFO office. Some people were depressed, unable to function, sleeping all day, staying in bed. Others became abusive, even physically violent, but "very often people who had been around for a long time wouldn't deal with it," in part because "there was this sensitivity and consideration given to the person who was being abusive because that person had really been through a helluva lot, suffered a lot, had been beaten and jailed, so they were not disciplined verbally and restricted." Later that fall Cunningham wrote to Constance Friess that "an atmosphere must be created in each project that will allow a person to take a day or so off when he is not feeling well or when he feels that he must relax." During the summer, MCHR volunteers had opened the temporary rest and rehabilitation center at Tougaloo. The nurses in the field knew the problem demanded a more substantive solution, and throughout the winter pushed the MCHR office in New York to respond.[18]

Josephine "Jo" Disparti grew up in a working-class family in an Italian section of Niagara Falls. Unable to afford anything but a local college, she enrolled in Niagara University and became interested in a nursing career. After graduating with a degree in nursing in the late 1950s, she became a public health nurse because she found the routine of hospital work "too confining." While working with black families in the public housing projects, Disparti first became interested in the race problem. "I got involved in their lives, with their kids' problems . . . It seemed to me they were treated unfairly. I had a different understanding knowing them as a nurse than I did growing up." Future jobs in Boston and in Ann Arbor confirmed her growing belief that racial discrimination in health care "was true everywhere in public health nursing."[19]

Jo had moved to Ann Arbor to start graduate work in nursing at the University of Michigan, but she learned that she lacked the necessary experience in the field and took a job at the public health department instead. In Ann Arbor she met young radicals like Tom Hayden and joined the local chapter of CORE. A local newspaper picture of Jo marching in a civil rights demonstration led to strained relations with her employer, who warned her "not to do anything so public." She received the same message upon her return from the 1963 March on Washington, and the following year she quit her job and went to Mississippi, arriving in the early fall, after the Atlantic City convention. CORE sent her to Holmes County and arranged for her to stay with local activist Hartman Turnbow.

Holmes would play an important part in the MCHR program. Located about eighty miles north of Jackson, it is mostly rolling hills. The eastern sector, however, is rich Delta farmland, and there in the early 1940s a group of black sharecroppers purchased their own farms as part of the New Deal's Farm Security Administration program. These men became economically independent, and they also possessed a freedom of mind and spirit rare among rural blacks. When the movement came to Mississippi, farmers like Ralthus Hayes and Hartman Turnbow were ready. Turnbow's grandmother had left him her farm, which he had worked for most of his fifty-nine years. A short, solidly built man, Turnbow was famous for his malapropisms (he referred to SNCC as the "Student Violent Non-Coordinated Committee") and for his fierce independence, backed by an impressive arsenal of weapons. He was the first of a group of fourteen residents of the Delta town of Tchula to attempt to register in the spring of 1963.

A month later, two white men threw three Molotov cocktails into Turnbow's living room and kitchen while he and his family slept. "My wife and daughter jumped up and run out, and the first thing they met was two white fellas in the backyard," Turnbow recalled. "I got my rifle, pushed the safety off, I got it into the shootin' position, and then I run out. The first thing I met was those two white fellas. They start to shootin' at me, and I start shootin' at them. So they run off, and then we come back and put the fire out." Later, county officials formally charged *Turnbow* with arson.[20]

Disparti remembers Turnbow as "very entertaining, charming, but also very intimidating." At meetings, "when things weren't going Hartman's way he would pull out a gun and put it on the table, and then he'd say, 'Let's vote!'" She had been staying with the Turnbows for little more than a week when night riders shot into her bedroom, and here she had her first encounter with southern justice. The sheriff and an FBI agent came by "and asked me all these questions and tried to get something on me. They searched my room, closets, luggage, anything. They were trying to find liquor. They had no interest in who shot into the house. They asked personal questions. It was my introduction to the FBI."

Disparti left the Turnbows and moved in with a local black woman named Lila Forte, who was active in voter education. "I would wake up in the morning at six o'clock and she'd already have somebody at the table learning to read the questions and rehearsing an answer," recalls Disparti. "She was such an inspiration, a quiet woman who had the courage to take in a civil rights worker." The young nurse began working out of a new community center, built and donated by a white northerner. The center was in Mileston, a Delta hamlet so tiny that Jo drove through it twice before she realized she had found it. In residence at the center were Henry and Sue Lorenzi, two white northerners who had come down at the end of the summer to work as community organizers.

Holmes County was one of the poorest in Mississippi. Of its twenty-seven thousand residents, more than two thirds were black, with a median annual family income of $895, less than a third that of whites. Housing was dilapidated and overcrowded; over half the homes lacked running water and indoor toilets. Blacks were reluctant to patronize the two county hospitals and two public health clinics (all segregated) because they usually did not have cash up front to pay for hospital services. Those who did seek help at the clinics were often treated badly. There was no black doctor in the county. Sharecroppers needed the plantation owner's permission to see a designated white doctor (a "quack," Disparti opined), who ran a private "hospital" of two or three rooms where surgical and medical patients were mixed in together. There were many stories of black people going into this hospital "with something minor and not coming back."[21]

Disparti's experience as a public health nurse eased the transition to this harsh environment. "I had worked in communities before, done lots of home visits, and I'd been a school nurse. So I felt comfortable working with people, visiting in the home, setting up meetings." She made it a point to seek out local women to ask if they knew people who needed health care. Through them, and with the help of the Lorenzis, she got the word out that a certified nurse who would make house calls was at the center—a task not so simple as it might sound. As a white outsider, now known to the sheriff and the FBI, she had to be careful. When a sick farmworker needed attention, someone would drive her out to the plantation at night. Sometimes she had to hide on the floor of the car. Then, before trespassing on the white owner's property, "I'd put a bandana on my head so my hair wouldn't show. They would just slip me in for my own safety, and for the safety of the people whom I was visiting. I was not afraid—I was very foolish."

She dealt with a range of health problems, but early on discovered an alarming number of high-risk pregnancies among poor black women who had no prenatal care. In rural Mississippi most black babies were still delivered by midwives, who were supervised by white public health nurses. Disparti met with the black midwives who worked in Holmes County and won their trust. They told her about their periodic meetings with the public health nurses, who humiliated them by having them sing little songs like "This is how we wash our hands, wash our hands . . ." Midwives were not supposed to take any high-risk pregnancies, but given the paucity of adequate health care, together with the widespread distrust of the white medical establishment, they often had to deal with serious prenatal problems. Midwives were unfairly targeted as the major cause of the high infant mortality rate in Mississippi. Not surprisingly, their numbers were decreasing.

After a month in Mississippi, Disparti began to feel isolated. She had intentionally avoided close contact with COFO, now experiencing serious problems in Holmes County. A September 13 report noted that "illness, police harassment, staff migration, and the cotton harvest have disrupted the local project." Relations were also strained with the black community. Strong local leaders like Turnbow became resentful of the young outsiders, who at one point were asked to leave. (COFO reluctantly moved its headquarters to the other side of the county to the hill town of Lexington.) Part of that resentment spilled over against Disparti, despite her distancing herself from COFO, and she found herself spending much of her time working to gain the trust of local blacks. With no black medical presence, she was "a nurse in Holmes County with no backup." Then when she read a newspaper story that Jack Geiger and Count Gibson were in Mississippi as part of a new organization, she called Geiger and told him how glad she was that they were involved. About a month later, in mid-October, Geiger asked her to work full-time for MCHR as a nurse and health organizer in Holmes County.[22]

Disparti's presence in Holmes, along with the existence of the new community center in Mileston, fit perfectly into a project MCHR leaders had been developing since the end of the summer. They recognized the need for the Medical Committee to have a permanent presence in Mississippi to

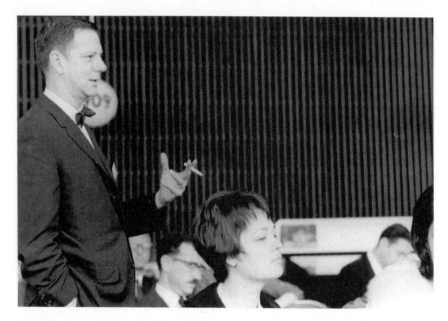

Count Gibson speaking at an MCHR meeting. (Charmian Redding)

challenge the perception that "well, we were here in the summer and wasn't that great and then good-bye." Employing public health nurses was but a first step for Geiger, who envisioned a maternal and child health clinic staffed with nurses and serving the rural black community. He persuaded Luke and Ruth Wilson, who had inherited the Woodward and Lathrop department store fortune, to fund the clinic with a thirty-thousand-dollar gift. The Delta Ministry kicked in by purchasing a Ford Econoline van and transforming it into a "healthmobile" (this was the heyday of the *Batman* TV series), a "radio-equipped ambulance-rescue vehicle outfitted to double as a mobile health center." Not only could it transport injured or seriously ill rural blacks to the University Medical Center in Jackson, it could also provide direct medical care to blacks who did not need major attention. Geiger and Gibson announced this project at the annual meeting of the American Public Health Association the first week of October, and the *New York Times* ran a story on the proposed center shortly thereafter.[23]

Although the Medical Committee had assumed that Holmes County blacks would rejoice at the idea of a center and a health van in their community, it proved to be a harder sell than anticipated. To begin with, the nurses had reservations about the proposed clinic and the van. On October 12, Cunningham wrote that "I still feel very strongly . . . against setting up a 'Public Health Service.' " She believed the proposed clinic would only "antagonize the Board of Health. I realize that Mileston is to be a pilot project, but a pilot project for what? I don't think we can possibly have similar projects all over the state of Mississippi." For Cunningham the project could only be justified if "the set-up is taken over by the local community and eventually be totally in the hands of the local community."[24]

Disparti believed that Holmes County blacks were not ready for the MCHR-sponsored clinic. She feared the mere presence of the van would exacerbate existing turf battles between COFO and Holmes County activists, and reported "some criticism of our initial idea to bring in a mobile health unit." And more than one local black leader was uncomfortable with the idea of "a nurse alone in a mobile unit." She agreed with Cunningham, then, that any "planning for the clinic's activities should be done with local people, who will be responsible for choosing programs. The mobile unit should be introduced only when the community is ready for it." (The van, when it arrived in mid-December, was stationed at the Delta Ministry office in Greenville, not in Mileston.)

Only eight people showed up in late November when Disparti called a meeting to form a countywide health association, but interest soon developed, and within three months the Holmes County Health Association was meeting regularly at the Mileston community center. Like Cunningham, Disparti wanted to develop political awareness of health care issues as well as provide local people with medical advice. She set up operations in two rooms in the center, one for her office and the other as an examining room. Disparti would see people with problems, "give them a little first aid, find out what was wrong with them," and refer the serious cases to Dr. Smith in Jackson. "It wasn't really a clinic" back then, Disparti recalls.[25]

The nurses also had issues with their employers. First, they felt patronized by the New York office, which required that all bills, from payments for eyeglasses for civil rights workers to local doctor bills to car rentals, be submitted to treasurer Moldovan, who would write the checks from his office. MCHR was the only civil rights organization operating in Mississippi with such an accounting procedure, and it created problems of credibility for local staff. Moreover, although the nurses were *the* MCHR medical presence in Mississippi, they did not have a direct voice in the policy decisions affecting their work. They did get strong support from Geiger and Des Callan, both of whom spent a good deal of time in Mississippi that fall and winter. But there was also the example of the doctor who lauded "the grand work being done by our little maids in Mississippi." That doctors had historically treated nurses as second-class citizens was nothing new. But in the context of the Medical Committee's work in Mississippi these long-standing attitudes adversely affected both policy and program.[26]

Throughout November and December, activists in New York discussed and debated the MCHR's program as it related to Mississippi. Aaron Wells, the organization's elected chair, was not an aggressive leader. (Tom Levin remembers him more as "a figurehead.") Major day-to-day decisions in the New York office fell to Moldovan and Esther Smith, their part-time fund-raiser whose influence extended into the area of policy making. Thomas and McKenna of the Delta Ministry were increasingly prominent in MCHR affairs. As the major funding source for the Mississippi project, the Delta Ministry was growing impatient with the Medical Committee's failure to define its role there, and so in late November of 1964 Thomas called for a meeting in Mississippi to "explore on the scene problems of MCHR program, personnel and direction," as well as its relationship to the Delta Ministry.[27]

The MCHR delegation included Geiger and Gibson, who was the director of the community health department at Tufts. They were co-chairs of MCHR's program committee. Another member, Sidney Greenberg, was working closely with Bob Smith to try to persuade officials at Tougaloo College (unsuccessfully, as it turned out) to commit to an ambitious health care outreach program on its campus. Also in the MCHR contingent was Des Callan, who in a short time had developed a passionate commitment to improving health care for black Mississippians.[28]

Desmond Callan grew up in an environment markedly different from most other MCHR leaders. He was born in Boston in 1925. His mother's family had been prominent in church and business life since their arrival in the Massachusetts Bay Colony in 1630, while his father had grown up "on the east end of London on the docks" and was a musician in the British army before studying for the Episcopal ministry and moving to America. A "very charismatic person with a phenomenal drinking problem," the elder Callan served for a time as chaplain of Wellesley College. Callan's parents divorced when he was seven. A child of wealth and privilege, Des attended Milton Academy before enrolling at Harvard in the fall of 1943. At the end of his first semester he was drafted into the army as an infantryman. His division arrived in Europe in late 1944, just in time for the Battle of the Bulge. Like thousands of other GIs surrounded by the Germans, Callan became a prisoner of war, and for the next few months he was moved from one prison camp in Germany to another, under trying conditions. "We were not beaten, but food was scarce, sanitation was nil, and so we were in a pretty weakened condition." Callan shoveled coal in a factory in Silesia, and was later part of forced retreats as the Allied troops advanced through Germany. On one of the marches he became very ill, suffering from malnutrition, beriberi, and dysentery. Fortunately, a Polish doctor singled him out and sent him back to a hospital at the main camp. Shortly thereafter, in the spring of 1945, Soviet troops liberated the camp.[29]

A year later, after months of recuperation, Callan entered Columbia University to study history, and he soon became involved in student political life. Although raised in a Republican family ("at age eleven I was militantly for Alf Landon"), by now he had shed his conservative roots and identified with the program of the left. He helped organize the American Veterans Committee (which opposed President Truman's aggressive policy toward the Soviet Union), joined the Progressive Party in 1948, and briefly dropped out of school to work full-time as an activist. By the time he returned to finish his history degree in 1950 he was married, needed work, and had decided to pick up on some of his army training and study electronics at a trade school. A job at the neurosurgical research laboratory at Columbia led to his decision to become a doctor, and at age thirty-one he entered Columbia Medical School, graduating in 1960. After his internship, Callan served as acting director of the neurology clinic at Columbia-Presbyterian Medical Center in Manhattan.[30]

From the time he entered medical school until his residency, Callan, now raising a family, was largely inactive politically, but in 1963 he joined the Physicians Forum and there met Walter Lear, who was putting together the Medical Committee for Civil Rights. Callan was in that small group of physicians who picketed the AMA meeting in Atlantic City. "I was not prominent in this [demonstration] at all," he recalled. "I felt very much alone in the glare not only of the sunshine but in the glare of attention that our small group in front of the photographers was getting. I was not one of the spokesmen." Callan had met Bob Smith at Atlantic City, and when the call came a year later to come to Mississippi he was an eager volunteer. Two trips to the state before the December meeting with the Delta Ministry convinced him that MCHR needed to develop a health program for poor blacks. He became a champion of the nurses, as his long, encouraging letters to Cunningham and Disparti attest. They saw him both as their contact person in New York and as a source of support and inspiration. He was now working late into the night on Mississippi problems, frustrated that the national office seemed unconcerned about the difficulties facing the nurses. Callan welcomed another trip to Mississippi as an opportunity to meet with people who shared a common vision.[31]

Callan, Greenberg, Geiger, and Gibson arrived in Mississippi on December 11. Their purpose was to gather information about the MCHR operation there and its relation to COFO, and to discuss the possibility of setting up a health care program in Mississippi with the financial backing of the Delta Ministry. In Jackson they met with the three staff nurses (Cathy Dahl would soon resign her position), who made their case for autonomy and for greater support from the national office. Specifically, they wanted a larger voice in the making and implementation of policy, a bank account to take care of bills locally instead of sending them to New York, and educational materials appropriate for a population lacking much formal education. The visiting physicians agreed, later reporting that "our group felt unanimously that far more of the weight of our work would have to be in backing, recruiting, and listening to the nurses," who should be "essential to any larger scale activities in the state, including those of short-term visitors from the North and West." Following the nurses' suggestion, the physicians recommended that these visits "be temporarily suspended until a stronger setup in Mississippi is arranged."[32]

Along with Smith, the group met with black physicians Matthew Page in Greenville and Anderson and Britton in Jackson. They all stressed the need for facilities to train black nurses and doctors, pointing out that the University of Mississippi Medical Center had yet to enroll a Negro medical or nursing student. The local doctors urged MCHR to press the federal government to desegregate these institutions, so heavily dependent on federal money and so obviously in violation of Title VI of the Civil Rights Act. The delegation left this cordial meeting with "the conviction that further personal and professional relationships with the Negro physicians of Mississippi are essential to our work."[33]

While they held no policy meetings with COFO leaders on this trip, the group did have a productive session with Muriel Tillinghast, who had succeeded Morris as manager of the Jackson COFO office. MCHR could no longer afford to pay all the medical bills for COFO activists, and Tillinghast agreed that in the future the committee would be responsible only for medical treatment approved in advance by Dr. Smith or one of the nurses. The visiting physicians recommended "that certain types of chronic or stress illnesses be handled out of state where we have better contacts or actual [MCHR] members," and they pledged to work with COFO in arranging for a health insurance plan for civil rights workers. (Three days later MCHR wrote a memorandum to COFO project directors announcing this clarification of policy.) Discussion then turned to the summer of 1965. Although SNCC had vetoed the black belt project as a whole, COFO had decided to recruit volunteers for another Summer Project in Mississippi, and Tillinghast asked MCHR to help screen applicants in northern cities.[34]

Thus it was in an atmosphere of guarded optimism that the delegation of northern physicians and Smith sat down to talk policy with their Delta Ministry counterparts that night in Greenville. Thomas and McKenna got right to the point. They wanted the Medical Committee to develop a health program for the Delta Ministry. The first priority should go to placing more full-time nurses in the field and "setting up a fully effective Jackson office with a strong director," as well as hiring an executive director in New York to support the Mississippi program. The Delta Ministry would pay 85 percent of the salaries and program expenses for the statewide activities and underwrite the salary of the New York director "to the extent that his time is spent on support of these activities." The Delta Ministry had plans to rent an abandoned black college campus in Mount Beulah, in central Mississippi, to be a training facility for groups of young activists who would become part of the "Freedom Corps." The Medical Committee would assist with this program, and could use part of the campus for its projected rest and rehabilitation program for activists who needed time off. The physicians endorsed the Delta Ministry proposal.[35]

Discussion turned to the larger problem of providing health care for poor blacks. The situation had not changed much over the past century. The small number of black doctors could not begin to serve nearly a million black Mississippians, white physicians operated Jim Crow offices with "cash-up-front" policies, hospitals were segregated, with inadequate services for black patients, and black physicians were still denied hospital privileges. Public health clinics across the state, while available to blacks, provided no transportation, often inadequate treatment, and no community outreach. Their major function was immunization, not treating sick people. So even if the Delta Ministry–sponsored program worked perfectly, it would do little or nothing for the vast majority of blacks who needed health care. But what about Mileston? Might not MCHR set up similar health clinics across the state, where blacks could get diagnostic and acute care for free? Geiger, who was most responsible for the Mileston program, did not think so. Having tapped a private source, the Wilsons, he knew that the idea that "you had to go out and find philanthropists" for every operation was not practical. Mileston, then, was "an incomplete idea and it wasn't replicable."[36]

But it was at that late night session that Geiger realized there was a model that might be "replicable," and that was the health care experiment he had seen firsthand in South Africa a decade earlier, where he had studied under two young physicians, Sidney and Emily Kark. The Karks had developed a concept called community-oriented primary care and applied it in the university's two health centers, which served blacks living in a public housing project in Lamontville and in the rural tribal reserve of Pholela. Everyone in these defined areas was considered to be a patient. Staff members collected information about health problems and developed a comprehensive plan of attack, including health services, nutrition programs, preventive medicine, and even environmental interventions. Once he made this connection, Geiger had an epiphany of sorts. "A good northern medical school ought to come down here and run a comprehensive teaching health center, properly funded and the whole works—health, community organization and social change." The group discussed the concept, but the hour was late and it didn't go further. The next day on the trip back to Boston, Count Gibson turned to Geiger and said, "Let's do it."[37]

Gibson, the only southern white physician prominent in MCHR, was born in Covington, Georgia, in 1921, and he believed that "the country owed African-Americans a particular debt for the legacy of slavery and segregation." A devout member of the Byzantine Church, he was fluent in several languages. He received his medical degree from Emory University, served a year in the army, and then worked at the Columbia-Presbyterian Medical Center in New York and the Medical College of Virginia. Gibson joined the faculty of the Tufts University School of Medicine and in 1964 became chairman of the Department of Preventive Medicine. He was in the first wave of physicians who worked in Mississippi, and like Geiger and Callan, he returned to the state several times during the fall of 1964. Now, after the Greenville meeting, Gibson realized he could use his position at Tufts to help make the dream of a comprehensive community health center a reality. He told Geiger he would ask the dean of the medical school to sponsor the project, and he offered the young Harvard faculty member a full professorship at Tufts on the spot so that he would have a base from which to operate.[38]

Geiger and Gibson became a team, traveling back and forth between Boston and Mississippi and Washington, gathering the resources they needed. They found their funding source in the new Office of Economic Opportunity (OEO), now in the process of awarding grants to agencies established to combat poverty in impoverished urban and rural areas throughout the country. Within a short time the OEO had awarded a grant to Tufts for two comprehensive health centers, one in Columbia Point, a Boston public housing project, and the other at an undisclosed site in the South. Gibson took on primary supervision of the Columbia Point center, which opened in late 1965, while Geiger turned his attention to the South in search of a rural location, a Pholela to complement Columbia Point's Lamontville. He would find it in the all-black town of Mound Bayou. (For an account of the development of the health center in Mound Bayou, see chapter 10.)[39]

Des Callan came away from the Greenville meeting convinced that MCHR had a role to play in creating a health program for the entire state of Mississippi. He believed that a statewide health conference should be called to create the basis for a health action movement, which would press state and federal officials to expand and equalize medical services. He later formalized his thinking in a paper, "A Mississippi Health Program: A Modest Proposal," which he hoped that the Medical Committee would take seriously.[40]

Two days later the MCHR executive committee met in New York and heard the report on the Mississippi meetings. There was general agreement, if not overwhelming enthusiasm, for the proposed alliance with the Delta Ministry. Some expressed pessimism over the prospect of finding a black physician to run the Jackson office. The committee was interested in the Delta Ministry's suggestion that MCHR employ a full-time executive director to run the national office. Ed Barsky's nomination of Esther Smith, however, did not resonate with other members of the committee. Al Moldovan announced that the organization's financial status was "fair," with outstanding debts of sixty-five hundred dollars.[41]

As the year ended, MCHR activists could look back with a good deal of satisfaction over what they had accomplished in only six months. They had demonstrated their presence and goodwill in Mississippi during Freedom Summer and made provisions to continue their relationship with COFO, while establishing a permanent national organization with affiliated local chapters. They agreed to hire two key people: a full-time medical director in Jackson and an executive director in New York, as well as three more nurses to work in Mississippi. Still, there was no consensus on program and direction. Members were willing to go along, for a time, with the efforts by Geiger, Callan, and others to do something to improve the health of indigent black Mississippians. For most, however, direct assistance to civil rights workers remained their priority. But by the beginning of 1965 it was clear that the civil rights community was no longer united, and COFO itself seemed to be coming apart. These developments did not bode well for an organization like MCHR, which was tied so closely to the program of a movement in transition, one that gradually, almost imperceptibly was heading toward Black Power.

CHAPTER 4

Selma and Jackson

At the end of Freedom Summer, Des Callan observed that "we must know by now that most of us are not very good civil rights organizers. On the other hand, we should also know that most civil rights workers do not make very good doctors or nurses." Callan had learned that "most civil rights organizations per se know rather little about health: especially about how to fight for it in their own programs. It is time for their great energies and resources to be thrown into the battle for better health for the deprived Negroes of the South and North." At the MCHR executive committee meeting in February of 1965 Callan presented his paper, "A Mississippi Health Program: A Modest Proposal," which began with the assumption that the "scandal" of "Negro health in Mississippi" was "at least as much a circumstance and product of political and economic exploitation as of direct absence of good medical care." While he believed the state government should be held accountable—the Medical Committee "should not let Archie Gray off the hook"—the situation was so bad that the federal government had to respond with "political and economic measures of a radical dimension." Specifically, Callan proposed convening a statewide conference on "Negro health status, care facilities, professional resources, and training opportunities." MCHR would be the catalyst for the conference— and constitute its medical subcommittee—but the major players would be black Mississippians: civil rights leaders, educators, and professional people and organizations. These delegates would determine the most urgent health care needs and how to address them.[1]

For Callan, it was evident that "while outside money (mainly federal) is essential to any basic change in the health status of Mississippi Negroes, even if available, these funds would not mean much of significance" if channeled through state agencies, which were controlled by segregationists. Therefore, the conference should constitute itself as a permanent body, "legally empowered to apply for, receive, and spend federal money." A year earlier such a proposal would have made little political sense. But Lyndon Johnson's ascension to the presidency brought with it a commitment to wage a war against poverty, providing federal grants directly to such local projects as the Community Action Programs. Callan endorsed Geiger's idea for "federally endowed health maintenance centers" to serve Mississippi blacks, and to provide training opportunities to encourage young African Americans to pursue careers in nursing, medicine, and other health fields. But, unlike Geiger, Callan advocated close cooperation with the new Mississippi Freedom Democratic Party, the political arm of the Mississippi movement. Finally, Callan recommended that the delegates to the MCHR national convention in Washington "declare Mississippi a health disaster area" and initiate a permanent lobbying effort in Congress to promote health care issues. Congress was now considering new areas of health education, such as Medicare, and MCHR could provide valuable input into the shaping of these programs.[2]

Callan's "modest proposal" met with enthusiastic support among the nurses working in Mississippi, the staff of the Delta Ministry, and civil rights leaders. With its emphasis on direct participation by local people, the plan was consistent with the movement's grassroots approach to problem solving, and it presented civil rights activists with the opportunity to establish their own health care program, a need heretofore unmet. On paper, at least, Callan's proposal appeared to be a godsend for the Medical Committee. COFO activists had made it clear that whatever health problems they suffered were minor in comparison with the needs of hundreds of thousands of poor blacks in Mississippi. And while they welcomed medical presence at demonstrations and physical examinations by physicians, they were no longer interested in entertaining doctors touring the state for one- or two-week sojourns. By supporting black organizing at the local and state levels, and using its prestigious sponsors to lobby for federal support for these initiatives, MCHR could have a real impact on health care provision in the nation's poorest and most backward state.[3]

Those attending the February executive committee meeting responded cautiously to Callan's proposal. While no one attacked the proposal directly, several board members expressed reservations about MCHR's participation. Charles Goodrich argued that "we should not jeopardize our tax exemption by engaging in lobbying." Al Moldovan stated that while the proposal was "very fine," he wondered where the funding would come from. He suggested that the members present come up with a concrete proposal for the first step in implementation. None was forthcoming. In truth, the physicians who founded the Medical Committee were still by and large committed to "being the medical guardians of demonstrations," as Callan later cynically put it. "The resistance focused really on the notion that the major task of MCHR was to provide medical presence and protection" for civil rights workers. It was his opinion that Esther Smith, Moldovan, and Ed Barsky, the triumvirate running the national office, were "not enthusiastic at all about getting staff into the South or getting involved in health programs." In the end, Jerome Tobis's motion that Callan's proposal be placed on the agenda of the national MCHR conference in Washington was approved unanimously. At that national meeting, Callan's program did not get serious attention from the delegates, who were still basking in the reflected glow of the Medical Committee's performance in Selma, Alabama.[4]

Aaron Wells had met with Martin Luther King in mid-February 1965 to discuss the Southern Christian Leadership Conference's move into Selma to dramatize the need for a law guaranteeing blacks the right to vote. King told Wells then that he saw no immediate need for a medical presence there, but that would soon change as racial tensions escalated in the Alabama community. After the murder of a young black man, Jimmie Jackson, by a white state trooper, SCLC decided to stage a protest march from Selma to the state capital in Montgomery, almost sixty miles away. On Friday, March 5, SCLC's Hosea Williams contacted Wells, requesting that MCHR doctors and nurses accompany the marchers on their journey. The following day MCHR sent six physicians and three nurses to Selma. Heading the delegation was Al Moldovan.[5]

A first-generation American whose parents had immigrated from Hungary, Moldovan was born in the Bronx, attended New York public schools, and graduated from City College. The day after Pearl Harbor he enlisted in the air force, and after three years as a radar officer came home with the rank of captain. He enrolled in Chicago Medical School, and while there became "very interested in the left-wing movement," serving as the national public relations officer for the Association of Internes and Medical Students (AIMS) in the months before it was red-baited out of existence. Returning to New York in 1954, he opened a practice in Spanish Harlem, his professional home for the next half century. He joined the Physicians Forum and there got to know "a number of very wonderful left-wing physicians, including Ed Barsky." As the organization's treasurer, Moldovan was one of MCHR's most influential figures during its early years.[6]

On Sunday morning, March 7, in Selma the medical team set up a clinic in the dining room of the small parsonage next to Brown Chapel, the AME church and the movement's command center. Consisting of a table, a bureau, and a mattress, the clinic contained only basic medical supplies. Moldovan and his group had come down with the expectation that MCHR's main contribution to the march would be moral support and perhaps some minor medical aid. But late Sunday morning he learned that Alabama state troopers were carrying tear gas. Shortly before they left, Moldovan told the marchers assembled in Brown Chapel that if they were gassed, "Don't panic. Don't rub your eyes. Wash them with water, if you can. And we'll be on hand to help." He later recalled, "And when I said, 'If you get knocked unconscious make sure you have somebody with you,' the whole place broke up in laughter!"[7]

There was something of a festive air in downtown Selma that day. One MCHR observer noted that by noon, an hour before the march was to begin, the streets were clogged with traffic, "mostly local white citizens driving around the center of town—many of them with the whole family in the car." It was a new kind of outing for parishioners leaving church on a pleasant spring Sunday. That afternoon nearly six hundred marchers left the church and headed through downtown Selma to cross the Edmund Pettus Bridge on the road to Montgomery. Four ambulances (three of them hearses from local black funeral directors) accompanied them at intervals, with Dr. Moldovan and two MCHR nurses in the "real" ambulance bringing up the rear. Police stopped all four vehicles at the bridge, refusing to let them cross with the marchers, stating that the bridge was closed to traffic.[8]

About ten minutes later the stranded doctors and nurses heard screams coming from the other side of the bridge. Roy Reed of the *New York Times* wrote about what he saw:

> The troopers rushed forward, their blue uniforms and white helmets blurring into a flying wedge as they moved. The wedge moved with such force that it seemed almost to pass over the

waiting column instead of through it. The first 10 or 20 Negroes were swept to the ground screaming, arms and legs flying, and packs and bags went skittering across the grassy divider strip and on to the pavement on both sides.

John Lewis, the co-leader of the march, recalled that "the first of the troopers came over me, a large husky man. Without a word, he swung his club against the left side of my head. I didn't feel any pain, just the thud of the blow . . . And then the same trooper hit me again. And everything started to spin."[9]

People were rushing back to the ambulances, carrying limp bodies in their arms. There followed the hysteria, panic, and confusion accompanying the exploding canisters of tear gas bombs. When Moldovan finally received police permission to drive across the bridge, he found the highway littered with hats, overnight bags, umbrellas, and other items the marchers had brought with them for the trip. "It was a horrible sight," he recalled. "I remember driving up to the bridge, and seeing people streaming back over the bridge—bloody—and crying from the tear gas. The gas was still so thick I started crying." Moldovan and his team—nurses Virginia Wells and Linda Dugan, and a local black physician—found several people still lying in the road, semiconscious. They got them into the ambulance and took them back to Brown Chapel, where the little medical clinic, now "looking like a MASH unit," was swamped by people in distress. In all, nearly a hundred of the six hundred marchers required medical care. The attending doctors reported fractures of skull and limbs, scalp lacerations, and multiple abrasions and contusions. The most common injuries, such as conjunctivitis and gastritis, were caused by tear gas poisoning. While there were no fatalities, the gassing and beatings took their toll on the victims psychologically as well as physically.[10]

Martin Luther King had not led the march. He was in Atlanta, claiming that he needed to preach the Sunday sermon at his home church. In fact, he was dissuaded from participating by his aides because they feared for his safety. King returned to Selma the day after the violence at Edmund Pettus Bridge and joined the debate that was under way between the SCLC activists and SNCC's Jim Forman about what to do next in Alabama. King favored resuming the march, and asked federal judge Frank Johnson—who was sympathetic to the cause of civil rights—for an injunction prohibiting the state of Alabama from interfering with the marchers. Johnson was unwilling to issue a restraining order until a full hearing could be held later in the week. The judge asked SCLC to post-pone the march, threatening to issue an order barring it if the leaders in-sisted on going ahead. King had never violated a federal injunction and did not want to do so now. Forman and other activists insisted that he march. The movement's most important figure had supported but not at-tended the first bloody march. Now he must stand up and be a man. With his reputation on the line, King reluctantly agreed to a second march on Tuesday, before the hearing.[11]

The Medical Committee volunteers responded to the news by mov-ing their clinic to a bigger space in the First Baptist Church, in anticipa-tion of the thousands of expected marchers. On Tuesday morning the ambulances fell into line, and police once again prevented drivers from ap-proaching the bridge. Earlier in Selma, King had received death threats his advisers took seriously, and they had arranged with MCHR to have a doctor at King's side the entire time he was in public view. Moldovan served as King's personal physician, and when the line of marchers set off to cross the bridge the second time he stood just behind King, along with nurse Virginia Wells, who carried first aid gear in her outsized handbag and a twenty-pound gas mask over her shoulder hidden under her coat. As it turned out, all the precautions proved unnecessary. Instead of a con-frontation with Alabama state troopers, King and the marchers stopped on the bridge, prayed, and then turned around and headed back to the black section of Selma. It appeared that King had reached an agreement with Alabama officials that if the marchers would turn back, the police would not attack or arrest them. Back at Brown Chapel there was much confusion among the hundreds of protesters who had just arrived in town, with no place to stay. Some left for home; others heeded King's call to remain in Selma in anticipation of another march to Montgomery.[12]

Among those who stayed behind was the Reverend James Reeb, a white minister from Boston. Tuesday evening he and two other pastors were attacked by local whites in downtown Selma. Reeb suffered a deadly blow to the head—a full swing with a baseball bat—and was taken to the black-owned Burwell Infirmary, where a local physician examined him. Reeb never regained consciousness. He died two days later. Demonstra-tors gathered outside Brown Chapel on Wednesday to protest the attacks on the ministers. There a state trooper confronted MCHR volunteers Jack Geiger and Richard Hauskenecht and took them to the county court-house, where the doctors were interrogated by representatives from the Alabama State Medical Society. Douglas Benton, the administrator of the

State Board of Licensure, warned them that because they were not licensed to practice in Alabama, they would be arrested if they even gave basic first aid to people in need. He told Geiger and Hauskenecht that had they been present at the beating of Reverend Reeb they would have violated the law by treating him. (This, despite the fact that Alabama had a "Good Samaritan" law permitting unlicensed doctors to administer first aid in emergency situations.) After being grilled for about a half hour, the two men were released.[13]

For the rest of the week, while King and his followers awaited Judge Johnson's decision, most of the activity in Selma centered around Brown Chapel, where the police restrained demonstrators from marching downtown. Geiger requested that the medical van be brought over from Mississippi, and nurses Jo Disparti and Phyllis Cunningham arrived during the middle of the week. Several carloads of SNCC workers also made the trip from Mississippi to Alabama, outraged at what they had seen at Selma bridge. They were angry at local white racists, at the federal government, and at Martin Luther King. SNCC had originally refused to endorse the march (John Lewis had participated on his own), believing that it was a waste of energy and resources and would detract from the work its Alabama staff had been doing in Selma before SCLC and King came to town. But after "Bloody Sunday" all previous reservations were swept aside. SNCC activists were upset when King equivocated on marching in violation of a federal court order, and they became furious when, unbeknownst to them, he cut a deal with authorities to avoid a confrontation at the bridge on Tuesday. Forman denounced King's conduct as "a classic example of trickery against the people," and announced that SNCC was shifting its operations from Selma to Montgomery. Forman had organized undergraduates at Tuskegee Institute and Alabama State College to launch a series of protests at the state capitol. These students were more aggressive than the Selma blacks in King's campaign, and more violence seemed inevitable.[14]

When Forman asked the Medical Committee to send a team of doctors and nurses up to Montgomery, the physicians in Selma responded. The SNCC leader had been a key supporter of MCHR since its founding. That Forman was more radical politically than King did not deter the dozen MCHR physicians who joined the SNCC-led activists in Montgomery. There they found law enforcement officers, if anything, even more brutal than their counterparts in Selma.[15]

With Montgomery public schools and many northern colleges in spring recess, the area surrounding the SNCC headquarters was teeming with local black youth and visiting college students. On Monday, March 15, police and demonstrators clashed near the state capitol. That night President Johnson, responding to the national outrage over Bloody Sunday and James Reeb's murder, went on national television to call on Congress to pass voting rights legislation, concluding his speech by invoking the anthem of the movement. "Because it is not just Negroes, but really it is all of us who must overcome the crippling legacy of bigotry and injustice. And we *shall* overcome." This was the high point of federal support for the black freedom struggle, and it did not go unnoticed in Alabama. But as if to underscore the distance still to be traveled, the following day Alabama police and sheriff's deputies attacked a group of young protesters at the capitol. After the police began pushing the students aside, several of the youths responded with rocks, bricks, and bottles. That brought on the mounted police with billy clubs and cattle prods. One newsman watched an officer begin clubbing the demonstrators. "Several still refused to move, and the man's nightstick began falling with great force on their heads." Then, following a "moment of freakish near-quiet, when the yells all seemed to subside at once," the officer "struck hard on the head of a young man. The sound of the nightstick carried up and down the block."[16]

Doctors on the scene led by Les Falk and Douglas Thompson moved in to assist the victims; an MCHR nurse, Robert Dannenburg, was arrested and jailed. Earlier the Medical Committee had established liaison with two local Catholic hospitals and set up a medical station near SNCC headquarters, stocking it with basic first aid supplies. At the scene of the police beatings they performed triage functions, providing first aid, arranging for hospitalization, emergency room care, and visits to physicians' and dentists' offices. MCHR also paid the medical bills for many of those needing treatment. The doctors visited the protesters who had been jailed, hoping that their presence would serve "as a deterrent to mistreatment by authorities." Other demonstrations followed in Montgomery on Wednesday and Thursday, with more police violence and arrests, filling the jails to overflowing. Yale Medical School professor Richard Weinerman, who headed up the MCHR contingent in Montgomery, later reported that while it was "hard to gauge the usefulness of our medical presence, the local Negro citizens and the student demonstrators seemed delighted to have the doctors around." In Montgomery as at Edmund Pettus Bridge, MCHR volunteers provided essential services at a time of immediate need, putting their bodies on the line while providing aid and comfort to civil rights activists at the mercy of angry and unrestrained police officers.[17]

Meanwhile, in another part of Montgomery, Judge Frank Johnson handed down a decision that approved the march from Selma to Montgomery. Immediately people from all over the country began to descend on Selma, including many health care professionals eager to be part of the unfolding drama. Aaron Wells became a member of the SCLC team planning the march. Medical preparations included provision of sanitary food and water for the marchers, portable restrooms along the march route, first aid facilities, and a plan for the evacuation and treatment of wounded individuals should another violent outbreak occur. David French, a surgeon who taught at the Howard Medical School, was in charge of acquiring medical supplies, and he paid in cash from his own pocket when the only local supply house refused to accept an MCHR check. The doctors did not screen the marchers because SCLC decided that any resident from Selma could participate. But they did give physical exams to those volunteering for the march, and they recommended that several with chronic health problems not make the journey. Apparently most of these people ignored the doctors' advice, including Jim Leatherer, a one-legged man on crutches who became an inspirational figure along the road to Montgomery.[18]

On Sunday, March 21, more than three thousand people gathered in black Selma to begin the historic march to the state capitol. Enthusiastic MCHR doctors and nurses from New York, Boston, Washington, and other big cities joined the throng. Their purpose was once again to provide medical presence, but unlike in Mississippi the previous summer, here the supply of doctors greatly exceeded the demand for services. "Everybody wanted to do something. Marching was wonderful. But we didn't have a role or a mission," recalled Tom Levin. Most of the more than one hundred MCHR medical volunteers served mainly to swell the crowd on the final days of the march. Those who staffed the makeshift medical centers along the way and drove the vans and ambulances had to deal with only minor ailments. Fortunately, there was no violence on the march, and no serious illnesses among the marchers.[19]

Portable health facilities were set up along the route of the march, including a huge, well-equipped mobile hospital provided by the International Ladies Garment Workers Union. Local black undertakers again donated hearses to serve as ambulances, and nurses Cunningham and Disparti were aboard the MCHR health van. "We drove slowly in the march," recalls Disparti. "We soaked feet. When people were tired we'd bring them into the van for a while and take care of them. We slept in the mud in our sleeping bags." In addition to maintaining a cafeteria and clinic in the basement of the First Baptist Church in Selma, at each stop MCHR set up tents (on one a cardboard sign read THE DOCTOR IS IN). "We would set up a little corner of a tent as a first aid station," June Finer remembers, "and a lot of it was dealing with people's feet." Many of the participants were older residents of Selma, whose shoes were not made for marching. One physician saw "teenage girls marching who had cloth around their feet with cellophane wrappers. They didn't have shoes." Few were used to such strenuous exercise. Athlete's foot, as well as blisters and bruises, were the major ailments. For Tom Levin, this was something of a religious experience. "I was down on the first aid line, cleaning the feet of the sharecroppers. I felt the Christian notion: better to take care of the feet of the poor at their feet than to tell them how to run their lives." Dr. Finer's recollection was more prosaic. "I remember a podiatrist on the march who was incredibly useful."[20]

The doctors and nurses were busy the last night of the march, when thousands of people "jammed into a field, ankle deep in mud and in the darkness," to hear a concert headlined by Harry Belafonte and Sammy

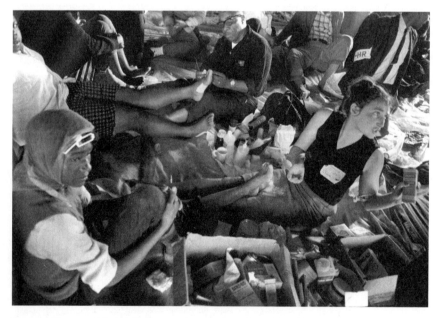

Dr. June Finer on Selma-Montgomery March. (Matt Herron/Take Stock)

Davis Jr. "We had people who had passed out from the heat, from the pressure, whom we had to get out of the crowd, into the tent. A few people dehydrated," recalled volunteer Alvin Poussaint. "We were just running that whole night." About a dozen marchers were sent to St. Jude's Hospital, and at least twice as many were treated in the field by MCHR doctors.[21]

The following day was warm and sunny as the swelling crowd walked through the streets of Montgomery to the capitol, where they heard Martin Luther King's words of encouragement and inspiration. By now it was a foregone conclusion that a strong voting rights act would pass Congress, and that thousands of black people in Selma and across the South would win the franchise. For many of the MCHR volunteers who heard King that day this was the high point of their affiliation with the civil rights movement. They returned home exhilarated.

There was, however, one serious problem that emerged from the Medical Committee's presence in Selma. Throughout the march the MCHR physicians all but ignored their black counterparts in Alabama, intensifying racial divisions that would soon plague the civil rights movement as a whole. A black physician on the march cynically observed that the MCHR doctors believed they had discovered discrimination in the delivery of health care. As one white activist doctor conceded, "There was a presumption that nobody had done anything until we got there." The Medical Committee volunteers in Selma assumed that they would take charge of providing medical presence and health care for the marchers. Although the National Medical Association had supplied funds to its affiliate, the Alabama State Medical Association, Alabama's black physicians were not consulted in the MCHR planning sessions, even though this was their home turf. MCHR got all the national attention, including articles in the *New York Times*, and SCLC gave it the prestigious responsibility of looking after Martin Luther King in Selma.[22]

All this grated on NMA president Montague Cobb, who was in Selma and became "very upset" with MCHR's dominating presence. Although Cobb had been among the first to protest against racial discrimination in the AMA, he was little known in the white medical community. Now he and his organization were marginalized in Selma, while whites who were newcomers to the civil rights struggle seemed to be everywhere. Cobb observed that MCHR doctors "came to us as missionaries, wanting to tell us what to do," and he found the Medical Committee's slogan— that it was "the health arm of the civil rights movement"—to be "both surprising and absurd." His views were shared by others, and at one point the Alabama NMA members on the march asked the MCHR volunteers to clear out of the state. Tom Levin later recalled that "we weren't attentive to the NMA. I saw black separatism develop. I understood it and appreciated it."[23]

Back in New York, MCHR leaders engaged in damage control. Wells said that the internal conflicts between MCHR and the NMA should be resolved immediately, and invited Cobb and his fellow NMA members to the MCHR national gathering in April. Wells believed that "while our relationship with the Alabama Negro physicians might have been damaged by the action of some of the members of [MCHR], I do not think it was destroyed completely." He said he would write letters to "many of the Alabama physicians, complimenting them for their work during the March, and letting them know how grateful we were to them for their participation, etc." Wells was also in contact with Leonidas Berry, the president-elect of the NMA.

Born on a tobacco farm in North Carolina in 1902, Berry graduated from Wilberforce University and received his M.D. degree from the University of Chicago. A successful internist and a social activist, Berry was an MCHR member and attended the Washington convention as a delegate from Chicago. There he told Wells that he was eager for the two organizations to work together on racial matters, and he suggested that MCHR hold its first meeting of the national governing council in Cincinnati in August—to coincide with the NMA's annual meeting—so that members of both boards could get to know each other. Berry renewed his request in a letter to Wells. Aware that MCHR did not enjoy much support from the NMA rank and file, he suggested that initially he and Wells should "play down any reference to affiliations" until there had been time to "soften up relationships." Then, later in the week, members of both groups would "draw up a proposal of cooperative relationship between the two organizations, defining areas of activity which would prevent conflict of interest and promote cooperation." For the white members of the MCHR board, then, this would be a unique opportunity to socialize and talk shop with the leaders of the black medical establishment.[24]

The meeting never took place. At the cocktail party that marked the end of the Washington convention, MCHR leaders decided to hold their first governing council meeting in New York in June, to coincide with the AMA convention. The argument that the board really needed to meet before August made sense, but the idea of confronting the AMA in front of the cameras in New York no doubt held more appeal for these health care activists than having drinks with their more conservative black colleagues in Cincinnati. Wells let Berry's letter sit on his desk for a month before responding. After begging forgiveness "for the long delay in answering your letter," Wells explained why the governing council meeting would not be in Cincinnati and promised to try to recruit his white MCHR colleagues to the NMA meeting. When the NMA met in Cincinnati in August, Berry announced "an energetic campaign to recruit white members. We cannot remain a segregated society when we are pressing for integration ourselves." But no white MCHR governing council member attended the convention. In electing Berry as president and then choosing Mike Holloman to succeed him, the NMA was responding to the spirit of the times, which demanded that black professionals take a stand against racial injustice. Its campaign to attract white members was short-lived. The onset of Black Power was less than a year away and would affect both organizations, with activist black physicians working within the NMA, trying to radicalize it.[25]

Self-conscious about belonging to a civil rights organization that was overwhelmingly white, MCHR members elected African Americans— Aaron Wells, Mike Holloman, and David French—as its first three chairmen. And shortly before the Selma campaign, MCHR hired its first full-time staff person, appointing a twenty-eight-year-old black man named John Parham as its executive director.

Johnny Parham was born and raised in the shadow of the Atlanta University complex. At Morehouse College he was part of a group that challenged Jim Crow seating on buses—before the Montgomery bus boycott. Later, as a graduate student in the Atlanta School of Social Work, Parham joined with Morehouse undergraduates Lonnie King and Julian Bond to attack segregation in local businesses as part of the Atlanta student movement, and he was present at the founding meeting of SNCC in 1960. After working briefly in California, Parham and his wife moved to New York, where he became director of the Brooklyn branch of the Urban League. There he and other local activists took on discrimination in the building trades. (He recalls that Urban League chairman Whitney Young "threatened us with disaffiliation" because he took his board of directors to walk a picket line.) When Parham received a call from Wells offering him the director's position, "I was completely unaware of the Medical Committee."[26]

It did not take the new executive director long to get his feet wet. He spent the first day on the job in Mississippi, meeting with Cunningham,

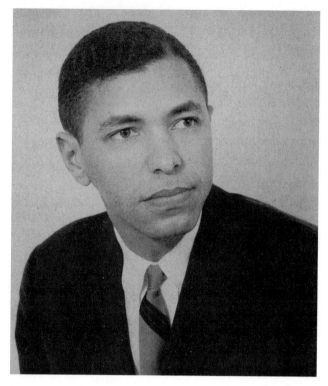

Johnny Parham. (Institute for Social Medicine and Community Health)

Disparti, and Geiger. Returning home he learned about the police beatings at the bridge in Selma, and for the next two weeks his office was in an uproar. Looking back on that time, Parham remembers the Medical Committee as "a volunteer crisis-based organization where everything was just flying all over the place. All we were doing was reacting." After only a week on the job, Parham wrote that "we must have a clearly defined organizational structure before we can begin to develop programs for a national movement." He wanted to centralize MCHR business in his office and for the executive committee to determine policy "relating to every official involvement of the organization," thereby preventing "the responsibility for policy from resting with individual members" of that central committee.[27]

Parham sensed this would not be an easy task. Most of those working in the office were volunteers whose previous experience had been in organizations like the Physicians Forum, which operated without a paid director. And because they were working for free, they often freelanced. "There were never any really defined roles," Parham recalls. "Everybody had developed their alliances. There were some who would say, 'This is what we are going to work on today. This is the crisis of the day!' Esther [Smith] would go in this direction, and there was a secretary who would go in another direction." Parham's natural allies were people like Callan, Geiger, and Gibson, the public health professionals who "may not have gotten extraordinarily excited about Selma, but who had a broader vision" for the organization, one that stressed programming in the North as well as the South. Parham too believed that "we needed to broaden our emphasis, because it was in a sense contradictory to have volunteers flying over inadequate health care in New York to go down to Mississippi."[28]

These and other matters were the subject of discussion and debate at MCHR's first national convention, held at Howard University in Washington from April 23 to 25, 1965. At the opening session an audience of about 150 people heard Joseph P. Resnick, a liberal congressional representative from New York, speak about race and health care. The major task of the delegates was to write a constitution. They agreed to elect a governing council comprised of four representatives from each chapter to be the governing body, which would meet at least once a year. An executive committee, elected at each annual meeting, would carry out the council's policies, and in effect run the national organization from New York. The question of fund-raising and dues was more contentious. Treasurer Moldovan wanted the chapters to send all dues money to New York, and he would return 60 percent to the chapters. He also believed that the national office should approve local fund-raising campaigns and events. The chapters insisted on more autonomy and got it. They would send only the national offices' portion of dues to Moldovan. They were free to raise money for their own projects, but they would need national approval for any fund-raising efforts or medical projects outside their metropolitan area. The issues of fund-raising and chapter autonomy would loom large in the months ahead.[29]

After the constitutional convention had completed its business, a series of workshops convened, covering such nuts-and-bolts issues as "chapter structure and membership" and "fund-raising and recruitment." Other sessions dealt with government programs, local activities, and "health projects in the South." Although keynote speaker Martin Luther King had to cancel, representatives from all the major national civil rights organizations spoke, including Jim Forman of SNCC, James Farmer of CORE, Aaron Henry of the NAACP, and James Bevel and C. T. Vivian from SCLC. In his presidential address, Aaron Wells proudly recalled MCHR's work from Freedom Summer through Selma. He called attention to continuing discrimination in the medical profession and the AMA, and he concluded by challenging his audience to deal with "the inadequate health facilities of the many 'Harlems' of the North."[30]

The Medical Committee's first convention was a success. Cities other than New York were well represented, and for the first time MCHR had a sense of identity as a national organization. Holloman, whose career as an activist physician preceded his picketing at the AMA meeting in Atlantic City in 1963, was a popular choice to succeed Wells as president. The executive committee added representatives from Pittsburgh, Chicago, Washington, and Baltimore. Although most agreed that the Medical Committee should expand its work into northern ghettos, the delegates left the convention committed to working in the South, and they were pleased to hear that MCHR had hired a young black psychiatrist, Alvin F. Poussaint, to become its first southern field director.[31]

Al Poussaint was born in East Harlem in 1934, one of eight children. He attended Peter Stuyvesant High School, where he was a classmate of future SNCC leader Bob Moses. Poussaint attended Columbia College on a state Regents' Scholarship and from there enrolled in Cornell Medical College. After graduating from medical school he moved to California, doing his internship at the UCLA Medical Center and then entering the UCLA Neuropsychiatric Institute. Poussaint was chief resident in Psychiatry when his old friend Bob Moses told him his talents were needed in Mississippi.[32]

Jack Geiger flew out to Los Angeles to interview the young psychiatrist and persuaded him to come to Mississippi for three or four days to look the place over. Except for a brief visit to a brother attending Hampton Institute in Virginia, this was Poussaint's first trip south. He and Geiger stayed with Bob Smith, who showed him around the community, took him to COFO meetings, and introduced him to nurses Cunningham and Disparti. Poussaint saw that MCHR needed someone full-time "to organize, to get it going. Bob Smith was trying to do it all, but couldn't. Not only did he have his own enormous practice, but he was also providing free health care for civil rights workers." Poussaint returned to L.A. still undecided, but he was leaning toward accepting the Medical Committee's offer.

Then Selma exploded, and Poussaint agreed to MCHR's request that he join Disparti and Cunningham in the medical van accompanying the march. For the young psychiatrist, this was his baptism into the movement. "I remember Al Poussaint on that march," Disparti recalls fondly. "Al hadn't been in the mud too often, and he hadn't been in the South. What courage it must have taken for him. But often he did not know what to do, whether it was safe or not. And here we were, white nurses with a black man, going places together, oblivious!" Poussaint recalls walking down Highway 80, "carrying an attaché case filled with every medicine imaginable. Every night when we pitched camp we would hold a clinic. During that week I met a lot of people. There was a lot of camaraderie, and we felt a loss at the end of the march. After that I was more determined that I would take the job, after finishing my training in June."[33]

Having made his decision, Poussaint was at first surprised and then dismayed at the reactions of his psychiatric colleagues at UCLA. "Their attitude was something like, 'Why do you want to put yourself in that situation, and risk being killed?'" It soon occurred to Poussaint that they were trying "to diagnose me, and interpret what I was doing as representing some psychopathology. I mean they said everything, like, 'You're showing something self-destructive, you have suicidal thoughts, you must be depressed, you should see the psychoanalyst'—all because I want to go to Mississippi." This experience stayed with Poussaint, and "gave me a new understanding about the role that psychiatry and psychology play in our society in controlling and manipulating people under the camouflage of therapy and psychological theory." Poussaint ignored his colleagues' advice and dire predictions and began planning his move to Jackson.[34]

Mississippi was beginning to change. Freedom Summer and the attendant national publicity brought grudging compliance with the new civil rights act and the peaceful desegregation of a handful of schools. White Mississippi was no longer monolithic on the race question, and voices of moderation, silent for a decade, once more were being heard. Yet the forces of reaction remained firmly in control at the statehouse, and the Ku Klux Klan was still doing its work, often assisted by local authorities. By the spring of 1965 the movement was also in a state of transition. Increasingly, veteran activists were rejecting integrationist goals and embracing what soon would be called Black Power. When Poussaint opened the MCHR office on Farish Street in Jackson he was dealing with a different environment from that encountered by the medical volunteers less than a year earlier. He relied heavily on Dr. Smith's advice as he began to make himself known in the community.

Bob Smith was living in a world of increasing pressures. He remained MCHR's most important contact in Mississippi, working with the nurses, treating civil rights workers, patiently mentoring the doctor volunteers who came down to help, flying to New York to board meetings, all the while maintaining his own practice and serving as the Tougaloo College physician. Aware of his importance to the organization, MCHR had given him an award at its convention and offered him the job of southern field coordinator before Poussaint came onto the scene. Smith had become more politically active. He marched at Selma, and he was a member of the steering committee of the Mississippi Freedom Democratic Party. As a black professional activist he had visibility in the white community and was subjected to continuing police harassment. He had been arrested on trumped-up speeding charges three times in early 1965 before his arrest on the same charge on March 10. At the police station, after he questioned the legality of his arrest, an officer grabbed him. Smith wrenched himself free and warned, "If you touch me again you'll have to kill me." The officer backed off. Smith refused to pay the fine and was thrown in the jail's drunk tank. Aaron Wells then wrote to Assistant Attorney General John Doar, demanding that the Justice Department "do all in its power to investigate the harassments." Earlier in the year Smith had seriously considered leaving Mississippi. He was to be married to Audrey Forbes, an Illinois pediatrician who was less than enthusiastic about moving to the Magnolia State, and living in Chicago had its appeal for Smith as well. In the end, he decided to remain in Jackson. He was there in the early summer of 1965 when black Mississippians experienced their own version of Selma.[35]

The Mississippi Freedom Democratic Party's plans to launch an intensive voter registration campaign were sidetracked when in mid-June Governor Paul Johnson called the Mississippi legislature into special session to repeal the state's discriminatory voting laws. Less flamboyant than his predecessor, Ross Barnett, but equally as committed to maintaining white supremacy in the Magnolia State, Johnson had undergone no eleventh-hour conversion to the cause of racial justice. Aware that in the wake of Selma, Congress was sure to pass a voting rights bill, Johnson told legislators he wanted to bring Mississippi's registration and voting requirements into line with those of northern states to pave the way for a court test once the new suffrage measure became law. If that failed, having no discriminatory voting legislation on the books might keep federal registrars out of the state. He was also aware that repealing the discriminatory statutes might undermine the FDP's challenge to the seating of Mississippi's congressional delegation (on the grounds that because blacks were denied the vote, the white delegation had been elected illegally).[36]

FDP strategists saw the special session as an opportunity to generate publicity and support for the congressional challenge. Applying the same arguments to state elections, the Freedom Democrats claimed that since the overwhelming majority of blacks had been denied the vote, the legislature was illegally constituted and thus the special session violated federal law. On the morning of June 14, FDP chair Lawrence Guyot led five hundred demonstrators out of Morning Street Baptist Church to begin a mile-long silent protest to the state capitol. Nearly half of the marchers were in their teens; about seventy-five were white summer volunteers in the state less than a week. Halfway to the capitol, Jackson police halted the march and began arresting participants for parading without a permit. They crammed demonstrators into paddy wagons and large caged trucks and delivered them to the state fairgrounds nearby, where they were deposited into two large buildings used for industrial and agricultural exhibits. The 482 people under arrest had literally been herded into cattle barns.[37]

Although the whole world had watched the beatings at Selma, in Jackson the police waged their war against peaceful protesters out of camera range, inside the fairgrounds. Phyllis Cunningham accompanied the demonstrators on the first march, intent on providing medical presence and administering any necessary first aid. Police arrested her along with the others for parading without a permit, shoved her into a crowded van, and put her into one of the fairground buildings. In this compound she saw police beating prisoners—"I tried to stay toward the center to avoid their nightsticks"—and then administered first aid to a man bleeding from the forehead, having been clubbed by a police officer. Also in the same compound was Linda Dugan, a nurse who had recently joined the MCHR staff in Mississippi. She was bandaging the wound of a woman who had also fallen victim to a nightstick. Police "were goading people with their clubs into a very compact group," reported Cunningham. It was hot inside the building and people were having difficulty breathing. Several had fainted, and "some of the taller people were lifting up the shorter people so that they could breath easier." Police then began segregating prisoners by race and sex. Along with the other white women, Cunningham was taken from the fairgrounds to the city jail.[38]

During the demonstration Jo Disparti was driving the MCHR van, "trying to get closer to the action" when an officer stopped her and told her not to go any further. "I said, 'I need to go there,' and he said, 'You can't go there,' so I said, 'Okay, Officer,' and he left me and I drove closer to the marchers. And when he saw me again he arrested me." Disparti was taken directly to jail. Ruth Steiner, a volunteer nurse who had come to work in Mississippi for an extended stay, was also arrested.[39]

The Jackson demonstration made the front page of the *New York Times*. More FDP supporters from across the state converged on the capital city to continue the demonstrations. Jackson had not seen such movement activity since the turmoil following Medgar Evers's funeral two years earlier. Smith and Poussaint, who had just moved to Jackson, provided medical assistance to demonstrators who had been beaten or released from jail. Police refused to let MCHR personnel inside the fairgrounds, so June Finer decided to get arrested and see for herself. Dr. Finer had stopped off in Jackson prior to opening up a permanent MCHR office in Selma. On the march "the pretty, thirty-year-old Chicagoan" was photographed comforting a five-year-old black boy, Anthony Quin. A "beefy, suntanned Mississippi highway patrolman" had just wrested an American flag from his hands, an unforgettable image captured by SNCC photographer Matt Herron. "The little boy was scared, and I just put my arm around him," recalls Finer. The officer arrested Anthony, his mother, McComb activist Aylene Quin, and Finer. Finer was taken to jail, not to the fairgrounds, and because her handbag contained prescription medicine as well as aspirin and bandages she was subjected to a thorough investigation before being released on bail. Mississippi health officer Archie Gray had hoped to find narcotics in her bag.[40]

As the demonstrations continued, a ritualized pattern of police brutality bordering on torture emerged from the fairgrounds compound. Teenagers and old people were among the victims. Annie Mae King, a Sunflower County activist well into her sixties, recalled that "they put you in those paddy wagons and they packed us in so tight until you couldn't get breath, you couldn't move. It was so hot we was just about to suffocate." Mrs. Alma Carnegie, sixty-eight, one of the stalwarts of the Holmes County movement, was kicked on the hip by a police officer while she was washing her plate. "He said I was out of line." An officer grabbed sixteen-year-old Bernice Crosby by the neck and began choking her. Then he threw her to the ground, grabbed her by the legs, and dragged her away. Female prisoners were subjected to lewd and suggestive remarks, including promises of release in return for sexual favors. Phil Sharp, a CORE worker from Jasper County, saw several policemen pick a young black man out of a line. "One ran a night stick between his legs and rolled it back and forth across his testicles. I saw the guy some hours later. His shirt was covered with blood and he was still bent over."[41]

Male prisoners reported having to run the gauntlet between rows of club-swinging policemen. The inmates slept on bare mattresses (if they had any) without blankets. During the day they had to sit on the concrete floor, with mattresses lying only a few feet away. Each day a machine fumigated the buildings with "a choking, eye-smarting cloud of gaseous fumes ten to fifteen feet high that rolled through the compound." The prisoners' daily diet consisted of grits and syrup for breakfast and string beans and hominy for the other meals. An investigating team from the National Council of Churches described the stockade as a "concentration camp . . . designed to break the spirit, the will, the health, and even the body of each individual."[42]

In such an environment many of the jailed demonstrators badly needed health care. Jackson city officials denied both Medical Committee personnel and the prisoners' personal physicians access to the fairgrounds. The city-approved doctor gave intimate physical examinations to black women with white male policemen gawking on. One woman suffering from pain stood in line to see the "jail doctor," but dropped out when she heard him ridiculing some of the other women about having syphilis and gonorrhea. When the doctor did prescribe medicine it was often not delivered. When news of the mistreatment of the prisoners reached New York, members of the MCHR executive committee sent telegrams to the Justice Department and to President Johnson, demanding that "the Federal government take serious, sustained action to ensure the safety of defenseless citizens confronted by sadistic law-enforcement officers." They wrote Mayor Allan Thompson of Jackson, asking that "M.C.H.R. teams be permitted to make rounds in the jails in the morning, evening, and immediately following arrests," a request Thompson once again denied. In Washington, Mary Holman and Robert Mishell of the D.C. chapter contacted the congressional office of Representative Charles Ryan of New York, who scheduled a briefing for other House members. Cunningham and Finer flew up to Washington to give firsthand reports, along with four Freedom Democratic Party members who had been jailed. The following day Finer was again arrested in a Jackson demonstration, although she identified herself as a physician and "was *not* indulging in civil disobedience."[43]

Sensing that the Jackson demonstrations had the potential to become another Selma, FDP's Guyot issued a call to "concerned citizens across the

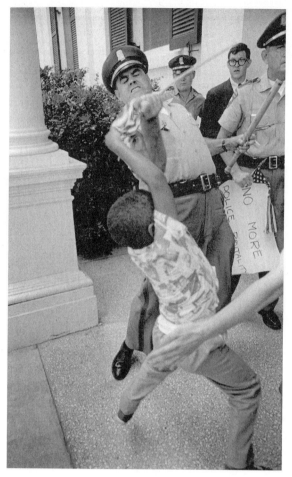

Police officer taking American flag from Anthony Quin. (Matt Herron/Take Stock)

country to come to Jackson to continue demonstrating against the state's denial of the right to vote." By the end of the first week, 859 marchers had been jailed, most of whom remained incarcerated in the compound. Yet Jackson was not to be Selma. Although a few clergy answered the call, there was no outpouring of support for the Mississippi campaign. The marches continued, and another 170 people were arrested over the next two weeks. But the supply of people who were willing to subject themselves to the harsh conditions in the compound was limited. Bail bond money was hard to come by; the national media had lost interest. FDP turned its attention once again to Washington and the congressional challenge. When the Mississippi legislature adjourned after passing the governor's repeal package,

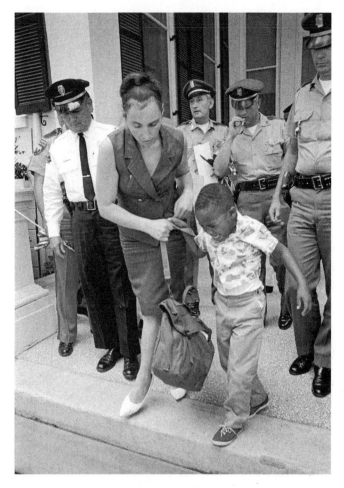

Dr. June Finer comforting Anthony Quin during the demonstrations in Jackson, Mississippi, summer 1965. (Matt Herron/Take Stock)

few white officials believed their action would delay enforcement of a new federal voting rights law.[44]

Members of the Medical Committee for Human Rights, so eager to jump on planes headed for Selma in March, stayed at home when Jackson exploded two months later. The small southern MCHR staff needed help. Poussaint reported that throughout the summer the MCHR office in Jackson "was operating nearly totally as a first aid and triage clinic. Emergencies abounded, the phone was constantly ringing from all over the state, and traffic through the office was hectic." In addition, "quite a number of psychiatric problems were handled by our office." Overall, MCHR estimated that two hundred volunteers would be needed during the summer of 1965 for projects in Mississippi, in Selma, in Bogalusa, Louisiana, where CORE demonstrations were under way, and in parts of Georgia, Florida, and South Carolina, where civil rights leaders were requesting MCHR assistance. On June 10, four days before the first FDP march in Jackson, Johnny Parham sent a grim warning to chapter presidents. "Our summer recruitment program is in desperate need of volunteers and funds. We do not have the funds to underwrite travel expenses for students, interns, residents and nurses, and the number of doctors expressing an interest in going south is extremely limited." Two weeks later, as the Mississippi demonstrations intensified, Parham notified all chapters of the "urgent need for doctors from Thursday to Sunday in Jackson." No one answered the call.[45]

Given the enthusiastic response to requests for medical personnel in Selma and in Mississippi during Freedom Summer, how does one account for this apparent lack of interest in southern fieldwork for the summer of 1965? No doubt for some physicians the Selma march satisfied their desire for personal involvement. They now had a sufficient trove of war stories with which to regale their colleagues and neighbors. But this cynical explanation ignores more substantive issues. First, the "white backlash" against the movement began five days after passage of the Voting Rights Act, when the black ghetto of Watts in Los Angeles exploded in violence, destruction, and loss of life. White liberals in the North—including physicians—began to question their support of a more militant movement where they themselves were increasingly the target of angry young blacks.

At the same time a debate was under way inside the Medical Committee over its program and mission. At the first meeting of the new governing council, held while the FDP demonstrations in Jackson were at their peak, Des Callan decried MCHR's "inability to decide on a clear order of program priorities at the convention or at any meeting since then." While the southern program of medical presence "has brought us fame and new members," Callan warned that "we must balance that against its high cost and question whether it truly meets the needs of the movement or ourselves. The civil rights movement today increasingly needs specific skills and programs, [but] MCHR's approach is symbolic rather than medical in its significance." Callan pointed to the fledgling health clinic in Holmes County as "a successful model that has the potential for reduplication in both the South and the North."[46]

MCHR appeared to be at a crossroads. Should it continue as "the medical arm of the civil rights movement" or shift its focus to develop programs that specifically addressed the health care needs of black and poor people across the country? The differences between the civil rights and public health factions, papered over during Freedom Summer and Selma, now resurfaced. With a southern field director and an executive secretary both fresh on the job, MCHR began its second year not without optimism, but with more questions than answers.

.

Summer 1965

By mid-1965 the civil rights movement was in transition, both in Mississippi and throughout the South. In the aftermath of Selma, black and white activists launched campaigns in cities like Bogalusa, Louisiana. Lobbyists in Washington pushed Congress to pass a voting rights law and, as part of President Johnson's Great Society, to enact social programs that were beneficial to African Americans. Down in Lowndes County, Alabama, however, a quiet revolution was under way. A group of SNCC organizers led by Stokely Carmichael had moved into Lowndes and they were working with local people to form an all-black political party with a black panther as its intimidating symbol. The Medical Committee for Human Rights tried to come to grips with these developments as it expanded into new territory.

There were now fifteen MCHR chapters in eight states. It had affiliates in the largest cities, but there were no southern chapters. Organizing in the nation's most conservative region proved difficult, for there both black and white physicians were reluctant to identify with left-wing practitioners from the North. New York was the largest MCHR chapter. Of its 250 paid members, more than 100 were physicians, dentists, and psychologists; 78 were registered nurses; the rest were social workers, lab technicians, researchers, and chemists.[1]

Organized in January of 1965 by some of the same people who had founded the Medical Committee seven months earlier, the New York MCHR suffered from a split personality. It was operating in the same market that supplied the national office with most of its income, so turf battles over fund-raising were inevitable. Its monthly newsletter, with a circulation of

3,500, and a membership campaign, "which will soon reach 25,000 health professionals in the New York area," provided a broad base of potential donors. Local members gave "numerous cocktail and house parties," sponsored a "Sunday Dansant" at the Village Gate, and printed 25,000 raffle tickets, with the lucky winners receiving "a color TV set and other valuable prizes." The national office was to receive a seventy-thirty split of the proceeds of these events. Philip Stewart, chairman of the New York chapter, complained that national fund-raiser Esther Smith was uncooperative, scheduling events in the city without informing him. When he contacted Pete Seeger about a benefit concert for the chapter, Stewart was embarrassed to learn that the folksinger and activist had appeared at a national benefit in New York only two weeks earlier. The problems of "duplication of effort and overlapping resources" between New York and the national office were never satisfactorily resolved.[2]

The New York branch needed money to underwrite one of MCHR's most important projects, Rest and Rehabilitation (R & R) for civil rights activists, the program begun by Trudy Orris in the summer of 1963. Directing it the following year was Sam Siegel, one of the few dentists to spend time in Mississippi during Freedom Summer. He returned to New York to organize a dentists' group within MCHR and arrange for "SNCC kids who were having trouble with their teeth to drive up here" for treatment. Working with Trudy Orris, Siegel formed a Professional Courtesy Committee of local doctors, dentists, and psychiatrists to give free treatment to visiting civil rights workers. The New York MCHR paid transportation costs and housed the workers. Some of them simply needed dental work or basic medical treatment, but others, suffering from burnout, required professional counseling away from the battle zone. During the summer of 1965 nearly forty southern movement activists came to New York as part of the R & R program, which continued into the following year. Not only was the New York chapter the most active in MCHR, it was also the most radical. Its members were among the most vocal opponents of the Vietnam War, and in ensuing years they embraced much of the agenda of the New Left.[3]

After New York, the Chicago area had supplied the most Freedom Summer medical volunteers. Its chapter evolved from the Committee to End Discrimination in Chicago Medical Institutions. Black physician Arthur Falls was the first chairman, ably assisted by Quentin Young, a forty-year-old doctor whose private practice served a racially mixed clientele in Hyde Park. The Chicago MCHR continued the work begun by the CED, demanding that local hospitals integrate and award staff privileges to black physicians. It joined forces with the Coordinating Council of Community Organizations in a number of marches protesting de facto school segregation. At each demonstration a doctor or nurse was present, and when Martin Luther King held a mass meeting in Grant Park on a hot, humid July day, fifteen MCHR doctors and twenty-two nurses were on hand to provide care for the estimated thirty thousand people in attendance. More than a thousand protesters were arrested during the subsequent demonstrations; the MCHR doctors made jail visitations and helped raise bail money. The Chicago branch, next to New York, was the most directly involved in the southern freedom movement. In 1965 the chapter made it possible for June Finer to work several months as the coordinator of the Alabama and Louisiana projects, provided total financial support to two medical students, Fitzhugh Mullan and Steven Cohen, to spend their summer in Holmes County, Mississippi, and recruited Helene Richardson, a registered nurse, to work in the Mileston clinic.[4]

Under the leadership of Howard University Medical School professors David French, Fredric Solomon, and Robert Murray, the Washington, D.C., chapter became national MCHR's Capitol Hill lobbyist, an effort led by its treasurer, a white southerner named Mary Holman. A nurse with family roots deep in Mississippi, Holman had close ties with the MCHR nurses and with Al Poussaint. She worked with the Mississippi Freedom Democratic Party and its congressional challenge, arranging housing and medical care for five hundred FDP supporters who came to Washington from Mississippi to plead their case. When the police arrested hundreds of demonstrators in Jackson during the summer of 1965 and housed them at the fairgrounds "concentration camp," the D.C. chapter arranged for several of the victims to come to Washington to tell their stories to influential congressmen such as John Ryan of New York. Fred Solomon, who sat in on the hearings, boasted that "MCHR commands greater attention from Federal officials than any of the civil rights organizations, at least in Washington." As the War on Poverty opened up new opportunities and challenges, the Washington MCHR lobbied Congress to allocate OEO funds for health care and to desegregate southern hospitals by enforcing Title VI of the 1964 civil rights law. Ideologically, however, Washington was one of the more conservative chapters, with its members less outspoken on issues like Vietnam.[5]

Most MCHR chapters were located in East Coast cities with medical schools and schools of public health. In Boston, much of the leadership came from Harvard and Tufts professors, most notably Gibson and Geiger. New Haven had a chapter because of Yale, headed by medical school professor Richard Weinerman, also a member of the National Executive Committee. Philadelphia's chapter was founded in 1965, and Walter Lear, now deputy commissioner of the Philadelphia Department of Public Health, drifted back into the movement he had initiated with the Medical Committee for Civil Rights in 1963. Down through the years Lear would remain one of the pillars of MCHR, in both good times and bad. Pittsburgh had a small but strong chapter under the leadership of Leslie Falk and the city's leading African American physician, Earl Belle Smith. The West Coast was represented by the San Francisco chapter and by a group of physicians operating under the banner of the Los Angeles Physicians for Social Responsibility (LAPSR). They cooperated with the newly formed Student Medical Conference to initiate health care projects in Watts after the riots in 1965. Medical and nursing students assisted Mexican migrant workers and Indian families on the Tache reservation, provided medical examinations for Head Start children in several locations, and worked in Mississippi and Louisiana during the summer of 1965.[6]

The center of black protest activity moved from Mississippi to Louisiana, which became the nation's hot spot in the summer of 1965, with CORE activists battling white supremacists in the Ku Klux Klan. The Klan's major stronghold in the state was Bogalusa, a mill town sixty miles northwest of New Orleans, across the Pearl River from Mississippi. MCHR volunteers who came to Bogalusa found an environment even more threatening than that in the Magnolia State in 1964.

Northern capitalists founded Bogalusa in 1906 as a center for the manufacture of paper and pulp products. By the early 1960s, the Crown Zellerbach plant employed more than half of the town's working people. Although about 40 percent of the population of twenty-two thousand was African American, blacks comprised only about 12 percent of the Crown Zellerbach workforce, with little chance for promotion from the low-level jobs they held. Black workers did have their own union, however, and a good number of black farmers owned their land, providing both groups with a degree of protection against white economic retaliation for civil rights activities. As a result, by the summer of 1965 Bogalusa was home to "arguably the most militant [black movement] in the entire South," according to historian Adam Fairclough. Direct action protests led to white retaliation, and the Ku Klux Klan spread like kudzu. Journalist Paul Good concluded that Bogalusa "has more Klansmen per square foot than this writer has encountered or heard of anywhere in the South."[7]

The direct action campaign started in January 1965 when the local Bogalusa Voters League (BVL) invited the Congress of Racial Equality to send in organizers. Founded in the 1940s, CORE had been operating in Louisiana since 1960, and shared with SNCC a commitment to grassroots community organization. The local Klan determined to expel the CORE outsiders and suppress the local BVL, led by Crown Zellerbach worker A. Z. Young. In one confrontation the police stood by as "Klansmen hurled bricks and bottles from car windows at black pedestrians; they assaulted blacks in cafes and gas stations; they flagged down cars and attacked their occupants." To counter the Klan and offer protection the police refused to provide, Louisiana blacks founded the Deacons for Defense and Justice in Jonesboro in the summer of 1964. A chapter in Bogalusa was formed the following February, with the endorsement of the BVL. Armed Deacons patrolled black neighborhoods, served as bodyguards for movement leaders, kept tabs on the police, and accompanied all demonstrations. They "soon became a legend in the civil rights movement."[8]

As summer approached, with Bogalusa now an armed camp, Dave Dennis of CORE asked MCHR to provide medical presence "in the same manner as [it] did last summer for COFO." June Finer had volunteered to be the southern coordinator for the summer, and in early June she rented the second story of an old residence in Baton Rouge, the state capital, about an hour's drive from Bogalusa. This "cock-roach infested place" next door to the CORE office served as the Louisiana state headquarters for MCHR. Finer then took off for Mississippi—the Jackson demonstrations and fairgrounds jailings had just begun—and left the Louisiana office in the charge of Hilda Braverman, an unpaid volunteer from Newark who was about to enter medical school. By mid-June more than one hundred CORE volunteers, most of them white northern students, had arrived in the state to participate in their "Freedom Summer." In Bogalusa this meant voter registration work, picketing downtown merchants who refused to hire black clerks, and daily mass marches to the city hall.[9]

Throughout June and into July, MCHR doctors and nurses worked with CORE activists, local BVL leaders, and the Bogalusa Deacons for Defense in their daily confrontations with the Klan. On July 8, four hundred local blacks and a small group of white CORE volunteers were returning from a march to city hall when a black teenager named Hattie Mae Hill slumped to the ground, clutching the side of her face. She had been hit by a rock and was bleeding profusely from her head. Volunteer Frank Lossy, a physician from Berkeley, came up from his station at the rear of the march to attend to her, and then asked Leneva Tiedeman, a registered nurse also from California, to take the girl back to the Union Hall, the march's staging area. As Tiedeman was helping Hill to a car (owned by BVL president Young) a twenty-five-year-old white man named Alton Crowe screamed "white nigger" and "bitch" at Tiedeman. The two women then ran for the waiting car, where driver Henry Austin, a twenty-one-year-old air force veteran, sat ready to take off and Milton Johnson stood outside waving them in. Both Johnson and Austin were members of the Bogalusa Deacons. As Tiedeman was scrambling to get in to the car, Crowe grabbed her and Johnson jumped him. Angry whites then attacked Johnson and Austin, while the women sought cover in the backseat.

In the ensuing melee Austin shot Crowe three times in the chest. Dr. Lossy (who was licensed to practice medicine in Louisiana) rushed up to offer assistance, telling police officers now on the scene that the MCHR van ambulance was available to transport the white victim to the hospital. The police ignored the MCHR physician, who then returned to the march, where he was threatened by white bystanders who believed he had refused to treat Crowe. Tiedeman and Hill made it back to the staging area, where an MCHR doctor treated the girl's wound. Police arrested both Austin and Johnson and took them away before local whites could have at them. Tiedeman and Lossy underwent hours of interrogation at the police station before being released.[10]

A black civil rights activist shooting a white attacker in the middle of a demonstration was unprecedented in the history of the movement, and suddenly Bogalusa was famous. Given the militancy of Bogalusa blacks and a local Klan that the police either could not or would not control, racial tensions were bound to intensify, and MCHR needed more personnel. "We have an urgent need for volunteers in Bogalusa, where we presently have only three doctors," stated Johnny Parham in a telegram to chapter presidents. During the July 8 demonstration the Medical Committee had become more visible, and as a result the police took steps to limit its participation. MCHR vehicles could no longer accompany a march and volunteer doctors were denied access to injured demonstrators who had been jailed. Medical volunteers continued to accompany the marchers and provide first aid for demonstrators who were beaten or hit by rocks and bottles.

Dr. C. H. Wright, an African American volunteer, reported that every day he treated "traumatic injuries sustained by civil rights workers at the hands of Bogalusa whites." The escalation of protests attracted federal attention. Representatives of the Community Relations Service tried to mediate, and John Doar, the Justice Department's top civil rights lawyer, came down to investigate. The result was a series of federal suits against the Bogalusa police force, city restaurants violating the Civil Rights Act, and the Ku Klux Klan, all of which had the immediate effect of decreasing, but not eliminating, acts of violence against local blacks.[11]

Since there was no African American physician in Bogalusa, local blacks came to MCHR doctors and nurses for treatment. Dr. Wright and other volunteers made house calls, took care of minor ailments, and referred more serious cases to the public hospital. Wright treated all civil rights workers, but if a patient was not "recognizable as a participant in the civil rights movement, verbal evidence was requested of their family's participation. This was my fee." Wright added that "I believe this spurred the community's interest in the project."[12]

Medical Committee personnel delivered birth control lectures to young boys and girls, visited CORE projects to talk with staff members about local health conditions and facilities (with an eye toward forcing local hospitals to comply with Title VI of the Civil Rights Act), and began a program to provide rest and recreation facilities for CORE workers. MCHR set up local health committees, and even arranged to have sewage lines extended to black sections of Jonesboro. They were heartened by the response from a number of black Louisiana doctors. By the end of the summer a New Orleans physician and nurse had agreed to visit Bogalusa each Tuesday.[13]

The summer program in Louisiana had been a success, with nearly thirty volunteers—including doctors from New Orleans—participating. Hilda Braverman summed up the committee's work in a letter to Parham in mid-August:

> We have provided physical presence at demonstrations, at picket lines, at mass meetings. But more important, we have made our physical presence known to the people throughout the state. They know that there are sympathetic medical people who can help them with their sewage problems, with their birth control problems, with ever spreading venereal diseases, and help them to obtain more adequate medical care.

Braverman urged MCHR to maintain its office in Louisiana beyond the summer, for "now that we have motivated a number of Negro communities to initiate health programs and have made ourselves known to the medical community of Louisiana we cannot in good conscience leave the state." Nonetheless, on September 1 the Medical Committee closed its Baton Rouge office, never to return, despite pleas from CORE and local people to remain. The MCHR governing council cited financial problems as the reason. It was true that contributions were down substantially from the previous year. However, for all but a handful of MCHR members, working in the South had lost its attraction. As for the national MCHR office, it paid remarkably little attention to the volunteers in and around Bogalusa.[14]

Much the same could be said for the Alabama project, which June Finer initiated after leaving Louisiana. The decision to open an Alabama office came shortly after the Selma march, and the first volunteers arrived in April. Early in the summer a temporary headquarters opened in Montgomery, staffed by Peter Schnall, a third-year medical student from the University of Southern California who was recruited to spend the summer in Alabama. In mid-July, Finer met with Schnall and Jeannette Badger, an African American nurse volunteer, to plan activities. Finer, who agreed to work in the South the entire summer for living expenses, moved the MCHR office to Selma to be close to the center of civil rights activity, and rented a three-room house to serve as both headquarters and dormitory for MCHR volunteers and staff.[15]

During July and August the Medical Committee volunteers worked with both SNCC and SCLC organizers in Alabama and marched behind demonstrators in towns like Greensboro, where the Klan had responded to a voter registration drive by bombing black churches. Police assaulted and arrested black protesters during their daily marches to the courthouse. MCHR personnel accompanying a demonstration late in July "were tear-gassed on all sides, cutting off every exit." The MCHR team treated the victims and taught the demonstrators how to respond to future attacks. That night June Finer and social worker Robert Jacobson stayed in Greensboro, "for trouble was forecast during the mass meeting and all-night vigil. We slept outside with the other vigilers, ready for emergency first aid treatment and also showing that the medical committee was with them."[16]

MCHR was also busy in Lowndes County, where SNCC organizers led by Stokely Carmichael worked with local people to found the Black

Panther Party, which would contest the fall elections. It was a turbulent time. Finer recalls that after a visit to jailed activists she and a colleague were chased out of town by a carload of whites "riding behind us, and then running parallel and dropping behind us again." That "scary ride" occurred shortly after a young white seminarian named Jon Daniels had been gunned down in cold blood at a Lowndes grocery store.[17]

During the summer, Finer and volunteer doctor Willis Butler made an unsuccessful effort to connect with local white physicians, including the president of the county medical society, Walter Greene. In a written report, Butler expressed his opinion that Dr. Greene's "physical resemblance to Gov. Wallace is matched by his philosophical affinity," and he was "one of the few men I know who seems to STRUT while sitting down." In the course of the conversation, Greene threatened legal action against MCHR for practicing medicine without a license, and spoke as though MCHR was a "great conspiracy aimed at his beloved southland." At one point, attempting to defuse the tension, Finer said something to the effect that she didn't want these things to become the subject of a quarrel, whereupon Dr. Greene replied with a leer, "Honey, I couldn't quarrel with *you* about anything." As they left he told Butler it was smart for him to have brought Finer along because if it had just been the two of them it would have been "knock down and drag out." (Butler later wrote that "June Finer remained cool and showed finesse" in conversing with this "white doctor who is almost overtly paranoid.") Greene's final piece of advice, that it would be "pointless" for MCHR to meet with the County Medical Society as a group, seemed almost redundant.[18]

The Medical Committee's relations with black physicians were less cordial than they had been in Louisiana, perhaps as a result of the fallout over resentment of MCHR's ignoring black doctors during the Selma-Montgomery march. Ultimately, this sense of isolation led MCHR to downplay its civil rights credentials in hopes of improving its image with local physicians, black and white. On October 5, after the wave of summer demonstrations, Finer asked Parham "to draw up a new brochure, avoiding our civil rights role as far as is compatible with minimal candour and your conscience, and stressing medical education in poverty-stricken areas," adding somewhat cynically that "a photo of a kindly, dedicated-looking doctor teaching a class of kids would be appropriate."[19]

Jewish volunteers worked to cultivate the "80 souls" who made up Selma's Jewish community. The local B'nai B'rith had disbanded over the national organization's call for support of the civil rights movement. After a visit to services at Temple Mishkan Israel, physician Zanvel Klein spoke with Rabbi Lothar Lubasch about racial matters. Despite his escape from Germany before the Holocaust, Lubasch failed to acknowledge any comparison between his experience with the Nazis and the plight of Selma blacks. Perhaps fearing another outburst of anti-Semitism (two years earlier there had been bomb threats directed against the temple) Lubasch "responded with every cliché in the book, from Negro irresponsibility to 'would you marry one?'" A week later, after services, two members of the Barton family, mother and daughter, invited Klein, along with doctors Finer and Robert Goldberg to their home, "which was really a brave act," Finer recalled. Mr. Barton was in the hospital suffering from severe depression. His wife had been running the family shoe shop, but a successful boycott by blacks of downtown Selma merchants had driven her out of business. The Bartons' experience illustrates the bitter irony of many in the southern Jewish community—sympathetic yet vulnerable, and in the end victimized if they did not play their cards right.[20]

Near the end of the summer, as civil rights activity declined, volunteers spent more time in the black community, treating minor ailments and dispersing nonprescription medicines, conducting door-to-door health surveys, and meeting with local people in small groups to talk about health problems. They showed films at these gatherings about subjects ranging from hookworm to syphilis, and a drama, *Palmour Street*, which portrayed a black family's problems. Visiting health care workers reported that they were well received by local blacks, in part due to the impact of Finer's presence. One volunteer expressed admiration bordering on awe for her "rapport with the Negro community." The MCHR house, open every evening until eleven, was a place where civil rights workers found "sympathetic listeners." MCHR hosted parties for the activists (a small R & R endeavor) every Thursday, and made plans to meet semiformally with local teenagers once a week.[21]

Thirty-seven volunteers came to Alabama in the summer of 1965 to work in the MCHR project, including six nurses, eight psychiatrists, and four psychologists. As was the case in Louisiana, everyone—MCHR staff and volunteers, movement workers, and local people—wanted to keep the Alabama office open during the winter. Johnny Parham asked SCLC's Andy Young for funds for MCHR to operate in Alabama, noting that organizing people around their health needs and demanding improved health services ought to be a priority for civil rights organizations. Although SCLC had requested the MCHR's assistance on several occasions, its response was negative. Finer stayed until October, and after that volunteers ran the office until Leneva Tiedeman arrived from Louisiana to take charge late in 1965. Unlike in Louisiana, the Alabama MCHR project stayed afloat, in large part because in the summer of 1966 nurses from Mississippi, including Cunningham, moved over to Selma to work full-time. Alabama would be MCHR's last southern outpost.[22]

Mississippi remained at the center of the Medical Committee's work in the South. When the national office hired Dr. Alvin Poussaint as southern field director it made good on its pledge to civil rights activists to initiate a full-time operation in Mississippi. The four-room headquarters on Farish Street in the heart of black Jackson was next door to the state office of the Mississippi Freedom Democratic Party and just down the street from the three civil rights law groups operating in the state. The office had an examination room that contained "a generous shipment of supplies and drugs" from the World Medical Relief Foundation.[23]

By the summer of 1965 the civil rights movement in Mississippi was in trouble. Escalating tensions between the more strident organizers in SNCC and CORE and members of local branches of the NAACP, who were growing increasingly impatient with the lifestyles of the young black and white activists, led to a decision in the spring to disband COFO, the organization that for more than three years had represented the black freedom struggle in the Magnolia State. Led by Lawrence Guyot, the Mississippi Freedom Democratic Party attempted to fill that void, but met with only limited success. The Democratic Party's failure to seat the FDP challengers at the 1964 convention disillusioned many SNCC and CORE organizers, including Moses and Dennis, both of whom had now left Mississippi. Guyot's attempt to re-create the Selma campaign in Jackson had failed despite the hundreds of people who voluntarily went to jail, and except for a major organizing campaign in Natchez, civil rights activity was not nearly so intense as in Louisiana and Alabama. As a result, MCHR attracted only a handful of physicians to Mississippi. Its program was enhanced, however, by a small group of medical students who came down for the entire summer.[24]

Inspired by the student participation in the civil rights movement and by MCHR role models, medical students across the country began to organize on their campuses. In 1965, Bill Bronston and Michael "Mick" McGarvey formed the Student Medical Conference in California and began working in economically depressed areas in and around Los Angeles. Seeing medical students as an untapped resource, MCHR made plans to send a contingent to Mississippi beginning with a week-long orientation session in Pittsburgh. The resource people at that session were a who's who of MCHR's Mississippi operation: physicians Geiger, Smith, Falk, and Poussaint, and nurses Cunningham and Disparti. The students learned about Mississippi history and culture from a young historian named David Montgomery. Bob Smith presided at a session on "The Medical Picture in Mississippi," which included a general discussion of "public health, doctors, dentists, hospitals, morbidity, mortality, etc." The students got a crash course on preventive medicine, including basic hygiene, sex education, and malnutrition, subjects all but ignored in their medical school curricula.[25]

Only nine volunteers showed up for the orientation: five medical students, two teachers, a nursing student, and one physician, Leon Kass. The relatively poor turnout stemmed mainly from problems in the national office and its communication—or lack thereof—with local chapters. In mid-June, Richard Weinerman of the Yale Medical School complained to Parham of "severe handicaps in recruiting students for the various summer projects, since all of this material was received by us after the end of our term, and after the vast majority of our students had departed for home." Parham wrote back (a month later) apologizing for "the lateness in approaching the summer students' project," and promised that next year "the chapters will be more involved" in planning the student program.[26]

Despite their small number, the medical students who spent the summer of 1965 in Mississippi made their presence felt. Assigned to both urban and rural districts, they lived with local black families. Poussaint, their supervisor, was also new to Mississippi, so the students "for the most part had a great deal of autonomy and flexibility." They served as health and welfare consultants to civil rights groups, investigated health facilities regarding compliance with Title VI, taught health classes, and became instant community organizers, recruiting small groups of people into local health associations. Volunteers in South Mississippi included medical student Jay Brown in Laurel, nursing student Mary Ellen Garfes in Hattiesburg, and sociology teacher Gretchen Pfeutze on the Gulf Coast.[27]

Most of the students (and Dr. Kass and his wife, Amy, a teacher) spent the summer in Holmes County. Jo Disparti had been organizing in the Delta section of the county, and had recently been joined by Helene Richardson and Pat Weatherly. The summer volunteers spent their time in the hills section in areas that had not received a lot of attention from civil rights activists. Harvard medical student Beach Conger was assigned to Lexington. He recalls that "I was full of grandiose concepts about what I was going to do as a medical civil rights worker but wound up working on voter registration and school integration . . . It was a remarkable experience." Steve Cohen, from the University of Chicago, was stationed in the northeast rural hill country. Another Chicago student, Fitzhugh Mullan, worked in Second Pilgrim's Rest, a hamlet near the "urban" area of Durant, population twenty-five hundred.[28]

Fitz Mullan was a New York blueblood whose family was listed in the social register. His father was a Park Avenue psychiatrist. Educated in private schools, Fitz "grew up in relative racial seclusion" and attended a New England boarding school where the words "nigger" and "coon" were common. After he entered Harvard in 1960 he began to take an interest in racial matters. Mullan had majored in history, taking only the bare minimum of science courses, so when the University of Chicago Medical School admitted him in the spring of 1964 it was on the condition that he attend summer school to make up his deficiency. That was Freedom Summer, and while Mullan's two roommates at Harvard were volunteering in Mississippi he was studying embryology at NYU. The following spring at Chicago when he heard Quentin Young speak about MHCR's sponsoring

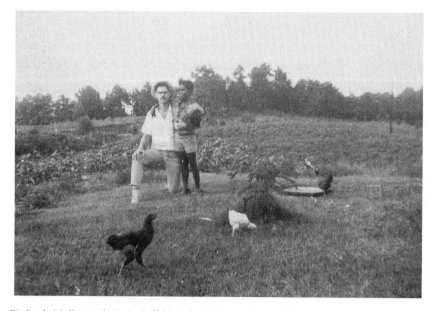

Fitzhugh Mullan with Rosie Saffold and chickens in Second Pilgrim's Rest, Mississippi, August 1965. (Fitzhugh Mullan donation)

medical students to work in Mississippi, offering to pay for transportation and twenty dollars a week, Mullan jumped at the chance.[29]

After attending the orientation sessions in Pittsburgh and meeting with doctors Smith and Poussaint in Jackson, Mullan was pretty much on his own once he got to Holmes County. He lived with the family of a black schoolteacher named Magnolia Reed. Her son, Cat, age sixteen, was Fitz's "driver, bodyguard—he looks 25—and passport into the black community." Mrs. Reed's mother also lived with the family, as did Magnolia's four-year-old grandson, Joel, who, to her consternation, insisted on humming freedom songs during shopping trips to the white part of town. Magnolia Reed's salary did not carry over into the summer, and the family depended on Mullan's stipend to put food on the table. The young medical student thrived in this environment. In his memoir, *White Coat, Clenched Fist,* Mullan wrote that "the Civil Rights Movement was so much more real, so much more compelling" than the "contrived and dull" medical school.[30]

Mullan immersed himself in the black community. Although the "baby doctor" (a reference to both his age and medical student status) did not practice medicine, "local people took satisfaction from the presence of a medical person in their midst. It gave the community a status it never had before." More active in the movement than the short-term volunteers, the "*doctor* civil rights worker" participated in a variety of protests, including the desegregation of the local movie theater. Accompanied by a dozen black teenagers, he bought tickets at the "white" window and they sat in the white section—the ground floor. It was a long evening. "It couldn't have been a worse movie—'Hush, Hush, Sweet Charlotte'—which showed blacks only as domestic servants," recalled Mullan. "And it was extremely scary, which we didn't need at all." A sullen white crowd was waiting outside, but the group "marched triumphantly back to the Negro section with white cars following along beside us." Later that night a cross burned, and an attempt made to burn down the church at Second Pilgrim's Rest. The following evening Mullan sat up all night with two local blacks, guarding the church.[31]

He had learned, as had other volunteers before him, that it was impossible to separate civil rights activity from health care advocacy. At the Pittsburgh orientation meetings the student volunteers were encouraged to form health associations, so he sent out word in Durant that there would be a meeting to discuss health concerns, to be held at the home of Mrs. Viola Winters, a respected elderly black woman. At first people were

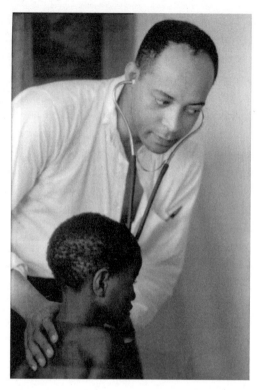

Physician examining child in CDGM center, Second Pilgrim's Rest, Mississippi, 1965. (Matt Herron/Take Stock)

reluctant to talk. This was, after all, the first civil rights meeting held in the town. (Stokely Carmichael once referred to Durant as "a place routinely to be avoided by black folk at high noon much less after dark.") But then a woman broke the ice with an angry outburst about her recent experience as a patient at the local hospital, and from that point on "people heatedly traded stories about the hospital and the local physicians." Blacks resented the segregated facilities in doctors' offices and in the hospital. They were particularly upset at the white physician (there were no black doctors in the county) who refused to treat patients who had outstanding bills.[32]

After a few meetings the newly formed Durant Health Association sent a delegation to confront the hospital administrator, demanding that the segregated wings be merged. He responded that the hospital had been arranged the way it was "so that everybody would be happiest." He told Mrs. Winters, who led the delegation, that "this civil rights talk has your head all confused." To which she retorted that the "civil rights talk" was here to stay and the next time they would bring an NAACP lawyer with them. Despite making no immediate progress, the members of the delegation found the confrontation empowering, and at the next meeting of the Health Association each member told her version of the story "to the mirth of all present." The group persisted and brought in a lawyer, but it would take two years before the hospital desegregated.[33]

Now a familiar and trusted member of the community, Mullan went to a neighboring town to talk about sex education to a group of teenagers. He arrived at the home of the young woman who invited him "equipped with a condom purchased at a local drug store and a half-used pack of birth-control pills borrowed from a civil rights worker," to find a "giggling group of girls" age eleven to twenty. As he broached the subject of birth control and began "passing my gadgets around the group," the father of his hostess pulled up a chair and began to listen. Immediately the mood changed. Mullan worried whether the man believed that he was encouraging the girls to be promiscuous—or teaching black genocide. The girls quickly drifted away, the meeting ended, and Mullan "taught no more sex education classes after that and my half-completed birth-control lecture still remains to be finished." Like Phyllis Cunningham before him, Mullan had learned that this topic, which touched the nerves of both religious fundamentalists and black power advocates, was dangerous territory, particularly if the teacher was white.[34]

As the summer wound down, Mullan joined a group of local activists in a door-to-door effort to persuade black parents to send their children to the previously all-white schools, and on registration day he stood with parents and civil rights workers at a barricade outside the school in a show of support. He also participated in Freedom Democratic Party voter registration drives, and took time off from medical school in the fall to fly to Washington to join a Holmes County delegation headed by Mrs. Winters, which met with five officials from the Department of Health, Education, and Welfare (HEW). Their accounts of the appalling state of health care in Mississippi laid the groundwork for a congressional hearing on discrimination in health and welfare programs in the South. Mullan returned to Holmes County during his Christmas vacation, renewed friendships, and was pleased to see that the Durant Health Association he founded was flourishing, with biweekly meetings drawing nearly thirty people. As a result of the fall conference with HEW officials, federal funds were withdrawn from two hospitals in the county, and an "abusive" welfare case worker was fired.[35]

The other volunteers had similar experiences that summer. Their lives had been changed by their work in Mississippi, and they returned to their medical schools radicalized, committed to developing a health care system that was both universal and color-blind. Soon they and others would form the Student Health Organizations, a national federation that worked with MCHR chapters while staking out their own independent course of action in communities across the country.

The federal government was becoming a stronger presence in Mississippi. The Organization of Economic Opportunity (OEO), the cornerstone of Lyndon Johnson's War on Poverty, created the Head Start program in the summer of 1965, providing poor children with preschool training, medical care, and two hot meals a day, as well as employment at decent wages for hundreds of local people who served as teachers and paraprofessionals. The OEO awarded its largest grant of nearly $1.5 million to the Child Development Group of Mississippi (CDGM). MCHR's Tom Levin worked with OEO program analyst Polly Greenberg, education specialist Jeannine Herron, and the Delta Ministry's Art Thomas to hammer out a proposal for the preschool program. During its initial seven-week run CDGM served nearly six thousand children in eighty-four centers in twenty-four counties.[36]

Medical services were an essential component of Head Start. Each child was to receive a physical examination, complete laboratory tests (including hearing and vision), and necessary immunizations. Most of these preschoolers had never seen a doctor. Levin's MCHR experiences in Mississippi the previous summer had taught him that local white physicians would be reluctant to participate in any Great Society program. Knowing that the few black physicians could not handle the additional work of examining thousands of children in a two-week period at the beginning of the program, he called on MCHR for help. In early April the executive committee agreed that MCHR should have a "consultative role" in CDGM, and a week later sent Levin a three-page protocol for the Head Start examinations. As the summer drew nearer and Levin asked for more specific kinds of assistance, opposition surfaced in the committee. At the June meeting, Ed Barsky and Marvin Belsky argued that because MCHR was basically a civil rights organization, its role in Head Start should be "strictly consultative." On July 2 Tom Levin and Bob Smith, who had signed on as CDGM's medical director, wrote to chair Mike Holloman requesting that MCHR send down two physicians to each of the five

CDGM districts. These ten doctors would supervise the work of health aides, analyze the recommendations for further treatment on the completed health forms, develop priorities for the treatment of medical problems, and "contribute to the future over-all health and educational aspects of the project."[37]

The letter produced a disappointing response. An angry Johnny Parham accused Levin of trying to "reroute" physicians planning to work with MCHR in Mississippi to the CDGM central office at Mount Beulah, and warned him to "avoid competition for personnel." Levin immediately apologized and offered to "pay MCHR medical personnel up to $150 a week to assist in the health program" (with the understanding that the stipend would be donated to the MCHR treasury).[38]

Jack Geiger was also put off by the way Levin was running CDGM's medical program. In a letter to the Delta Ministry's Warren McKenna in early May, Geiger expressed alarm over the possibility that CDGM would ask MCHR doctors to perform the Head Start physicals ("grossly illegal and in violation of state licensing laws") or to "train local people to do physical exams . . . which is the nuttiest idea of all." Part of the problem was personal. Levin later bluntly stated that "I fought with Jack a lot. I didn't like Jack." The two men embodied the conflicting factions in MCHR. Geiger's goal was to improve the health care of black Mississippians by working through the system, while Levin saw his primary role as that of political agitator. He envisioned the Child Development Group of Mississippi as an arm of the movement, and provided jobs for local civil rights workers in Head Start centers. With a curriculum that included civil rights history and reflected "the cultural heritage and values of the Negro population," CDGM set out to develop a generation of young blacks who would challenge Mississippi's white supremacist power structure. Geiger's fear that Levin would violate state law and medical ethics proved unfounded, but his distrust of Levin's operation resonated throughout MCHR's leadership. Whatever the reason, the Medical Committee missed an opportunity to play an important role in a program that would have a positive impact on black children in Mississippi.[39]

In the end, those local black doctors who had been most active in the Mississippi civil rights movement—Smith, Shirley, and Anderson—did most of the medical work for CDGM, assisted by black physicians in communities where CDGM was operating, and by a handful of white physicians like Jim Hendrick, who served as chair of the Jackson Medical Committee for Head Start, a role that did not endear him to the state's medical establishment. Although MCHR participation was minimal, one important exception was psychiatrist Josephine Martin, who, with her husband, economist Bob Schwartz, spent much of their summer in Mississippi working with CDGM.[40]

Josephine Diaz was the daughter of a Spanish cigar maker in Tampa. The family moved to New York, where she attended elementary and high school. Contracting tuberculosis as a teenager, she spent two years in a sanitarium, where she met and married Earl Martin, a fellow patient. After graduating from Hunter College and working at various medically related jobs, she entered medical school in her thirties, divorced Martin, and married an Englishman, Cedric Belfrage, one of the founders of the leftist *National Guardian*. Belfrage was deported for his political views, and "Jo" accompanied him to London (where she treated W. E. B. DuBois for a heart ailment). She returned to New York, entered a psychiatric residency at Bellevue Hospital, divorced Belfrage, and married Bob Schwartz, a Wall Street economist who shared her commitment to human rights. (She once observed that "all my husbands were wonderful men, each appropriate for his time.")[41]

Jo Martin's trip to Mississippi in 1965 initiated a lifelong commitment to the southern freedom struggle. She and Bob Schwartz toured a dozen Head Start centers and were impressed with what they saw. "As a result of the local participation, and especially with the active involvement of their parents, these children are not only experiencing the warm acceptance of the community, but are also seeing their parents in a new light of dignity and responsibility in planning their life." They were discussion leaders at a meeting of the Delta Ministry's Freedom Corps, and on their drive home they stopped in Atlanta to spend time at SNCC's headquarters. Here Martin discovered her major value to the movement, that of counselor to civil rights activists experiencing the trauma of battle fatigue. Jim Forman, who had more than his share of adversity, wrote that Martin "helped me to unravel many of the conflicting tendencies, to bring focus and greater clarity to this head." Jo and Bob met Unita Blackwell, who would become a force in Mississippi politics (and the recipient of a MacArthur Foundation Fellowship), beginning a lifelong friendship. "She was something we had never seen before," Blackwell remembers. "She was the doctor who was on the battleground." Blackwell and Forman are but two of dozens of movement activists, including Stokely Carmichael, whom Martin helped guide through dark periods. She personified what was best about the Medical Committee, although she was not one of its leaders.[42]

As for CDGM, the OEO cited it as a model program, "one of the best in the country," and praised its parent involvement. But once Mississippi politicians woke up to see an ongoing federally financed institution operating independently and committed to black empowerment, they took action to destroy CDGM. Senator John Stennis led the charge. His investigations revealed that CDGM had paid the fines of staff members arrested in the Jackson demonstrations in June. Other funds were unaccounted for, but in the end the OEO disallowed less than $5,000 of the $1.5 million grant. The price for CDGM's continued existence, however, was the head of its director, Tom Levin. His management style was freewheeling, and at times he came across as arrogant. But his vision for CDGM, both as a preschool program and as an agency for social change, was what made it unique in Head Start. Pressured by OEO officials, the CDGM board removed Levin even before the summer program ended. CDGM continued its operations for the next three years, but it had to fight against the state and against a rival Head Start agency, Mississippi Action for Progress (MAP), which was more acceptable to the white political establishment. In 1968 the OEO cut Head Start funding, including a 25 percent reduction in Mississippi, a move dictated both by increasing demands for supporting the war in Vietnam and by a conservative backlash in Congress against the poverty program. All Head Start agencies, including what was left of CDGM, protested these reductions, but to no avail.[43]

Tom Levin resumed his practice as a psychoanalyst in New York. He remained active in social justice issues, but he did not return to Mississippi, and he drifted away from MCHR, the organization he as much as any other individual brought into being. As MCHR was entering a critical phase, others would have to make the case that the Medical Committee needed to retain a strong presence in the Deep South.

CHAPTER 6

The Last March

In the fall of 1965 the Medical Committee's activity in the South once again centered around the Jackson office, where Poussaint supervised a growing team of public health nurses. In addition to Cunningham and Disparti, three African American nurses joined the staff. Poussaint met and recruited Patricia Weatherly in New York, where she had been head nurse at Memorial Hospital for three years. Mississippi native Helene Richardson had worked in the surgical unit of Homer G. Phillips Hospital in Chicago and for the past six months had been a staff nurse in the psychiatric division of the Veterans Administration Research Hospital. Both were thirty years old and came to Mississippi in mid-July, shortly after Poussaint assumed his responsibilities. They were assigned to Holmes County. Jeannette Badger, another New Yorker who had been a summer volunteer in Alabama, began working out of the Jackson office in November. The Delta Ministry paid their salaries. Two other nurses were no longer with the program. Linda Dugan, the MCHR nurse, resigned, and Ruth Steiner, an effective volunteer nurse, finished her six-month commitment in September.[1]

Jo Disparti was growing increasingly frustrated in Holmes County. The demise of COFO in the spring did nothing to end internal bickering in the local movement. Disputes involving power and turf continued unabated. From the beginning Disparti had resisted MCHR efforts to dictate policy in Holmes, first with the gift of the medical van and later in the offer to open a community health clinic in Mileston. "I wanted things to come from the grass roots," she declared. By the middle of the summer she knew it was time to move on. "Somewhere along the way the balance shifted from not being able to quit the 'struggle' to not being able to stay in it," she wrote to Johnny Parham. "When I can leave, I will." A month later she made it official. "Working for the Medical Committee for Human Rights has been a crazy, unique, valuable experience but now, after a year, I believe it is best for me, both personally and professionally, to leave Mississippi." In September she moved to Boston to help Jack Geiger and Count Gibson organize the nation's first comprehensive community health center, at Columbia Point.[2]

Phyllis Cunningham was also growing restless. She had spent the year organizing neighborhood health associations in and around Hattiesburg, with some success. Yet by the summer of 1965 one of her groups had dissolved "when two of the members were informed that they would no longer receive allotments from the Department of Welfare, and others feared similar retaliation if they continued to try to change the existing situation." Later she wrote that "as an organizer, I constantly met with the reluctance of the community people to become aggressive in attempting to have a voice in the decisions which affect the basic necessities of their very lives." Knowing that historically "Negroes have been intimidated and have suffered retaliation" for speaking out did not make her job any easier. Poussaint wanted her to work out of the Jackson office, which she did, joining Jeannette Badger in the fall. There she continued working with

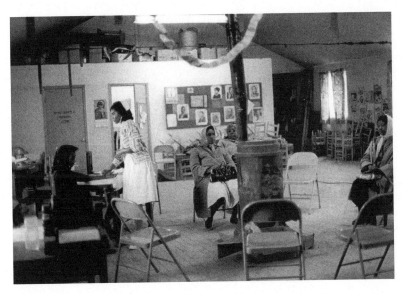

Nurse Helene Richardson at the Mileston clinic. (Charmian Redding)

community leaders in a number of counties. The two nurses also traveled across the state gathering evidence of racial discrimination in hospitals, all of which were in violation of Title VI of the Civil Rights Act of 1964.[3]

On November 10, the Dr. Irving W. Winik Health Clinic officially opened in Mileston. It had been over a year since Jack Geiger had secured funding from Luke and Ruth Wilson, who wanted to establish an appropriate memorial to Winik, a Washington, D.C., doctor who had been active in left-wing health organizations like the Physicians Forum. Before she left, Disparti had purchased equipment for the clinic and provided orientation for the new nurses, Weatherly and Richardson. They were welcomed by Holmes County blacks, in part because they were African American but also because they had not been caught up in the internal movement turf wars of the previous year. Members of the Mileston health association worked with them to paint, decorate, and add the rest of the equipment to the two-room clinic, part of the larger community center built by volunteers a year earlier.

The clinic involved local people in the decisions about its operation, including the payment of a three-dollar annual fee for participating families. Its purpose was to diagnose and screen women and children for health

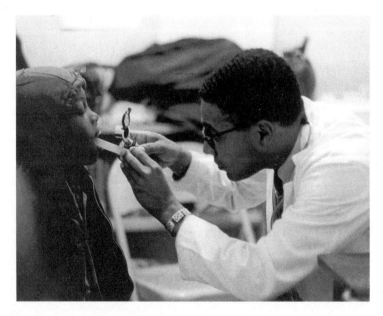

Dr. Alvin Poussaint examining a child with a sore throat at the Mileston clinic, 1966. (Charmian Redding)

problems. Throughout the week the nurses called on families to tell them about the new clinic and sign them up for examinations. Every Wednesday, Poussaint drove up from Jackson to perform physical examinations and do lab work for the patients, dispensing drugs and medicine where appropriate. More serious cases that required hospitalization or surgery were usually referred to University Hospital in Jackson, which was obligated by state law to treat indigent cases. At the end of each examination Poussaint talked with the patient in the consultation room as the nurses prepared the next patient. The nurses followed up with home visits, or met the clients at meetings of the health association. The clinic attracted the interest of local teenage girls, who assisted the nurses on "clinic day" by helping the patients fill out forms, taking weights and temperatures, and doing eye chart examinations. Seeing this interest, the nurses formed a Health Careers Club so that the young people might learn how they too might become health care professionals.[4]

The Mileston clinic was far from a solution to the health care problems of the poor. Weatherly and Richardson pointed out that for those demanding "quick and dramatic solutions to existing health problems, this type of work is likely to seem offensively trivial." And Geiger, who had come up with the idea, realized that while the Winik Clinic was "important, symbolic, and useful in making a difference," it could never be expanded "on a scale that would matter." But with their commitment to maximum community participation and involvement, their emphasis on preventive medicine as it related to the physical and social environment, and their operation within (while attempting to change) the existing structure of a society, these health care innovators learned it was possible "to reach people at the grass roots level, and to help them without destroying their self-reliance."[5]

The nurses in Holmes County carefully documented the segregation they observed in the local hospitals. As noted, in 1963 the U.S. Supreme Court had ruled against the "separate but equal" clause in the Hill-Burton Act, meaning that federal funds could no longer be used to build or maintain segregated hospital facilities. And Title VI of the Civil Rights Act of 1964 forbade discrimination in any activity receiving federal funds. After passage of Medicare and Medicaid legislation in 1965, southern hospital administrators began to squirm, for by continuing to discriminate they faced the possibility of losing millions of dollars of badly needed federal funds. Fortunately for them, however, the federal government appeared to be in no hurry to force compliance. Here the Medical Committee stepped in to play a major role in bringing about the desegregation of hospitals.

. From the time he took over as southern field director, Poussaint was determined to do something about institutionalized racism in the provision of health care. He joined the MCHR nurses (Cunningham and Badger crisscrossed the state visiting hospitals) and local black doctors in gathering information about discriminatory practices in Mississippi's hospitals and public health clinics. Poussaint designed a twenty-three-question form for MCHR workers and local people to use in their investigations. In some hospitals, such as King's Daughters in Yazoo City, the evidence was indisputable. Although built with Hill-Burton funds in 1953, King's Daughters had never admitted a black patient.[6]

More typical was the general pattern of segregation, discrimination, and humiliation found at Scott County Hospital in Morton. Although the county was nearly 50 percent African American, black patients in the county's general hospital had but three rooms with five beds and were housed on a separate floor; whites had eight rooms and thirty beds. If more than five blacks were admitted they were put on beds set up in the hall. Rooms for white patients had air conditioners and fans; rooms for blacks did not. The beds in the black section were hand-me-downs from the white ward. One bathroom served all black patients; every room on the white floor had a private bathroom. The "Negro rooms" had no bed lights, mirror lights, or night-lights. Black patients suffered further humiliations. The hospital provided them no wheelchairs, which meant that "a Negro patient who cannot walk and is leaving the hospital must be carried out by his people." Any black seeking emergency care had to wait until all whites received attention, even those who came in later. Fathers could not see their newborn babies because the ward was on the "white" floor, a common practice. St. Dominic's Hospital in Jackson, run by Catholic nuns, forbade blacks from trespassing onto the second floor, home of the maternity ward. In an act of kindness the sisters modified the policy in 1963 to allow black fathers to view their children, once, soon after birth. (St. Dominic's would be the first Jackson hospital to desegregate under the Title VI mandate.)[7]

Along with the NAACP Legal Defense Fund and the National Medical Association, MCHR filed hundreds of complaints against hospitals and public health clinics across the South, submitting them to the Department of Health, Education, and Welfare, the government agency then responsible for enforcing Title VI compliance. Throughout 1965 HEW took little note that few southern medical facilities had begun the process of desegregation. The columnists Rowland Evans and Robert Novak had written that "the ultimate racial weapon of Title 6 has been put in cold storage," concluding that "HEW no more wants to use the ultimate weapon of Title 6 than the State Department wants to use the hydrogen bomb." Reports from the field bore this out. Cunningham noted over the first five months of 1965 several Hattiesburg blacks had written to HEW to register complaints, but had "never received answers." Part of the problem was lack of staff. In January of 1965, HEW had fewer than twenty people responsible for Title VI compliance, and one man had sole responsibility for Title VI enforcement of health-related programs. Meanwhile, the government had to prepare to place nearly twenty million people under Medicare coverage, a process complicated by the AMA's opposition to the program. To push for the integration of all health care facilities, and to deny hospitals access to Medicare dollars if they refused, appeared to many in the government bureaucracy as an unachievable goal, particularly in light of the July 1, 1966, date when Medicare was to go into effect.[8]

Early in the fall of 1965, Poussaint met with HEW officials in Washington. While admitting "they were not following up complaints adequately," they begged off with the excuse that HEW "was *not* given additional staff to enforce compliance . . . and had no full-time investigators," which led Poussaint to conclude that "it appears that enforcement of Title VI has been left to the already overburdened staff of regional HEW offices." Behind the scenes, HEW officials were "confidentially seeking the assistance of MCHR members and chapters in filing complaints" and in publicizing them.[9]

All this came to a head on December 16 when MCHR chair (and president-elect of the NMA) Mike Holloman led a delegation, including representatives from the NAACP Legal Defense Fund, to meet with HEW head John Gardner. When Gardner failed to show up for the meeting and sent his assistant instead, Holloman was outraged, and the next day fired off a telegram to Gardner. "We note that you have met freely with conservative elements of the health profession. We wonder if your failure to meet with us has racial implications and may be symptomatic of the reluctance of your department to come to grips with the discriminatory practices in health care." He went on to say that the Medical Committee for Human Rights and the Legal Defense Fund planned to file complaints "against all hospitals which practice the least bit of discrimination." Holloman's message to Gardner was widely reported in the press. It proved effective, and in the days and weeks that followed HEW abruptly shifted its priorities, launching a massive investigative campaign to bring some nine thousand hospitals nationally into compliance with Title VI before the Medicare target date of July 1.[10]

Stung by criticism that HEW was indifferent to segregation in the institutions it supervised, Secretary Gardner took action. In response to a complaint Poussaint had sent to Robert Kennedy, Gardner assured the senator that HEW would "bring all of these institutions into compliance not only with the letter but the spirit of the law." Gardner noted that in December he created the Office for Civil Rights, headed by Peter Libassi, and had requested "full-time program staff" to carry out Title VI operations. The most demanding health care task, the investigation of hospitals, was now assigned to the Public Health Service, with a newly created Office of Equal Health Opportunity (OEHO), with Robert Nash, a former social worker from New Hampshire, in charge. HEW declined to go after the segregated private offices of physicians, claiming that because Medicare payments went directly to the patient, physicians' offices were not covered by the law. In truth, HEW had neither the staff nor the will to investigate nearly 150,000 doctors' offices, and as a result some white doctors in the South maintained segregated waiting rooms well into the 1970s.[11]

Nash had an overwhelming task, and early results were discouraging. By the end of the first week in May, only half of the 140 hospitals in Mississippi had responded. Of these, 65 replied that they did maintain segregated facilities, and only 5 had signed the compliance form. Other states showed similar patterns of evasion or defiance. Nearly 2,000 southern hospitals were not in compliance as of June 1. By then President Johnson had made it clear that he expected action from the federal bureaucracy, and that he would withhold federal money from hospitals that discriminated. In a speech on June 15 that singled out segregated facilities, Johnson warned hospital administrators that "the Federal Government is not going to retreat from its clear responsibility." The answer to the problem of discrimination is simple, he said. "It is for every citizen to obey the law." By that time Nash and the OEHO were blanketing the South with teams of investigators, who let local hospital authorities know that the federal government meant business.[12]

The OEHO assault on hospital segregation was, in the words of David Barton Smith, "something equivalent to a children's crusade that actually seemed to work." Secretary Gardner temporarily reassigned 750 people to OEHO from all areas of HEW. "There were bench scientists, veterinarians, local field managers from the Social Security Administration, Public Health Service nurses, pharmacists from the Food and Drug Administration, researchers from the National Institute of Health." Among the recruits was a young physician named Paul Plotz, who had come to the NIH after finishing his residency. While he did not consider himself "political," Plotz had led a successful protest against the NIH policy of automatically enrolling its researchers in the AMA, and had joined the Medical Committee after hearing Geiger speak at a meeting in Boston.[13]

Plotz was one of some two hundred investigators brought to Atlanta for an HEW-sponsored orientation session in mid-April. Both Poussaint and Cunningham attended the meeting as consultants. The plan was to send teams to check on those hospitals in the South (and some in the North) that had submitted forms stating they either were in compliance or were planning to comply with Title VI to become eligible for Medicare funds. MCHR documented examples of discrimination by more than two hundred hospitals, sixty-six of them in Mississippi, in the month of April alone. At Poussaint's suggestion, the investigators were asked to go into the black community the day before their visits to get firsthand accounts of the hospitals' practices. Poussaint feared, correctly as it turned out, that hospital administrators would resort to subterfuge to create the appearance of desegregated facilities, only to return to "normal" operations as soon as the investigators left town.[14]

In some larger cities black health care professionals and activists had been alerted to the visits, and were waiting for the investigators when they came to town. (Holloman was spending one day a week on the phone as an HEW consultant, calling black physicians he knew in southern cities to tell them about the oncoming investigations.) Plotz and his partner were assigned to visit small hospitals along the Mississippi Gulf Coast and several hospitals in Tennessee. Without contacts in the black communities, they designed their own system. After alerting the hospital administrator twenty-four hours in advance of their visit, they would "find the black part of town, stop in the middle of a big intersection, and roll down the window and tell someone who we were and say we wanted to find out about the hospital and what was going on." This direct approach worked. "Blacks were eager to talk." What they heard proved invaluable, particularly in the community where, upon learning of the visitation, the hospital had discharged all its black patients! Plotz and his partner talked to one of the black patients who had been kicked out. Then "we spent the next several hours learning the geography of the hospital and the names of the patients who had been discharged. We knew which wards had been closed. And when we went in the next day and got the official tour, we confronted them with what we knew."[15]

This kind of deception was common. At a large Catholic hospital in Nashville, the administrator, a nun, was assuring Plotz that the hospital did not discriminate at all, when her phone rang. It was the admissions office, asking where to put a patient. The administrator quickly replied, "Well, we have a white bed up on 5 West," and then sheepishly looked up at Plotz. On another hospital tour, after Plotz pointed out that the white ward had air conditioning while the black ward did not, his host cryptically replied, "*They* don't like cold air." HEW investigators in other cities found that hospital officials had taken down all the Jim Crow signs before the visitation, and in one case dressed a black janitor in pajamas and put him in a bed on an all-white floor.[16]

By mid-June, 360 HEW examiners were conducting nearly four hundred hospital visits a week. It was now clear to southern hospital officials that they would have to do more than simply sign a form to gain access to Medicare funds, and some used the visits to begin the process of compliance. Taking down signs, desegregating the lunchrooms, eliminating segregated entrances, and awarding hospital privileges to black doctors were all relatively easy steps. Integrating recovery rooms was quite a different matter. While the HEW guidelines did not require every room be integrated, they did say that rooms and wards should be assigned randomly. In her study of hospital integration in Greenville, Mississippi, historian Lynn Pohl found that "the primary dilemma with desegregation for whites centered not around doctors or nurses, but the patients' discomfort around other patients of a different racial background." A particular problem occurred with visitation, where "a white could be alone in a room with a group of blacks, in a position with no control or authority."[17]

Room integration was the sticking point for the many southern hospitals that had initially opted out of the Medicare program. As time passed and their financial situation deteriorated, many hospitals solved this problem—and received federal funding—by eliminating patient wards and converting multi-occupancy rooms to private rooms. New hospitals in the South built with Hill-Burton funds, like Hinds County General in Mississippi, had only private rooms. "The construction of hospitals with essentially all private rooms is not necessarily related to the problem of civil rights," concluded the surgeon general's office. It was, of course, *directly* related to the problem of civil rights. Conversion to private rooms meant fewer beds in many hospitals, and higher costs for patients. But most patients, black and white, preferred private rooms if given the choice. Black doctors by and large did not object to these changes, and MCHR and the other watchdogs did not make this an issue.[18]

The audacious decision to flood the South with hospital investigators in the early summer of 1966 caught segregationist opponents off guard, but by the fall several members of Congress—not all of them southerners—questioned both the pace and the scope of HEW's desegregation program and began a campaign to undermine the agency's work. Over the next year, efforts increased to reduce its authority to take strong action against segregated institutions receiving federal funds. A forced reorganization in the fall of 1967 led to resignations of key people like Robert Nash, and the demise of the Office of Equal Health Opportunity.[19]

The backlash against enforcement of Title VI (and against the civil rights movement in general in the fall of 1966) should not overshadow the work done by federal officials, volunteer examiners, and civil rights organizations like MCHR to ameliorate the effects of a century of segregation in southern hospitals. By the time the program began in July 1966, most hospitals were cleared for Medicare funds. Some, like Baptist in Jackson and Kings Daughters in Greenville, refused to desegregate for a few years, but by the early 1970s something of a revolution had taken place in southern hospitals, which were now the most integrated facilities in their communities. In contrast to the public schools, which whites abandoned for segregation academies, southern hospitals needed every federal dollar they could get, and in the long run defiance of the law was simply not a viable option.

The physicians and nurses of the Medical Committee for Human Rights deserve their share of the credit for this success. They uncovered horrible conditions facing black patients in "white" hospitals, supplied HEW with hard evidence of racial discrimination, and then worked with the agency in investigating hospital conditions to bring about compliance. Thirty years later Frank Weil, who in the late summer of 1966 had been put in charge of the hospital branch of OEHO, wrote to Alvin Poussaint, by then a distinguished Harvard professor. Weil noted that when he took over there were some five hundred complaints against hospitals on his desk, three hundred of which had been filed by MCHR under Poussaint's signature. The purpose of his letter, Weil said, was "to thank you very belatedly, but also very warmly, for giving OEHO a good start in the civil rights investigating business."[20]

While MCHR was assisting OEHO in desegregating hospitals, there remained the problem of getting senior citizens onto the Medicare rolls. Rural blacks in particular were hard to reach. Most had not heard of the program, had limited formal education, and were unsophisticated in dealing with government agencies. The Social Security office, in charge of enrollment, was dragging its feet. In Washington, Mary Holman created a one-page form to explain the Medicare program for hospital and physician care in language anyone could understand. At the end it said, "*To get both free Hospital Insurance and Doctor Insurance*: Write to Social Security Office, 'I want free Hospital Insurance and Doctor Insurance,' and your name and address." Holman sent the form to the MCHR's southern office, where staff members not only used it in their canvassing but also distributed copies to civil rights workers in five southern states. Holman later reported that the OEO had finally recognized the problem and had used her material as a model for the "low literacy leaflets" it began to distribute throughout the country.[21]

During the early months of 1966, while Poussaint and his staff were waging war against Jim Crow hospitals, the Medical Committee's national office was locked in an internal battle that threatened the very foundation of the organization. At its most basic, the fight was over money and power, and it pitted treasurer Al Moldovan against executive director Johnny Parham. But the divisiveness went much deeper.

When Evelyn Dupont signed on as the MCHR secretary and first full-time staff person in the summer of 1964 she found an office in chaos. "There was an atmosphere of hostility, secrecy, intrigue, and disruption. Every volunteer considered himself or herself an executive, undertaking responsibilities like opening mail and answering phone calls and handling committee business." Dupont soon quit her job, in part because she could not get along with Esther Smith. Smith had come to the office as a volunteer fund-raiser, and by fall she was working full-time as the director of special projects. Unofficially, she had become of the office manager, alienating Dupont in the process. Dynamic and dedicated, the forty-year-old Smith had been a union organizer and was active in the Women's Division of the American Jewish Congress. She got along well with Moldovan and the chair of the fund-raising committee, Ed Barsky. All three had long-standing Old Left connections and drew like-minded people to the office as volunteers. (Parham recalled that Moldovan "recruited a lot of women who came in as bookkeepers. Tom Levin referred to them as 'Al's Bolsheviks.' ")[22]

When Parham stepped into this scene in March of 1965 he found "a volunteer, crisis-based organization where everything was just flying all over the place. All we were doing was *reacting*." Nobody seemed to have defined roles, yet "everybody had developed their alliances." Although hired primarily to raise money and expand the chapter base, Parham grasped that MCHR needed "to put in place a framework, a structure, so we can say, 'Here is what the Medical Committee is all about.' " Over the next twelve months he tried to transform a voluntary organization formed in response to Freedom Summer into a more formally structured body resembling that of the Urban League, where he had come from. Parham failed to achieve his goal in part because of the MCHR's governing body's refusal to give him the authority he needed to hire his own staff and make needed operational changes.[23]

This growing factionalism in the national office directly impacted fundraising. Donations of nearly one hundred thousand dollars had poured in during and after Freedom Summer to assist the organization to carry out its stated program: to support the brave young activists risking their lives in Mississippi. That fall and winter Esther Smith attracted crowds to fundraising events featuring star attractions such as Sammy Davis Jr. and Dizzy Gillespie. The "annual dinner," which paid tribute to physicians Benjamin Spock and Paul Dudley White, and featured a dramatic reading by actress Ruby Dee, netted nearly twenty thousand dollars. (Celebrities like jazz musicians Gillespie and Miles Davis were recruited by their doctors and dentists in New York.) But the local chapters did not send much money to national, and individual physicians were not as a rule generous in their giving. Efforts to attract foundation support also came up short, so that by July of 1965, Moldovan could dramatically announce, "We are now bankrupt!" It was not quite that dismal, and MCHR limped along into the fall, but it was clear to Moldovan and his supporters that Parham was not a good fundraiser, a key part of his job description. Parham, on the other hand, had become alarmed over the shoddy manner in which the books were being kept.[24]

Al Moldovan, one of the hardest-working members of the Medical Committee, had volunteered to be the unpaid treasurer, a thankless job. He held that position for nearly two years. With no training in accounting, he relied on friends to come in and take care of the books and conduct the annual audit. As executive director, Parham was ultimately responsible for keeping track of the money, and when in the fall of 1965 he started asking questions about the upcoming annual report, Moldovan got defensive. To see that the Medical Committee's finances were handled in a haphazard manner did not require a degree in accounting. A "petty cash" budget operated as something of a slush fund, checks made out to cash had no receipts to substantiate them, and some employees' wages had not been reported to the IRS. As Parham pressed for more information, Moldovan became evasive. Parham then hired his own bookkeeper, who told key leaders that she was "appalled by the looseness of MCHR finances—in all the years I have worked as a bookkeeper I have never seen the likes of it."[25]

By early December the turmoil in the New York office had reached members of the executive council and the chairman, Mike Holloman. A social activist admired and respected throughout MCHR, Holloman had other pressing responsibilities and had remained on the sidelines as tensions and charges escalated. In a December 4 letter to Parham he admitted that "most of the criticism that has been leveled at me . . . during the past few weeks is entirely justified." To "assist more effectively in meeting the demands of the chairmanship," he asked Parham to supply him with copies of all correspondence coming into the office that "pertain to administration, policy, funding, and performance, including a monthly operational breakdown of the organizational expenses." Such information, Holloman added with remorse, would enable him to "be prepared to talk intelligently, as a good Chairman should."[26]

The charges and countercharges grew more heated in the new year. When Parham hired an accountant to conduct a separate audit of the MCHR books, Moldovan submitted his resignation as treasurer, agreeing to stay on temporarily until his successor was chosen. On February 4, Holloman sent a telegram to the governing council proclaiming that an "Emergency Situation Affecting Future of Medical Committee Human Rights Has Arisen," and summoning members to a meeting at his office two days hence. There Parham alleged "inconsistencies and improprieties in the finances of MCHR." Moldovan defended his bookkeeping. The council directed Moldovan to work with the finance committee to provide a full report to the MCHR governing body. It also appointed Walter Lear—who had not been a party to the infighting—to head a group to make recommendations concerning the future structure of the national MCHR office.[27]

But the damage had been done. Moldovan later recalled that "there was an inference that I was running away with money. I had to defend my reputation." On February 25, Esther Smith submitted a bitter letter of resignation, denouncing "the irresponsible charges made in an irresponsible manner. How was it possible for mature people—who knew of the selfless devotion of the National Treasurer of MCHR and myself . . . to condone unsubstantiated accusations?" That same day office secretary Hilda "Tuni" Berman also resigned, claiming that Parham had unfairly denied her a raise, and adding that "I feel very strongly that an injustice has been committed through the under evaluation of a primary department of MCHR—its fundraising department."[28]

It was only a matter of time—three weeks, to be exact—before Parham submitted his own resignation. In a letter stating that "my functioning as executive director has been greatly hindered, in part, due to an inability to perceive the role of professional staff," he reiterated his point that financial irregularities had "hindered my ability to propose a 1966 budget based on 1965 disbursements." Parham observed that raising these points at the emergency meeting had created "a greater degree of concern for the personalities that reacted to my having raised certain issues, rather than to the issues which should be of foremost concern." Parham's resignation left the national office in shambles, with no remaining professional staff or fundraisers, without a permanent treasurer, and with virtually no money in the coffers.[29]

Who was to blame? Did Al Moldovan and Esther Smith help themselves to the MCHR treasury? There is no evidence that they did, and no one ever made that charge directly. Moldovan had failed to employ sound accounting practices, but Des Callan was no doubt correct when he concluded that "the charges about how the books were kept were leveled more out of confusion and frustration than anything else." For Callan, the MCHR governing board deserved most of the blame because it "lacked structure." The executive committee (and its later successor, the governing council) failed to provide a clear sense of direction for MCHR and denied Parham the freedom he needed to develop his own staff and procedures. As a result the New York office remained a place where volunteers went their own way, and many of them resented Parham as a young outsider who was being paid too much ($15,600) to do his job.[30]

Race was also a problem in both the office and in the organization as a whole. Callan put it bluntly at the March meeting of the governing council. "This organization cannot accept Negro leadership." Expanding on this observation years later, Callan stated that "where black leadership [in MCHR] was compliant with what the majority of white leaders wanted, that was fine." But when Parham insisted on being his own man, he got into trouble. Parham did not see himself as a victim of racism per se, "but you really had a level of paternalism to the extent that you wanted to have some blacks around, but you didn't necessarily want them making too many moves without your absolute approval." Parham's lack of medical credentials also undercut his authority. "I did discover—and probably discovered too late—that you have a lot of egos among physicians." He found it comparable to the "preacher ego" that afflicted the civil rights movement, especially in the leadership of the Southern Christian Leadership Council.[31]

MCHR held its second annual national convention at the University of Chicago, a week after Parham resigned. Most delegates came to the meeting unaware of the infighting in New York or the Medical Committee's desperate financial situation. In a closed session the governing council attempted to resolve—or at least put the best face on—these contentious issues before the convention got under way. Moldovan's treasurer's report drew pointed questions from Jack Geiger concerning the bookkeeping involving his pet project in Mileston, and from David French, the incoming MCHR chairman. The council voted to send Moldovan's report to the membership, and assigned the finance committee to make a full investigation with recommendations.[32]

Next the board discussed the findings of the Special Administrative Review Committee headed by Walter Lear. Among other changes, the Lear committee recommended that the next executive director of the organization be a physician. There was some discussion of the report, but no action was taken. Given the current unresolved crises, no one was prepared to say, "This is how we must proceed."[33]

The convention itself was contentious. The Medical Committee had been founded as a civil rights organization to provide assistance to the black freedom struggle, but by the spring of 1966 most of the seventeen chapters had little contact with the southern program. To remind MCHR of its mission, Cunningham and other Mississippi staff members brought a number of poor blacks and civil rights activists like Annie Devine to the Chicago convention to provide the delegates with firsthand accounts of the medical and political problems facing blacks in the Deep South. She was surprised to find that the meeting's organizers, preoccupied with other business, were reluctant to give Mississippi a place on the program. "There was a real fight to let local people speak at the convention," she recalls. "We pushed and pushed to let them speak." Finally, convention planners agreed to put the Mississippians on the agenda, "but it was like cursory—'Yeah, let them speak, and then we'll entertain them.'" Cunningham also noted the irony that all this was going on at a convention where the featured speaker was Martin Luther King.[34]

The issue that split the convention apart, however, was a resolution from the floor demanding that the organization go on record in opposition to the Vietnam War. Since the summer of 1965, when President Johnson began the escalation of American involvement, the conflict in Southeast Asia had divided progressives. Most MCHR members opposed the war, but in the spring of 1966 a majority—including the leaders—did not want the Medical Committee to take a public position against a president who supported the civil rights movement and had initiated a war on poverty. For Moldovan and other fund-raisers, Vietnam was the kiss of death. The war was still "popular" among most Americans, even more so among the economic elite. "The ideology has nothing to do with it. It's strictly logistics," said Moldovan. "When I ask somebody for a thousand dollars to support the civil rights movement I can't also ask them to oppose the Vietnam War." Already strapped for funds, MCHR was courting disaster by taking on the war.[35]

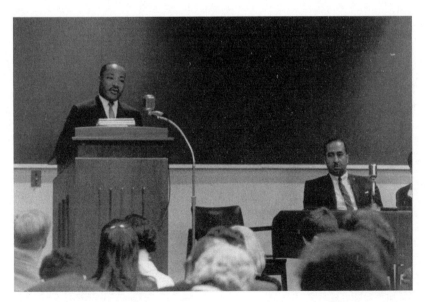

Martin Luther King Jr. addressing MCHR convention, Chicago, 1966. (Charmian Redding)

The antiwar resolution also drew fire from public health advocates, who regarded developing programs in the South and in the northern ghettos as MCHR's priority. They registered their opposition to the war in other organizations, but wanted to keep MCHR distanced from political controversies not directly related to health care. Paul Plotz believed that "it was destructive to take an organization that had a very focused mission, and simply because it was leaning in a certain direction to have it co-opted on some other issue. I didn't like that at all."

Black doctors were reluctant to oppose Lyndon Johnson, who in the past two years had pushed two milestone civil rights bills through Congress. Roy Wilkins and the national NAACP and Whitney Young and the Urban League were strong supporters of Johnson's foreign policy. Martin Luther King had not yet come out publicly against the war; only SNCC among the civil rights organizations had done so. David French, who would be the last black MCHR chair, believed that the black freedom struggle was what MCHR was all about, and he resented the "group of people who had an additional cause, which would supersede that mission. As far as I was concerned, the [Vietnam resolution] was a red herring and not in our best interest." Des Callan recalls that he was "totally convinced that if [MCHR] took a position at that point—before

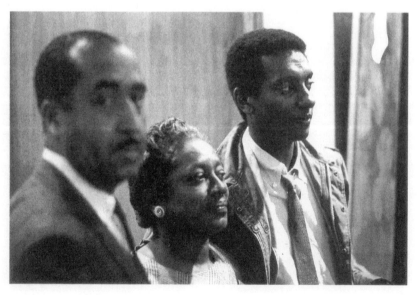

Mike Holloman (left), Annie Devine, and Stokely Carmichael at MCHR Convention, Chicago, 1966. (Charmian Redding)

King had taken a position—that the black doctors would resign en masse."[36]

Support for the antiwar resolution came mainly from younger physicians, nurses (such as Cunningham), and medical students, thereby splitting the Medical Committee along generational lines as well. For activists like June Finer, taking a position on the war was a moral question. "At that point it was overwhelmingly important to take a stand. We just couldn't continue to be just a medical civil rights group." In the end, the issue was too emotional to resolve on the convention floor. At its concluding session the governing council made the decision "that there be a mailing referendum to the membership concerning our Vietnam position"—the result to be announced at its meeting at the end of June. When those votes were tabulated, MCHR did go on record as opposing United States' policy in Vietnam, but it came with a price. After the debate in Chicago a number of the older members became inactive. They were no longer comfortable in the organization they had founded two years earlier to provide assistance to civil rights workers in the South.[37]

The Chicago convention resolved little. The southern program would continue, but without promises of additional funding its future was problematical. Many delegates left Chicago assuming that MCHR would now be centered in local chapters, with a national office acting mostly as a coordinating agency, but that decision too was put off to a later date. The New York office remained open, temporarily at least. Parham stayed on until June 1, replaced then by a short-term volunteer, Rosalie Ross.

When Parham returned from the Chicago convention a letter was waiting on his desk from Mary Holman, who "just wanted to remind you that you are a very smart, gifted fellow with a sterling professional record. You have done a lot of good, and suffered for the movement—which is an okay thing to suffer for." What Johnny Parham had not been able to do, Holman wickedly observed, was "to soothe the anxieties, fulfill the desire for status and power, and be both a papa and a puppet to a thousand physicians. Utter failure!"[38]

Al Poussaint returned from the Chicago meeting to his work in Jackson. Jeannette Badger was also there; Phyllis Cunningham had moved to Alabama to run the Selma office, assisted by Pat Weatherly. Helene Richardson remained to staff the clinic in Mileston. All the nurses and Poussaint were working on Title VI inspections as the deadline for Medicare compliance drew near. No one was prepared for the decision by the first African American graduate from Ole Miss to return to his state to stage a one-man March Against Fear.

At one forty-five P.M. on Sunday, June 4, 1966, James Meredith stood outside the Peabody Hotel in Memphis. Now thirty-two, Meredith had all but dropped out of sight since his graduation from Ole Miss three years earlier. He had toured Africa, moved to New York with his wife and son, and was now a student at Columbia Law School. Surrounded by a handful of supporters and journalists, Meredith stepped off toward U.S. Highway 51 to begin a 220-mile walk to Jackson "to challenge the all-pervasive and overriding fear" still prevalent among most black Mississippians and to convince them it was now safe to register and vote. Always a loner, Meredith had not discussed his plans with any national civil rights leaders, nor had he been in touch with movement people in Mississippi. He turned down Poussaint's offer to have MCHR provide medical presence, stating that if you have some doctors on the road then that implies it's not safe, thereby undercutting the central purpose of the march.[39]

On an uneventful first day Meredith walked twelve miles to within a few hundred yards of the Mississippi border and then returned by car to Memphis. On day two, just south of Hernando, a white man named Aubrey James Norvell stood up in the roadside brush, twice shouted out the name "James Meredith," raised his shotgun and fired three loads of buckshot. Horrified companions and reporters saw Meredith fall, struck by some sixty to seventy pellets in the head, neck, and body. About fifteen law officers who were "in the vicinity" quickly apprehended Norvell, an unemployed hardware contractor from Memphis, and rushed Meredith to a Memphis hospital.

Leaders of the national civil rights organizations gathered almost immediately at Meredith's bedside and won his endorsement to continue the march while he recuperated from his wounds (which, it turns out, were not all that serious). Martin Luther King and Floyd McKissick, the new head of CORE, were the first to arrive, followed by SNCC's Cleveland Sellers, Stanley Wise, and Stokely Carmichael. The three had left a SNCC project in Arkansas to drive to Memphis after they heard the news. Just a month earlier Carmichael had replaced John Lewis as chairman in a hotly contested election that signified a new direction in SNCC, one that stressed black consciousness and building independent institutions in the black community. At the meeting of the leaders in Memphis, a confrontational Carmichael had demanded that all whites be excluded from the march and that the Louisiana-based Deacons for Defense be invited to provide protection for the marchers. At that, both Roy Wilkins of the NAACP and Whitney Young of the National Urban League withdrew their organizations' support for the march and left town. Martin Luther King did not pull out, and he reached an understanding with Carmichael that both whites and the Deacons be included. King wanted the march to enlist support for Lyndon Johnson's new civil rights bill, which would make attacks on civil rights workers a federal crime. Carmichael, with support from McKissick, insisted instead that "the march serve as an indictment of President Johnson over the fact that existing laws were not being enforced." Despite their disagreements, King and Carmichael had arrived at an unspoken understanding. The press later exploited the two leaders' ideological differences, but without their cooperation and willingness to "agree to disagree" the march might never have made it to Jackson.[40]

When march organizers asked MCHR to provide medical presence, Poussaint and Badger drove up to Memphis for the planning meetings. The Medical Committee became one of six civil rights organizations endorsing the march. Meredith's original route led straight down Highway 51 to Jackson, but now the march leaders changed plans and veered off into the heart of the Delta, with its majority black population. Poussaint recalled that during the march he and the other volunteers "did our usual medical committee things. We did a lot of screening of people and put out notices that people who were ill or who had heart conditions should not march." They took steps to ensure a safe water supply and "even distributed stuff for the sun." Cunningham returned from Selma to the Jackson office, where she was in charge of securing additional medical supplies and arranging for their transportation to the march locations. Early on there were no outside MCHR volunteers.[41]

Bob Smith joined the march for a few days at the outset, and he served as Dr. King's personal physician. "I marched side by side with him down the road, with bushes and trees hanging all over, and I just knew Martin Luther King was going to be assassinated," he recalls. "We were about the same size and I just hoped that whenever it happened that they got the right person (laughs)." Smith—and local blacks—were inspired by King's presence. "There was really something charismatic about him, but nothing pompous. There were poor people in the Delta in these little towns, people who had been afraid to move, but as Martin Luther King moved through these little towns people walked off the plantations and joined the march." Smith remembers that many of them stayed with the march until it reached Jackson. "It was the most inspirational thing I have witnessed in my life: people walking off the plantation, joining the march, and not turning back. I don't know if some of these people ever got back home."[42]

The MCHR medical van accompanied the marchers. At night the staff treated those suffering from blisters, heat exhaustion, and other ailments. One day Poussaint got called to the rear of the march where a man "was short of breath. I sat him down in my car and saw that he was having some heart distress. And I pulled out my stethoscope and his lungs were just filled with fluid. Andy Young came up to the car and said, 'What's the matter?' And I said, 'He's going to die.' Which he did." Poussaint immediately informed King, who said that they would stop and hold a press conference. Poussaint was incredulous. "I said, 'What? A press conference? Why, they're going to attack *you* for letting this man march.'" King assembled the press along the road and "gave this blistering attack on the segregated health care system in Mississippi that had denied this

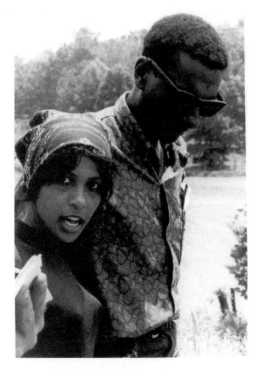

Nurse Jeannette Badger with Stokely Carmichael during the Meredith March, 1966. (Charmian Redding)

man adequate medical care. He was brilliant. The next day the headline was 'King attacks segregated health care.' "[43]

For the most part, the march moved peacefully through its first week. But as the demonstrators reached Greenwood, the center of much white repression of civil rights activity, the atmosphere became tense. The trouble began when police arrested Stokely Carmichael and two other SNCC workers as they defied a city order by putting up tents to house the marchers on the grounds of a black public school. They were hauled off to jail in handcuffs. The city backed down and allowed the marchers to spend the night on the school grounds. Six hours later an angry Carmichael, just out on bail, told an agitated crowd of six hundred—most of them local people—that "this is the 27th time I have been arrested—and I ain't going to jail no more." Then he shouted "We want black power!" The crowd cheered, and with each repetition grew more enthusiastic. "Now from now on when they ask you what you want, you know what to tell 'em. What do you want?" Stokely asked rhetorically, and the crowd roared back, time and again, "Black Power!" The nation would soon get the message.[44]

For most white Americans, the new slogan came as a shock. They quickly came to see Black Power as "racism in reverse," with violent implications. But veteran black activists knew that Carmichael's speech was no spontaneous outburst. SNCC had been moving in a nationalist direction since the 1964 Democratic National Convention in Atlantic City, burning its bridges with the white community, renouncing the philosophy of nonviolence, decreeing that integration was irrelevant. Malcolm X, not Martin Luther King, was the role model for these radicals, who were now imploring black Americans to turn their backs on white society and build up institutions in their own communities. During his Greenwood speech Carmichael had come close to a working definition of Black Power when he said that "we have to do what every group in this country did—we gotta take over the community where we outnumber people so we can have decent jobs." For black Mississippians this made sense. This had been a primary goal of their movement all along. Nonetheless, "Black Power" became the bogeyman for much of the media. Press coverage of the march turned negative, as attention focused on internal bickering and ideological differences, symbolized in the positions of Carmichael and King.[45]

While the main contingent of the march moved down through the Delta to Belzoni and through the hamlets of Midnight and Louise, about twenty marchers led by King then split off and drove across the state to Philadelphia to hold a service commemorating the second anniversary of

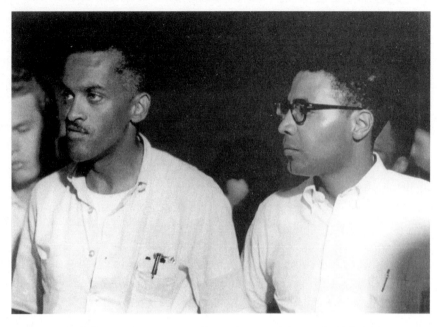

Owen Brooks (left) and Alvin Poussaint during the Meredith March, Philadelphia, Mississippi, 1966. (Charmian Redding)

the deaths of Chaney, Schwerner, and Goodman. About two hundred local people joined the Meredith marchers to walk from the Mount Nebo
Baptist Church to the county courthouse. Fearing that King might be attacked in Philadelphia, SCLC staff member Andrew Young had asked
Poussaint to keep close to King as he marched up to the courthouse. Prevented by the police from assembling on the courthouse lawn, the group
moved a block away to the county jail. Several hundred whites shouting
racial epithets surrounded the marchers. Owen Brooks of the Delta Ministry was "scared to death. We were just ringed with people who had all
types of armaments with them." "I just started trembling," recalled Poussaint. "I thought they were going to tear us up." After kneeling to pray, the
marchers began to work their way back to the relative safety of Philadelphia's black district but were attacked with clubs and bottles by a white
mob as local police and Justice Department officials and FBI agents looked
on. Poussaint later observed that "one of the things I felt that day with
King was the courage and bravery of that man. The fearlessness." As for
King, he later said that in Philadelphia that day he had "yielded to the real
possibility of death."[46]

That night Governor Johnson's highway patrol was out in force as the
main contingent of the march had closed to within twenty miles of their

destination in Jackson. About a thousand people greeted the marchers as they arrived at the Madison County Courthouse on the town square. As in Greenwood, the marchers planned to pitch their tents on the campus of a black public school. When Canton officials refused permission, a defiant Carmichael told the crowd that "they said we couldn't pitch tents on our own black school ground. We're going to do it now!" and he led a march from the courthouse to the school, about fifteen blocks away. There the crowd, now numbering about thirty-five hundred, was met by sixty-one state troopers lined up in full battle gear and carrying nightsticks, carbines, automatic shotguns, and pistols. Faced with this show of force, about a third of the people melted away into the twilight, but nearly twenty-five hundred remained to begin putting up the tents.

At eight forty P.M. a state trooper issued a warning. "You will not be allowed to erect the tents—if you do you will be removed." Two minutes later, after putting on their masks the troopers began firing tear gas across the field. The first volley scattered the crowd, but the police kept on firing and then waded in with their guns and billy clubs. Paul Good, a journalist on the scene, wrote that "they came stomping in behind the gas, gun-butting and kicking the men, women, and children. They were not arresting. They were punishing." Poussaint, who was at the scene, recalls the pandemonium. "You heard people being hit with rifle butts, you heard people being kicked with boots, young kids like two and three years old were running around, screaming that they were blind. People didn't know what was happening, whether they were being killed or gassed, so they were just screaming, rushing around. We went running out on the field because there were a lot of people lying on the ground unconscious." Poussaint found the driver of the medical van lying unconscious and a medical student writhing in pain from what turned out to be broken ribs and a punctured lung. He had been gun-butted by a police officer. Poussaint looked up to see Carmichael running across the field shouting, "You're killing my people!" and heading straight toward the line of state troopers. At that point, "four or five of us physically tackled Stokely and dragged him off the field and put him in a [beverage] cooler and told the workers not to let him out. He was totally out of control, and was going to get killed by the policemen."[47]

Aware that the small MCHR contingent was inadequate to the task at hand, Poussaint called Bob Smith in Jackson, who contacted Clarie Collins Harvey, the owner of a black mortuary and a political activist. Harvey sent her funeral hearses to Canton, where Smith and other local black physicians joined Poussaint in the field. "We set up a triage clinic," Poussaint remembers, "and we were seeing the people being brought into us, and some of them had bruises all over them and some of them had burns, and we decided which ones had to go to the hospital. We stayed up that whole night taking care of people."[48]

For Smith, the scene "was like a civil or national disaster . . . which of course it was." More people were gassed, kicked, and clubbed in Canton than at Selma bridge a year earlier, but the reaction in Washington and across the nation was now quite different. The next day Attorney General Nicholas Katzenbach merely said that he "regretted" the use of tear gas against the marchers "because it always makes the situation more difficult." He refused to condemn the police action because the whole matter was under investigation. Deputy White House press secretary Robert Fleming told reporters that Lyndon Johnson had "no specific reaction" to the gassing of the demonstrators, and the president refused to meet with a delegation of ministers who wanted a stronger federal response. The MCHR members scattered across the country may well have agreed with the ministers, but this time they did not jump on planes bound for Mississippi.[49]

Several factors account for the changing national mood. For the past two summers riots had erupted in many northern cities, actions universally condemned by the press and public. After passage of the two landmark civil rights laws, white Americans were asking, "What more did the Negroes want?" The war in Vietnam was now engaging tens of thousands of America troops in combat, and antiwar activity had become the priority for many white liberals. More immediately, Carmichael's cry for Black Power had already resonated, and the press was conveying a message that white people were uncomfortable if not unwelcome on this march.

As the demonstrators headed toward Jackson on the final leg of the march they proceeded down Highway 51 without further incident. Meredith, having recovered from his wounds, now led the marchers down to the friendly campus of Tougaloo College, just north of the capital city. That night nine thousand supporters, including Hollywood stars Sammy Davis Jr., Burt Lancaster, and Marlon Brando, attended a mass rally on the football field. The following morning the marchers pushed off into the city, and as they moved through black Jackson on the way to the state capitol hundreds of local people joined them.[50]

Bob Smith, Phyllis Cunningham, and Al Poussaint were "manning the medical outposts" along the march route. They had been the mainstays of the MCHR operation in Mississippi. Smith had been disturbed about the problems in the national office and the recent turmoil at the Chicago convention, but his focus was now on Mississippi. Active in the Freedom Democratic Party, he was also becoming increasingly vocal about racial discrimination in the delivery of health care. Cunningham's heart was still with SNCC. Black Power did not bother her. She was happy working in Selma, and hoped that the MCHR would make the commitment to keep that project open.[51]

Poussaint had undergone something of an ideological transformation since his arrival in Jackson, fresh from California, less than a year earlier. Cunningham remembers that at first Poussaint disapproved of her work with SNCC. "He thought I should be doing only Medical Committee things." Poussaint remembers Carmichael coming up to him in late 1965 and greeting him ironically with the exclamation "Here is the father of black nationalism!" But as he became more familiar with the depth of racism in the South and its impact on African Americans, Poussaint began to change. His high school friend Bob Moses, now no longer active in SNCC, had "become a guru for black consciousness. He was like a Pied Piper going through Mississippi." When he was in Jackson, Moses stayed at Poussaint's house, where he held meetings for movement workers. There "he was saying in his low-key way 'I bring you here because I think there is a new direction we have to go.'" At these sessions the problems between black and white movement workers, including white women activists, were discussed, which Poussaint documented in a paper that he presented two weeks before the march (and that, when published later in the year, would make his reputation). "The Stresses of the White Female Worker in the Civil Rights Movement in the South" graphically—some would say unfairly—analyzed the motivation of white women coming south to work in the movement. Here he coined the term "White African Queen Complex." His assertions hit home personally for two white women activists, Phyllis Cunningham and Jo Disparti, whose contributions had been essential to Poussaint's success in the Medical Committee's southern office.[52]

By the time the speeches got under way at the capitol late that Sunday afternoon in June, three weeks after James Meredith set out alone on his march against fear, about fifteen thousand people had assembled to hear Martin Luther King declare that the march and rally "will go down in history as the greatest demonstration for freedom ever held in the state of Mississippi." Representatives from all the sponsoring organizations spoke.

The overwhelmingly black audience cheered them all, including Poussaint, representing MCHR. "I'm a psychiatrist," he began, "and I am here to say that the civil rights movement is doing more for the mental health of the Negroes and of all Americans than any other force in this nation." He went on to comment on the brutality in Canton, "a vicious, sadistic attack by racists bent on preserving the unjust system of white supremacy." Warming to his subject, Poussaint observed that "for many years we have been singing 'We Shall Overcome,'" a song that "is almost obsolete and too passive. A new day is here," he thundered, "and we should begin to think, act, and feel that 'We Shall Overthrow!' We shall overthrow the vicious system of segregation, discrimination, and white supremacy!"[53]

From the standpoint of the Mississippi movement, the Meredith March was a success. Nearly four thousand blacks had been registered to vote, and an estimated ten thousand local people had marched at least part of the way. National attention had been concentrated on Mississippi for the first time since 1964, and the police brutality in Canton provided sobering evidence that white supremacy remained the central fact of life in the Deep South. But this was to be the last great march of the civil rights era. The country became polarized over Black Power, and many white liberals were no longer comfortable in this new movement environment.

This was certainly true for many in MCHR. Later in the summer, Rosalie Ross, the volunteer who was running the New York office, wrote to Cunningham that contributions were way down and that "there has been little interest shown by MCHR members since the Meredith March." The handful of medical volunteers had done good work in the South in the summer of 1966, but as members debated the organization's structure, program, and future, it became clear that the southern phase of the Medical Committee for Human Rights was nearing its end.[54]

CHAPTER 7

The War at Home

By the summer of 1966, the national MCHR was in shambles, the civil war in the New York office having all but destroyed the Medical Committee's ability to function as an organization. The southern program now generated little enthusiasm. The Meredith March and its demand for Black Power had alienated white liberals across the land, while the civil rights movement itself as a whole seemed cast adrift. Looming over all of this was the specter of Vietnam. With tens of thousands of American troops now on their way to Southeast Asia, antiwar protests erupted across the country. Younger activists in MCHR now viewed ending the war as their priority, and once the organization voted to take a stand in the spring of 1966, the Medical Committee never wavered in its opposition to the Johnson administration's Vietnam policy.

Despite the breakdown in New York, the southern staff carried on its summer program in 1966. Two dozen volunteers, most of them medical students and nurses, lived with black families and worked in local communities in Mississippi and Alabama. Their work included providing medical care for 150 displaced plantation workers living in prefabricated plastic houses in Greenville, Mississippi, and for inhabitants of another "tent city" in Alabama. Poussaint reported in mid-August that the health clinic in Mileston under the direction of Helene Richardson "is still going strong" and that MCHR was providing a medical presence for the SCLC-led demonstrations in Grenada, where white mobs had attacked marchers. Cunningham and Weatherly continued to work in Selma.[1]

In later years, MCHR veterans like Quentin Young and Walter Lear would maintain that the Medical Committee was "thrown out of the South"

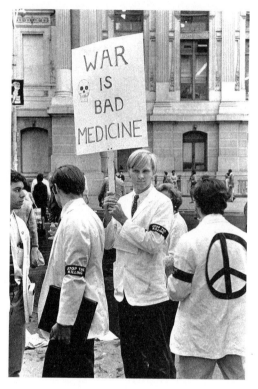

Antiwar protester, Philadelphia, Pennsylvania, 1970. (Bill Wingell)

by Black Power militants. That was hardly the case. Movement people still valued the work provided by the health care activists and wanted a continuing MCHR presence. As late as July of 1966, Poussaint was calling for more volunteers, expressing his disappointment that "the response to our appeal for volunteer medical workers in the South this summer has not been as good as we hoped it would be." The Medical Committee's internal problems and lack of financial resources, as well as a growing indifference among members to the black freedom struggle in the South, were in large part responsible for the decision to pull out. At its June 26 meeting in Chicago, the governing council voted to pay "all southern staff salaries through the end of August only," and that "no money from the general fund will be used in the South after September 1." Once again MCHR was broke, and it owed SCLC for its share of expenses incurred during the Meredith March. A fund-raising letter sent out after the march failed to garner support. Moreover, the National Council of Churches (NCC), a stalwart supporter of the civil rights movement, was now under fire from some of its more conservative denominations. The white backlash had set in among church people too. The NCC drastically reduced funding for the Delta Ministry, which in turn ended its direct subsidy to MCHR's southern operations.[2]

Phyllis Cunningham was determined to keep the Alabama office open. In early July she wrote to Cecile Boatwright, a volunteer in the New York office, that there was only seven dollars and eighteen cents left in the bank account. "Help! We need reimbursement funds . . . July rent is now due." She persevered, even after the September 1 cutoff of MCHR funds. "I would like to talk with someone before the governing council meeting in San Francisco," she wrote in mid-October. "I do hope someone becomes interested in the Southern Program at the meeting and will 'adopt' us." She tried to lobby her friends in the North to intervene. "Have you talked with Des yet?" she asked Pat Weatherly. "I haven't heard from anyone, not even Mary Holman. I really feel like we are all alone now."[3]

With the handwriting on the wall, the southern staff made other plans. Jeannette Badger had moved away during the first week of September. Helene Richardson got married and also left Mississippi that month. Alvin Poussaint took a job with the Tufts University Medical School. Only Phyllis Cunningham remained to shut down the Mississippi operation. "It was a bitch closing the Jackson office," she told a friend in early October. "It symbolized a whole lot—the closing. I am now back in Selma and the Jackson office is no more." The Mileston clinic, no longer funded, also shut down. But Bob Smith, Aaron Shirley, and James Anderson remained and, along with a handful of other physicians, continued the struggle to provide better health care for black Mississippians. At the same time, Jack Geiger and Count Gibson were organizing a community health center in Mound Bayou to complement their urban center now under way in the Columbia Point section of Boston.

All that remained of the MCHR presence in the South was the Selma operation, led by Cunningham and Weatherly, who were both working without pay. "We decided to continue our work regardless of the lack of financial support from the national organization," they wrote a potential donor. The two were joined in Selma by a volunteer nurse, Mary Ellen Garfes, who took a job at a local hospital to earn money for their rent and utilities. The nurses continued to cultivate the local health associations, organizing around health issues to persuade people to become politically involved.[4]

Here it should be duly noted that in the end it was the nurses who sacrificed and pleaded to keep MCHR's southern project alive. Since the fall of 1964 this dedicated group of health care activists had been responsible for most of the Medical Committee's success in the South. For Phyllis Cunningham this was a particularly difficult time. Not only had the Medical Committee pulled out of the South, but fundamental changes were occurring in the civil rights movement as well. Always first and foremost a SNCC person, Cunningham drove from Alabama to upstate New York in late November to attend an unforgettable SNCC meeting held at the estate of the black entertainer, Peg Leg Bates. There, after a heated debate that lasted nearly three days, by a narrow margin black SNCC members voted to exclude whites from the organization. Although Cunningham was comfortable with the concept of Black Power, her final SNCC meeting was traumatic, as black SNCC workers "kept coming over and saying, 'This doesn't mean you. You're the only nurse we have. You have a technical skill and we don't mean you.'" Finally, she'd had enough. "I said, 'I'm sorry, I'm white'—and I left." Lacking any financial (or spiritual) support from MCHR, she did not even bother to return to Selma to pick up her belongings. Cunningham enrolled in the graduate program in public health at the University of North Carolina, and then moved to New York. Weatherly and Garfes left Alabama early in 1967. Later in the year a grant from the New York Foundation temporarily revived the Selma project, under local control and without direct MCHR involvement.[5]

A week before the October 29 meeting of the governing council, David French, the new national chairman, wrote a letter to MCHR chapters that began, "We stand at the Crossroads. The MCHR exists in various stages of activity in 17 chapters throughout the land. The national organization has nevertheless ceased to be. It is essential that we make a firm decision about what the nature of our national structure shall be." A professor of surgery at Howard Medical School, and a commanding figure with a strong public presence, French wanted MCHR to retain its position as "a unified national liberal force in medicine" rather than become "a loose confederation of individual chapters, essentially autonomous, and with little or no national policy."[6]

More than forty MCHR activists came to San Francisco, including founding members Tom Levin, Mike Holloman, Des Callan, Jack Geiger, Count Gibson, and Leslie Falk. June Finer was there, along with young activists who had cut their teeth in the Student Health Organizations: Bill Bronston, Fitzhugh Mullan, Mick McGarvey, and Peter Schnall. That the

MCHR gathering coincided with the annual meeting of the American Public Health Association (the mainstream professional organization of choice for health care progressives) was no doubt a factor in generating the large turnout, but the delegates were responding to a sense of urgency. As the new vice chairman Quentin Young put it, melodramatically, "This meeting is the Valley Forge of our group."[7]

The conference began on a somber note. Callan, the new treasurer, announced that the national office had closed, a decision mandated "both by the lack of money and by the lack of activity to sustain the work of even one office worker," adding that "most furniture has been sold and supplies sold or given away." Only the organization's files remained, temporarily stored in a doctor's office. MCHR had outstanding debts of more than $11,000 and less than $2,500 in the bank. Although there were still seventeen chapters in major cities across the country, "the base of activity is in nine or ten chapters," and dues-paying members numbered fewer than five hundred. After French reported the closing of the Jackson office, the delegates voted to send letters of commendation to "Dr. Poussaint and the Selma nurses." A letter was read from Martin Luther King expressing his regret that MCHR had to curtail its activities in the South.[8]

The conversation then moved to the Medical Committee's program and structure. Earlier in the month council member Henry Kahn had written that the principal failure of MCHR, almost since its inception, was that "no one tackled the problems of formulating a concrete MCHR program that would keep the larger membership directly involved and move the concept of human rights in health beyond merely patronizing the civil rights movement. The idle national membership has quickly tired of supporting a token project far from home, and the Negro freedom movement has indicated it does not wish to be patronized. The prognosis for MCHR," Kahn concluded, "is grave." Simply stated, the problem was, "If you are no longer the medical arm of the civil rights movement, then what are you?"— a question that would haunt MCHR for the next decade.[9]

Delegates in San Francisco could not agree on a national program, but a consensus quickly developed that the focus of MCHR should shift from its national office to the local chapters, many of which were already addressing the health problems of poor people and minorities in their communities. The "Structure Committee" minced no words. "Should there be a national office? *Yes.* What for? *Scut and service—not policy.*" (The dictionary defines *scut work* as "a hospital term for unpleasant, especially trivial chores and paper work.") The job of the national office should be to maintain a roster of members and addresses, collect dues, and communicate with members through a newsletter. It would be housed in rent-free space and staffed by a half-time secretary and volunteers. MCHR, then, was to become an organization of autonomous chapters, "with national officers taking on only powers delegated by the chapters," and with the governing council meeting twice a year rather than quarterly. The annual budget would be well under $20,000, but even at this reduced level raising money would be difficult, for all the national fund-raisers had quit earlier in the year.[10]

The Medical Committee would continue to pressure the federal government to carry out health care reform measures, with the Washington chapter acting as liaison; demand more vigorous enforcement of Title VI regulations; and promote neighborhood health center programs, "particularly the new ones mandated by OEO legislation." Local chapters should exert pressure on medical and nursing schools to admit more minority students, particularly blacks. And the Medical Committee as a whole would actively recruit women and minority health care workers, especially those who were not M.D.s. To signify this new beginning, the governing council passed a resolution to change the name of the organization to the "Health Committee for Human Rights." (That did not happen. Members soon realized that a new name for the same organization would be confusing, and it would undermine the credibility that "MCHR" had built up over the first two years of its existence.)[11]

Delegates left the San Francisco meetings with mixed feelings. In many ways their organization had failed. It was in debt and without a fund-raising apparatus, both the national and southern offices had been shut down, and no common program remained to justify a strong national office. They knew that the organization's new commitment to do something about medical care back home in the North and to broaden the membership base would not sit well with many members. The delegates had, however, determined it was important that the Medical Committee survive, and they had taken steps to insure its short-term future, albeit in a very different environment. Soon it would experience a revival, attracting new and younger members, many of whom were drawn to the organization by its bold stand against the Vietnam War.

The Medical Committee's position on the war evolved in response to the increasing American presence in Southeast Asia. At its first convention in

April of 1965, Bill Bronston introduced a resolution that MCHR go on record in condemning the U.S. presence in Vietnam and the use of torture by the South Vietnamese army. Both measures were soundly defeated. There were fewer than thirty thousand American "advisers" in Vietnam. A year later a bitterly divided convention split over the war, resulting in the loss of members. Two months after that, President Lyndon Johnson approved a troop force of 431,000 to be reached by mid-1967. That escalation took a deadly toll, with the number of American casualties (killed, wounded, and missing) rising from 2,500 in 1965 to 33,000 by the end of 1966, and to a total of 80,000 by the end of 1967, including 13,500 killed in action. Vietnam suffered more. Between 1965 and 1967 American planes dropped more bombs there than it had during all of World War II. Napalm and toxic chemical defoliants such as Agent Orange destroyed millions of acres of land. By the beginning of 1968, American and South Vietnamese troops had killed 220,000 of the enemy. Some 415,000 Vietnamese civilians died during the ten years of American involvement in the war.[12]

At its May 1967 convention, the Medical Committee adopted a resolution opposing this "senseless and self-defeating" war, demanding that the government undertake "unilateral, immediate cessation of hostilities . . . negotiations with all belligerents [and make] arrangements for internationally supervised free elections" that would "recognize the right of the Vietnamese people to determine their own destiny." This strong statement went against public sentiment, for even as late as the spring of 1967 a majority of Americans favored staying the course in Vietnam. When Martin Luther King went public with his opposition to the war he was widely denounced, even within the civil rights community. King wrote to Quentin Young that he "was especially happy with the position taken by the Medical Committee on the peace issue. We must continue to raise our voices loudly and clearly to end this tragic war." MCHR joined with other medical groups that opposed the war—the Physicians Forum, Physicians for Social Responsibility, and Psychologists for Social Action—to form the Council of Health Organizations (COHO). Members also helped organize other professional antiwar organizations such as the New York Medical Committee to End the War in Vietnam.[13]

In addition to its public position, MCHR became more directly involved when it initiated a program to provide physical examinations for young men facing the draft. Participating doctors and psychiatrists were opposed to the war, believed that the draft was unfair, and knew that physicals for pre-inductees were often faulty. About 100,000 men were drafted annually between 1960 and 1964, but with the escalation of the war that number jumped to an average of 300,000 between 1965 and 1968. The Selective Service's examining physicians found it difficult to keep up. According to the comptroller general, between 1966 and 1970 more than 100,000 young men had to be discharged within one year after induction for preexisting medical and psychological problems that had gone undetected. While a physical exam by an MCHR doctor had no legal standing, the overworked military physicians could use the findings of private doctors in classifying draft-age men.[14]

For the activist physicians, what made matters worse was that the majority of those serving in the military—about 80 percent—were from poor or working-class families. And they were young. The average age of a combat soldier in the Vietnam War was nineteen, compared with twenty-seven in both World War II and Korea. Until mid-1968, students enrolled in college or graduate school programs received deferments. In 1969 a lottery was instituted, but even then those with good connections found ways, such as enlisting in the National Guard, to avoid combat. That year MCHR pointed out that "men whose parents can purchase exhaustive medical examinations for them may be found to have exempting conditions, while others less fortunate are denied this opportunity." Cooperating with local draft counselors, the Medical Committee initiated a national program to provide physical or psychiatric examinations to any young man "who believes he is ineligible for medical reasons but who lacks the means to obtain medical testimony to that effect."[15]

While sympathetic physicians had been performing pre-induction physicals for years, the Medical Committee's national campaign hit full stride at about the time that Selective Service ended deferments for most college students. The organization distributed copies of the "MCHR List of Medical Disabilities," a compilation of more than one hundred conditions and ailments that exempted draftees from the military. Volunteer doctors had instructions for composing a letter to the Selective Service. "It is probably best not to conclude that the registrant is unfit for military service, [but instead] to provide the physician at the pre-induction physical examination with the data necessary to make his judgment." The guidelines also encouraged solicitation of letters "from as many physicians as possible, preferably specialists," to bolster the case for deferment.[16]

Many military physicians received these letters with "contumely and hostility," a response that appeared to shock MCHR's Eli Messinger, who innocently proclaimed that "we're actually doing the military a favor by screening out those who have problems that would impair their ability to function in the army." Early in 1970, the General Accounting Office had suggested that private doctors be assigned to local draft boards to take care of the overload, but Selective Service director General Lewis B. Hershey rejected that advice, claiming that "an increasing number of 'resistance' physicians and psychiatrists [are] furnishing questionable medical statements to local boards." Hershey's charge had some merit. There were documented cases of fraud, such as the New York psychiatrist who wrote up to seventy-five letters a week to local boards (at $250 a pop!) certifying that her "patients" were medically unfit for military duties. MCHR directives made it clear that "our function is solely to discover or substantiate existing disabilities, describing them in detail." Still, there were cases that crossed the line, as when an MCHR dentist admitted, years later, that he had fitted a friend's son with braces to keep him out of the army. ("Any ailment that requires frequent treatment" was grounds for deferral.)[17]

Thousands of potential draftees took advantage of the services, most of them in major cities. In August of 1970, *Newsweek* reported that in New York and Boston "nearly two-thirds of the men taking pre-induction examinations are currently rejected, usually for medical or psychiatric reasons." Nationally the number of potential draftees excused for medical or psychiatric reasons had risen from 30 percent in 1968 to 46 percent in 1970. During that time deferments for college students had ended.[18]

Despite its ambitious program, MCHR failed to achieve its primary objective, "to combat present racial and class bias in the evaluation of draftees." Dr. Murray Abowitz, chair of the Los Angeles MCHR/PSR Draft Examining Panel, a group of more than one hundred physicians and other professionals, boasted in early 1970 that "Los Angeles leads the nation; no other community has such legal and medical aids for draftees so well organized and available to all, regardless of ability to pay." And yet, "despite our proud and glowing reports, doubts gnaw at our innards, increasingly." The problem in Los Angeles and in every other MCHR project was that "our services are sought mostly by white, middle-class and college youths . . . able to pay customary fees and very grateful for the service performed." The L.A. chapter had "made constant effort to make our work known to poor and minority youth," establishing contacts with draft counseling centers in the ghettos and the barrios and offering free physicals to anyone who needed one. When they made the offer, Abowitz recalled,

"We trembled with fear that we would be swamped, inundated, with demands for free service beyond our means to provide. Well, that has not happened at all."[19]

Two questions arise here. Why would affluent whites prefer to be examined by MCHR doctors rather than their own family physicians, and what factors kept black men from seeking this assistance? Many white youths, it seems, were reluctant to consult their family doctors—most were card-carrying members of the AMA and did not hold draft dodgers in high regard—unless their disability was so serious that any doctor would be comfortable signing off. The more liberal MCHR examiners, on the other hand, might be more sympathetic to listing personality disorders such as "antisocial behavior" or "repeated inability to adjust to peer groups" as justification for a 4-F exemption.[20]

On the surface it would appear that African Americans would be most likely to oppose the war and the draft. Their battles were being fought at home and, in the words of Muhammad Ali, "No Vietcong ever called me 'Nigger.'" Between 1961 and 1966, 12.6 percent of American soldiers in Vietnam were black, a figure that corresponded to the percentage of African Americans in the population as a whole. Yet in 1965 a record high 24 percent of U.S. combat deaths were black. Still, few black men sought out draft counselors or physicians. One MCHR doctor speculated that perhaps blacks were simply more patriotic than whites. Economic considerations were important. For many black young men, the military was the best job they could get. (Until 1966, blacks were three times as likely as whites to reenlist.) But by 1966 black leaders and organizations like SNCC and CORE had come out against the war, and in the late 1960s and early 1970s blacks became more reluctant to do military service. Their avoidance of draft counselors and free physicals is probably best explained by Elmer L. Sullivan, an Episcopalian priest who worked with conscientious objectors. "The whole Selective Service set-up is very cerebral, like a chess game," he wrote. "It's definitely a middle-class, educated person's game, and most poor people in the ghetto don't like to play games like that. It isn't their bag, this filling out of forms and personal appearances and appeals and whatnot." In 1968, at the peak of the draft, the medical disqualification rate for whites was one and a half times the rate for blacks.[21]

Eli Messinger, who along with his wife, Ruth, had organized a draft counseling service in the Bronx, told a *New York Times* reporter that "I'm concerned . . . that our services are being used by middle-class, sophisticated, better educated young men, but not by blacks, and in this way maybe unintentionally we're agents of social discrimination." A member of the Los Angeles panel of examining physicians questioned "the validity of our organization helping white middle-class kids avoid the draft when their places would be taken by poor and minority youngsters." The hard work, dedication, and successes of the hundreds of resistance doctors of course had no effect on the actual number of men called up in the draft. The bottom line was that for every middle-class white man in suburban Los Angeles they helped to avoid military service, a black man from Watts served in his stead.[22]

Antiwar medical activists involved with draft issues also had to contend with a problem closer to home, that of forced military service for physicians and nurses who opposed the war, a matter dramatically brought home by the case of Captain Howard Levy. Though not then an MCHR member, Levy fit the profile of the organization's founders. Born and raised in Brooklyn, from a Jewish and working-class family, Levy graduated from NYU and received his medical training and did his residency in New York. Although his early political views were "conventional, bordering on conservative," his experience working in the hospitals made him aware of the problems of racism and poverty. Under the Berry Plan, which permitted physicians to defer military service until they finished their residency, Levy was commissioned a reserve officer in the Army Medical Corps in 1962. By the time he entered active service in 1965 the twenty-eight-year-old physician was a staunch opponent of the Vietnam War.[23]

Levy was assigned to Fort Jackson in Columbia, South Carolina. A complicated man, he was difficult to fathom, and from the time he arrived at the base his behavior was unconventional, to say the least. Levy refused to join the Officers Club because he did not like golf, tennis, or officers, waved back at enlisted men when they saluted him, and lived off the base, where he devoted his spare time to working in an SCLC voter registration project in the black community. He was outspoken about the war and expressed his views freely to anyone, from officers and enlisted men to the patients at the dermatology clinic he ran. Already a marked man, Levy crossed the line when he refused to provide medical training to a contingent of the Green Berets called aidmen. Not medics in the conventional sense, they were members of a twelve-man "A-team" trained to conduct guerrilla warfare behind enemy lines. The aidmen took regular turns on combat patrols. Levy taught these men his specialty, but soon began to question his role. He concluded that he would teach dermatology to medics, whose job was to apply their skills on the battlefield wherever needed, under the supervision of military physicians. The aidmen, on the other hand, were taught to use their medical skills politically, to offer their services, for example, to civilian populations in return for information or loyalty. "It is medicine with strings," said one observer, "penicillin with bayonets." Levy put it bluntly. It was "Kill, kill! Cure, cure!" Gradually, Levy recalls, he began to realize the implications of what he was doing. "Finally, I just stopped."[24]

The army charged Levy with disobeying a lawful order and promoting "disloyalty and disaffection among the troops" through his antiwar proselytizing. His court-martial became a show trial, attracting media representatives from across the country at a time when opposition to the war was increasing. Levy's attorney was Charles "Chuck" Morgan of the American Civil Liberties Union. A Birmingham resident who became famous after a speech denouncing the white leadership of that city following the church bombing that killed four black girls in 1963, Morgan began his defense by citing the "Nuremberg precedent," connecting Levy's refusal to train Green Berets to the atrocities they allegedly committed in Vietnam.

Surprisingly, the presiding judge allowed Morgan to proceed along this line, stating that should he prove that the United States as a matter of policy had been committing war crimes in Vietnam, then Levy could be acquitted under the Nuremberg precedent. Morgan called three former Green Berets to testify, including Donald Duncan, a combat veteran whose writings had cataloged acts of brutality committed by allied troops. Duncan spoke of Americans standing by while South Vietnamese troops cut off the ears of slain Viet Cong guerrillas, and of orders to "get rid of" prisoners he captured while on patrol, meaning "to shoot 'em or stick a knife in 'em." His refusal drew a reprimand from his commander when he returned to the base. While these and other atrocity stories (including accounts of torturing POWs to get information) captured the headlines, the military commander in the trial concluded that the defense had not made its case. While Levy may have learned secondhand of "needless brutality in the struggle in Vietnam," there was no evidence to invalidate the order to train aidmen "on the grounds that these men would have become engaged in war crimes or in some way prostitute their medical training by employing it in crimes against humanity."[25]

Denied the Nuremberg defense, Levy brought in prominent physicians to testify on his behalf, including MCHR members Victor Sidel and Benjamin Spock, the popular pediatrician who had already achieved notoriety for his militant antiwar position. These witnesses argued that as a physician Levy's primary responsibility was "to his own interpretation of the ethical codes that govern medicine." They too would have strong reservations about training special forces troops, given that purely medical decisions were subject to political and military judgments. "Anything that makes medicine backslide into an agent of any ideology is bad for medicine," concluded one of the witnesses. Several other drafted physicians from the Fort Jackson hospital supported Levy, including Captain Ivan Mauer, Levy's replacement as chief of the dermatology clinic at the base. Mauer also said that he would refuse an order to train Green Beret aidmen. (The job eventually went to a civilian physician.) Such support from his base colleagues raised the question as to why Levy was being singled out for a court-martial, which could result in jail time, rather than a reprimand or reassignment.

One observer noted that "the trial brought into the open an undercurrent of anti-Semitism." Taking pains not to create another Dreyfus case, the army assigned a Jewish lawyer to prosecute Levy. Nonetheless, a South Carolina newspaper charged that a New York group endorsing Levy was dominated by Jews, and Levy's defense team received anti-Semitic mail. (His unsuccessful appeal argued that had he not been Jewish and involved in civil rights work off the base he never would have been charged.) The military tribunal found Howard Levy guilty and sentenced him to three years at hard labor. He was handcuffed and led away to the military stockade at Fort Jackson, then transferred to the federal penitentiary at Leavenworth to serve two years before his release on probation.[26]

The Levy case became a cause célèbre in the antiwar movement, especially among health care professionals. MCHR members accompanied Dr. Spock on a well-publicized visit to Captain Levy in the Fort Jackson stockade. The organization joined with the New York Medical Committee to End the War in Vietnam to form the National Committee for Howard Levy, M.D., and circulated a petition that concluded, "We as fellow members of the health professions applaud Captain Howard Levy's actions as being in the highest tradition of medical ethics." The Medical Committee also addressed the larger ethical issues raised by Levy with a call to end the military draft of health professionals and instead create "an independent Government financed Health Corps [to address] the needs of military personnel and their dependents." Administered by a committee of health professionals, it would be a voluntary service. Not surprisingly, the government did not respond to this suggestion with enthusiasm.[27]

Following his release from prison Levy continued to agitate against the war, now as a member of MCHR. He won the organization's support for a Medical Education Project at Fort Sam Houston in Texas, home of the Brooke Army Medical Center, the basic training site for all physicians inducted into the military. There five thousand enlisted men—including members of the Green Berets—trained to become field corpsmen or other health-related specialists. Antiwar coffeehouses had sprung up near military bases across the country, and Levy wanted to extend this concept by targeting medical personnel.[28]

The project got under way in the summer of 1971, led by Henry Kahn, a young New York internist and Harvard Medical School graduate. With him were Gordon Livingston, a psychiatry resident at Johns Hopkins Hospital in Baltimore, and a former navy nurse, Susan Schnall. A graduate of the U.S. Military Academy, Livingston had been sent to Vietnam in 1968 as a major in the medical corps. His "qualified support" for the war soon gave way to disillusionment. When he began to speak out against the war he was relieved of duty, sent back to the United States as "an embarrassment to the command," and then dismissed from the army.[29]

The daughter of a marine killed during the invasion of Guam during World War II, Schnall grew up with personal knowledge of the human suffering caused by war. An early antiwar activist, she enrolled at Stanford University and accepted a nursing scholarship provided by the U.S. Navy. She chose this career because she wanted to care for the troops who had been wounded in Vietnam. When questioned about her political views, she told her superiors, "I'm antiwar, and I'll take care of anyone who needs my services." Upon graduation in 1967, she received her commission and was stationed at Oak Knoll Naval Hospital. Schnall began going to MCHR meetings in San Francisco at the home of Philip Shapiro, a psychiatrist and a leading Medical Committee activist. When she learned in October of 1968 that two air force men were planning an antiwar demonstration, she decided to publicize the event on military bases in the Bay Area. Angered when her signs were ripped off bulletin boards at the Oak Knoll base, Schnall rented a two-engine Piper Cub and found a pilot. She and her husband, Peter, filled the plane with leaflets and then released them over two bases and the aircraft carrier USS *Ranger*. The press was waiting when they landed. Later she spoke at the demonstration while

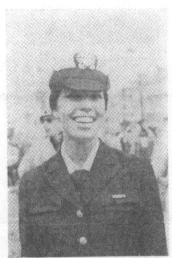

Navy Nurse Lt. (j.g.) Susan Schnall

Everybody's Sweeheart -- 20,000 times

She loves everybody and everybody loves her. Navy Nurse Lt. (j.g.) Susan Schnall, assigned to the Oaknol Naval Hospital, could also be termed "Miss Peace Bomb of 1968." She led her bombing crew on a mission of mercy, Thursday, October 10. The crew of four included Vietnam vet Jim Rondo, medical student Bill Gray, and Lt. Schnall's husband, Peter, also a medical student.

Mission targets were the aircraft carrier USS Ranger, Oaknol Naval Hospital, Treasure Island Naval Base, Presidio Army Hq., and Yerba Buena Island.

The mission was: hit the target with 20,000 leaflets telling about the October 12 GI march and explaining to all service personnel their rights should they choose to participate in the march. As Lt. Schnall put it, "We wanted them to know they had a right to participate and no one could stop them."

The leaflets were right on target. Lt. Schnall summed it up simply by saying, "The Leaflets opened up and it was beautiful." The men could be seen scrambling for them.

It was a success in more ways than one. West Coast newsmen rushed to Palo Alto airport for a post-flight press conference with Lt. Schnall and her crew. The story received wide coverage.

Navy nurse LTJG Susan Schnall, 1968. (Susan Schnall donation)

wearing her navy uniform. (She reasoned that "if [General] Westmoreland can wear his uniform while testifying before Congress in favor of the war, then I can wear my uniform while demonstrating against it.") For this act of insubordination she was court-martialed and found guilty of "conduct unbecoming an officer and a gentlewoman." No doubt because her "conduct" had gained widespread publicity—Schnall was interviewed on Walter Cronkite's network news program—she did not have to serve jail time. As a civilian she began organizing in San Francisco and started a coffeehouse for GIs in Berkeley before moving to New York to continue her antiwar activity with the U.S. Servicemen's Fund. Invited to Texas, she agreed to come for a short while to talk with nurses about the ethical problems facing medical workers in the military.[30]

Kahn rented an apartment just outside Fort Sam Houston, and he and Schnall prepared a leaflet to distribute at the base. When Schnall was caught and banned from the base, MCHR activists called a press conference to publicize the incident, and then initiated biweekly meetings featuring antiwar films and discussions. Nearly two hundred people showed up at a downtown coffeehouse on a rainy night to hear Schnall and Livingston talk about their military experiences. Levy also contacted activist Jane Fonda about staging "an anti-war alternative to Bob Hope's traditional pro-war entertainment." They called it FTA (Free the Army, in polite company), and with fellow actor Donald Sutherland, Fonda took the show to cities near large military bases. They performed in San Antonio before a crowd of three thousand GIs. The FTA show led to increased interest in the MCHR program, and attendance at the biweekly film showings and discussions doubled to around sixty participants. Kahn helped a group of enlisted men put out *Your Military Left*, a "good quality GI underground paper." Six physicians undergoing military training filed for conscientious objector status, and wrote a letter to the new student officers (all eight hundred of them) explaining their actions. The army did not stand idly by while this small group of agitators tried to undermine the nation's mission in Southeast Asia. The base became off-limits to all MCHR civilians, and the medical servicemen and women being trained there were warned to steer clear of these agitators.[31]

By the middle of August, Kahn, Schnall, and Livingston had left Texas; their job had been to get the project up and running. Before he departed, Kahn requested funds from the MCHR to rent a storefront meeting center near the base, employ two full-time staff members to continue the education campaign, and organize an MCHR chapter on the base. "Support of the Military Education Project is essential because of American militarism itself and because it's the most efficient, productive way to introduce MCHR and its ideas to a new generation of young health workers," Kahn argued. Shortly thereafter he reported that "despite a support resolution several months ago, MCHR hasn't responded in an organized way to this urgent organizational need." His plea had gone unanswered. The MCHR treasury once again was bare, and by then the campaign for a national health insurance program had become the national office's priority.[32]

The Medical Committee also supported one of its officers who engaged in an audacious act of civil disobedience. On the night of November 1, 1969, eight people broke into the Selective Service headquarters in Indianapolis and ransacked the office, destroying draft board records and scattering thousands of documents around the headquarters. Calling themselves the "Beaver 55" (a name they never explained) they left the following message: "We are not criminals ashamed of our action. We are sure the destruction of draft records has some of the qualities inherent in the actions of our founding fathers. We trust that the American people will vindicate us." Six days later five members of the group broke into the Dow Chemical Research Center in Midland, Michigan, and demagne-

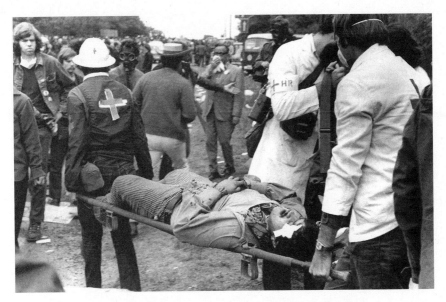

Casualty, antiwar demonstration at Fort Dix, New Jersey, 1970. (Bill Wingell)

tized computer tapes containing research and marketing information about Dow products such as napalm, nerve gas, and defoliants that later would be known as Agent Orange. Once again they were not caught, but on November 22 they held a press conference in Midland where they justified their actions. "We have done this because we will no longer tolerate this madness. We will no longer tolerate any form of conscription to kill." All eight were promptly arrested.[33]

Three of the Beaver 55 members were teenagers who belonged to the Young Christian Students. Another three were in their early twenties. Tom Trost, thirty-seven, was an ex-army sergeant who had been a national organizer for the Young Christian Worker Movement. The oldest member, and one of three women in the group, was Jane Kennedy, forty-three, a registered nurse with degrees from the University of Pennsylvania. At the time of her arrest she was the assistant director of Nursing Research and Studies at the University of Chicago hospitals. Kennedy was also a national officer of the Medical Committee for Human Rights and a member of the Chicago chapter's executive board.[34]

A federal jury in Indianapolis found all eight members guilty of destroying draft records. On June 19, 1970, Kennedy and the four men who entered the Midland Dow offices pleaded guilty to breaking and entering

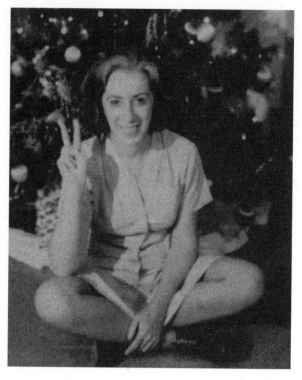

Jane Kennedy in prison, Christmas, 1970. (Institute of Social Medicine and Community Health)

and malicious mischief and received sentences numbering one to four years in prison. (The three teenagers were not involved in the Dow operation and did not serve time in jail.) The four men were immediately imprisoned in Detroit. Kennedy was sent back to Indianapolis to await sentencing.[35]

White, middle-class, and a devout Catholic, Kennedy was shocked by the appalling conditions in the women's prison of the Marion County jail. She wrote a letter describing what she saw and experienced and smuggled it out through a visiting friend. As a health care professional Kennedy was concerned that there were no drug detoxification, venereal disease, or rehabilitation programs at the jail. A doctor was available only once a week, and inmates with serious medical problems were routinely denied hospital care. Kennedy observed several prisoners dragged away to the "hole," solitary confinement. She suspected they were being punished for homosexual behavior, for the next day the jail superintendent "scathingly denounced 'sodomy' and pledged 'burning' and prosecution" for anyone caught having sex. A few days later all inmates were placed "on restriction," meaning they were denied contact with the outside world, including family members and attorneys. After twenty-four days, Kennedy was transferred back to the Detroit House of Correction. For her, "the last seven days I spent in the Indianapolis Jail were the most terror-filled of my entire life."[36]

A year later at a parole hearing Kennedy was asked if she regretted her crime or might "do it again." Any hopes for parole were dashed two days later when the *National Catholic Reporter* published the long letter she had written in the Indianapolis jail. From then on her treatment in the prison got worse (which she again recorded in a letter published in MCHR's *Health Rights News*). In early December Warden W. H. Bannon placed her in solitary confinement for a week. He refused to give her a reason, but he later told a reporter that Kennedy was "always involved in some mischief here . . . Every time she's told something to do, she always has to ask why. She's like a lot of those people who want peace and think they can tear up other people's property. I've been in prison work more than 40 years and I have never seen anything like her." In January the parole board again "decided to continue the case" of Jane Kennedy because of the "high probability of her further involvement in behavior which would constitute a violation of the law." By now all of the other members of the Beaver 55 were free. When the board told Kennedy it would not consider her case for another eighteen months, she became despondent. "I feel like someone who has lost his bearings," she wrote. "For now, for the first time, I think I may never leave prison." On April 18 Kennedy informed the parole board that "I can say now that I cannot see any value to be gained in performing any act which would menace society or the public safety." This general statement was enough for the board, which granted her parole on July 23, 1971.[37]

Throughout Kennedy's long ordeal she received support from the MCHR national office and especially from her friends in the Chicago chapter. A defense committee raised funds, and MCHR kept its members informed of all developments. The national office started a letter-writing campaign that targeted the Indiana and Illinois senators, her cause was favorably reported in the Chicago press, and an MCHR delegation met with the parole board chairman in the spring of 1971. Still, this was not a cause the membership as a whole embraced. An earlier attack on the Selective Service offices by Daniel and Philip Berrigan overshadowed the action by Kennedy and her allies. As one Chicago MCHR member noted, "A lot of us in MCHR are the first people to rush off and defend other political prisoners and issues. The Beaver 55 case and imprisonment has been brushed off rather lightly at the last few national meetings." MCHR members regarded Kennedy as a martyr and a hero, and they wanted to end the war. But as health care professionals most of them preferred to act within the mainstream of the antiwar movement.[38]

The Medical Committee had been interested in Dow Chemical ever since it received a gift of five shares of stock in March of 1968. As a stockholder, MCHR pressed the company to add the following proposal to be sent to shareholders in the proxy statement announcing the agenda for the 1969 meeting: "Resolved, that the shareholders of the Dow Chemical Company request . . . that napalm not be sold to any buyer unless that buyer gives reasonable assurance that the substance will not be used on or against human beings." Dow refused to send out the proposal, arguing that the production of napalm is "an ordinary business operation" and thus not a subject for discussion at the meeting, an argument supported by the Securities and Exchange Commission. Physicians and medical students from the Detroit chapter picketed at the annual meeting, and MCHR lawyers (at considerable expense) took the case to the U.S. Court of Appeals, which ruled that the napalm proposal was a "proper subject" for inclusion in the proxy proposals. When the MCHR resolution finally did make its way to the Dow shareholders it was of course overwhelmingly defeated. The action against Dow was an example of a tendency within MCHR to become involved in high-profile operations that attracted publicity, and that diverted scarce resources away from low-key projects, like organizing military health care personnel at Fort Sam Houston.[39]

Beginning in 1965 the Medical Committee discussed the feasibility of sending medical supplies to the National Liberation Front (Viet Cong) and to North Vietnam. *Health Rights* published an article, "Medical Aid for Vietnam" in its spring 1966 issue, which drew angry letters from a number of readers. Two years later, with members firmly on record opposing the war, MCHR sent a delegation headed by national vice-chair Paul Lowinger to meet with North Vietnamese officials in Paris. There the group pledged "medical reparations" for the civilian victims of U.S. bombing attacks in Vietnam. Over the next three years, MCHR supported a variety of efforts to supply North Vietnam with medicine and medical texts. In 1972 a delegation headed by Quentin Young and Mike Holloman left for North Vietnam to deliver medical supplies in person. They got as far as Laos before North Vietnamese officials turned them back, stating that their safety could not be assured because of the U.S. saturation bombing campaign in the North.[40]

After initial misgivings, the Medical Committee for Human Rights had participated enthusiastically in the antiwar movement, providing physicals and counseling for draftees, supporting Howard Levy and Jane Kennedy, organizing health care people inside the military, and ultimately reaching out to the "enemy" in Vietnam with symbolic shipments of medical supplies. Opposition to the war had become a primary organizational concern, as younger political activists replaced the old guard health care reformers in the MCHR leadership. It was during this period in the late 1960s that MCHR reinvented itself as an organization of the New Left, jumping in to assist antiwar protesters, the Black Panthers, and rebellious students. They also agreed to provide medical presence for Martin Luther King during his last campaign.

CHAPTER 8

The Medical Arm of the New Left

"Medical presence" remained an important part of MCHR's program long after it had left the South. Critics inside the Medical Committee argued that linking up with "whatever movement was most current or fashionable at the time" resulted in ego-tripping and kept the organization from developing its own ideology and program. But as requests for help kept coming, during the late 1960s and early 1970s individual chapters assisted groups engaged in a range of political protests from coast to coast. One such case was the Medical Committee's involvement with the Poor People's Campaign.[1]

In the months following the Meredith March, Martin Luther King found himself increasingly at odds with the Johnson administration. In addition to the war in Vietnam, King was disturbed over the president's apparent abandonment of the War on Poverty. A country that could provide jobs for the unemployed through the Works Progress Administration during the Great Depression, he argued, "can certainly do it now when we are sick with wealth." King told his staff that "we can't solve our problems now until there is a radical redistribution of economic and political power . . . We are engaged in [a] class struggle . . . dealing with the problem of the gulf between the haves and the have nots." His bold criticisms had made him persona non grata at the White House. Ridiculed by black power advocates for his refusal to abandon nonviolence as a philosophy, and criticized by moderate civil rights leaders for linking the antiwar and civil rights movements, he seemed almost desperate when in late 1967 he announced his plans for the Poor People's Campaign.[2]

King foresaw a multiracial army of the dispossessed descending on

Washington, taking up residence in a shantytown, and demanding programs to aid the poor, including a massive federal effort in the inner cities, a guaranteed annual income, jobs, and improved health care. The civil rights leader envisioned "a thousand people in need of health and medical care sitting in around Bethesda Naval Hospital so that nobody could get in or out until they got treated. It would dramatize the fact there are thousands of people in our nation in need of medical services." The threat of massive disruptions in the nation's capital did not sit well with most Americans, who had had their fill of civic unrest; nor did it initially garner much support among Southern Christian Leadership Conference staff members, who feared that a defeat here would have devastating consequences for the civil rights movement—and for SCLC. King was adamant, and his organization moved ahead with plans for poor people's caravans to converge on Washington in April.[3]

When King sent out the call for "doctors and nurses . . . to be helpful in whatever way you can," MCHR agreed "to provide first-aid care and comprehensive medical coverage for the entire population of the tent city for the duration of the march." The bulk of this support would come from the Medical Committee's Washington chapter. Mary Holman, who would play a key role in the MCHR effort, was pessimistic about the campaign's chances for success, and she hoped that King "would call it off in some graceful way or other." And, in expressing her reservations about staging the encampment in the spring, Holman proved prescient. "APRIL? Why April? The spirit may tell us to build arks. Did that preacher ever trench a tent, do you think?"[4]

For weeks the leaders of the Metropolitan Washington chapter of the Medical Committee had been preparing for the thousands of protesters who would descend on Washington for the PPC. In light of the Detroit riot of 1967, they had also been planning for any large-scale civic unrest resulting from racial disturbances or antiwar demonstrations in the nation's capital. In late February, physicians Arthur Frank, Jesse Roth, Sidney Wolfe, and Henry Metzger contacted government and community officials, including police, health, and civil defense workers. They made it clear that MCHR's role was nonpolitical: its sole purpose was to assist these agencies in an emergency. As the physicians later observed, "Government officials will not cooperate and may actually prove obstructive if they are convinced that the group consists of 'radicals' or 'a bunch of civil rights punks.'" MCHR received tentative permission from the police to visit inmates in jails and from local hospitals to coordinate activities in case of an emergency. Medical Committee physicians who worked at the National Institutes of Health and/or were licensed only in Maryland or Virginia were granted temporary licenses to practice in the District. The activists also met with church groups and representatives of the black community, and they formed a plan to locate temporary medical facilities in neighborhood churches.[5]

King, of course, never made it to Washington. Having spent nearly three months promoting the PPC, he took a side trip to Memphis to support garbage workers on strike for higher wages and better working conditions. There, on April 4, he was shot dead while standing on the balcony of his room at the Lorraine Motel. Almost immediately, blacks poured into the streets in major American cities. The worst violence occurred in Washington, where MCHR activists administered first aid to local blacks caught up in the middle of three days and nights of "vandalism, looting, and setting of 1,000 fires [that] caused more destruction than any recent big-city riot in the United States except for Watts and Detroit." There were 7,600 arrests and 13,600 troops deployed. Twelve people died, and hundreds more suffered cuts, beatings, gunshot wounds, exposure to tear gas, and trauma.[6]

Headquarters for the MCHR operation was the suburban home of Henry Metzger. Volunteers met at his house, and then traveled in groups to the affected parts of the city. Police advised them of the best routes to use and occasionally provided escorts. At scenes of disturbances emergency physicians examined hundreds of people. In addition to the predictable fractures, eye injuries, gunshot wounds, and head injuries caused by the riot, they treated patients suffering from epileptic seizures, asthma (attacks exacerbated by tear gas), severe hypertension, and acute anxiety and psychoses. Working mostly from temporary medical facilities, they went into volatile areas for emergencies, as when one physician saved the life of a severely injured soldier in cardiac arrest.[7]

The local medical agencies were usually cooperative. Paul Plotz at the NIH recalls that "I went to D.C. General Hospital and with the collusion of somebody on the staff gathered supplies, huge quantities of bandages, and other kit materials," then put together kits for people going into the riot areas. MCHR also recruited and transported twenty-seven nurses to an understaffed hospital, where they served for the next two days.[8]

The 7,600 D.C. residents arrested during the riot were held either at the city's fourteen precinct stations or in the two courthouse jails. These lockups, designed to hold prisoners for only a few hours, lacked medical care facilities and offered minimal food, water, bedding, and sanitation. Given the word from MCHR that doctors were available, four police precincts asked for immediate help and six others requested assistance later. Since most of the seriously injured had been taken to hospitals, the physicians at the jails were equipped to handle most of the medical problems they encountered. For many of those incarcerated this was their first arrest, and they were emotionally shaken, afraid, and depressed. They received some reassurance from the forty doctors working four- to six-hour shifts in the precinct and courthouse lockups.[9]

The Medical Committee also aided D.C. residents uninvolved in the disturbances. Physicians provided medical care in refugee centers set up by churches and other community groups. Not only were most doctors' offices and pharmacies closed in the riot areas, people who needed drugs or medical assistance were afraid to leave their homes because of curfews. MCHR headquarters established a hotline staffed by a physician twenty-four hours a day for five days. Callers were provided with information about which drugstores were open in the city, and they were assured it was legal to violate the curfew for medical emergencies. In several cases at the height of the riots, when people needing medication could not leave their homes, volunteers brought the drugs to them. (The Peoples Drug store chain provided free drugs. Ironically, several Peoples stores were looted and burned in the riot area.) About a hundred MCHR members participated in the medical relief effort and they were joined by an equal number of volunteer physicians, nurses, drivers, and office workers from the D.C. area. With the nation grieving the death of Dr. King, and clouds of smoke covering the Washington landscape, these health care providers worked under adverse conditions for nearly seventy-five hours. Most of the media ignored them—the big story was the looting and burning—but their dedication stands out in the midst of this tragedy.[10]

After Dr. King's funeral, the SCLC staff—now led by the Reverend Ralph David Abernathy—stepped up preparations for the Poor People's Campaign. Participants came from all over the country. Most were impoverished southern blacks, joined by poor whites from Appalachia, Native Americans and Mexican Americans, as well as some northern white college students who were not poor. Black youths from northern ghettos came as well, and would make their presence known. On May 12 Abernathy and the first contingent of marchers from Marks, Mississippi, arrived in an encampment designated as "Resurrection City," fifteen acres in West Potomac Park that bordered the Reflecting Pool from the Lincoln

Memorial to Seventeenth Street. An agreement with the National Park Service limited the population of the shantytown to three thousand, with a park permit that expired on June 16. Firearms and liquor were prohibited—as were the U.S. Park Police. Although they had jurisdiction, the Park Police agreed to stay out of the encampment unless invited. To provide security, SCLC organized a group of marshals, most of whom were young men from northern street gangs. "These young gang members . . . have always lived outside the system," explained SCLC staffer Albert Sampson. "Our idea was to bring them into the system, let them have a role in the functioning of Resurrection City."[11]

A coalition of medical groups calling itself the Health Services Coordinating Committee (HSCC) provided medical care in Resurrection City. Included in the coalition were members of the local black medical associations, students and faculty at the Howard Medical School, the National Medical Association, and the Medical Committee for Human Rights. Relations between the two national organizations had always been problematical, and MCHR chair Quentin Young went out of his way to appear cooperative and nonthreatening. In a letter to NMA chairman Lionel Swan, Young expressed "our willingness to collaborate with all concerned medical groups, especially the NMA . . . I think it is desirable that we synchronize activities as closely as possible, in order to avoid overlap and maximize our joint abilities to assist."[12]

MCHR was well represented in HSCC. David French was special affairs coordinator, Philip Askenase served as "medical chief" for the campaign, and Mary Holman oversaw the operation as administrator. MCHR set up its headquarters before the demonstrators arrived. Located at St. Stephens Church, about three miles away from the encampment, it was to become the nerve center of the medical effort. Holman was in charge of the operation, which was staffed twenty-four hours a day by volunteers. They sorted out the logistics of assigning personnel, gathering and distributing drugs and medicines, and responding to urgent calls for help within Resurrection City. By all accounts this was an efficient and effective operation. But after two weeks the *Washington Afro-American* accused Holman, "a white woman from Mississippi who lives in Silver Spring, Md.," of not utilizing available black personnel. A victim of racial, gender, and regional stereotyping, she resigned under pressure. (According to Holman, "I was fired from this volunteer position because black doctors from the NMA objected to having 'A Southern White Woman' as the administrator.") After this contretemps subsided, there developed a strong degree of interracial cooperation among the health care volunteers. Edward C. Mazique, the distinguished African American physician and D.C. resident, headed up the Health Services Coordinating Committee, and worked closely with MCHR committee members, including Sid Wolfe. Midway through the campaign Arthur Frank, the co-chair of the D.C. chapter, wrote to Quentin Young that "we're really cooperating well with the NMA and Howard MDs, etc. Maybe we can turn them on."[13]

The major obstacle to providing health care to Resurrection City was the District medical establishment. The overwhelmingly white D.C. medical society was opposed to the PPC, and few of its members volunteered their services. D.C. General Hospital had no interest in treating out-of-town patients, who were sent to the more welcoming and historically black Freedmen's Hospital. A problem arose when the Health Department refused to move its health van into Resurrection City. Citing lack of adequate plumbing and electricity on the site as the reason, it parked the van a half mile away. Even after such facilities were available the Health Department refused to go in, fearing loss of authority in the black-run camp. This prompted the HSCC to declare that "unless we can decide where the van stays we will ask them to remove their van from the operation." As the debate dragged on, the HSCC took the initiative and moved a health trailer provided by the Seventh-day Adventists into Resurrection City and staffed it with MCHR volunteers.[14]

The friction between health care volunteers and the D.C. medical establishment paled in comparison with the turmoil inside Resurrection City. The camp marshals who were recruited from urban street gangs used their authority to harass whites, particularly members of the press, who found it increasingly difficult to gain admission to the encampment to get their stories. Heavy rains turned the encampment into a quagmire, and living conditions, already primitive, now became intolerable. As the days passed, boredom set in and tempers grew short. Reports filtered out of heavy drinking by youths, which led to theft and physical assaults. The marshals had lost control of Resurrection City. Black electrician Alvin Jackson quit his job as deputy chief marshal inside Resurrection City, citing as his reason the escalating, uncontrolled violence. Men were "coming home from a day's picketing to find their belongings stolen or their wives raped . . . If the leaders don't do something soon this is going to be known as blood city instead of Resurrection City."[15]

Throughout the chaos, medical volunteers continued to provide health care for those inside the camp. In addition to the Seventh-day Adventist facility, two other vans were located just outside Resurrection City, each staffed round the clock by volunteer doctors and nurses. The services of dentists and dental students from Howard University were in such demand that the U.S. Public Health Service brought in a dental van from an Indian reservation. Two psychiatrists maintained a clinic seven nights a week. Once the D.C. Health Department got on board it provided immunizations, chest X-rays, and skin and blood tests.[16]

A key demand of the campaign was "the provision of adequate health care for all citizens." A trip through Resurrection City would have cleared up any questions about the quality of health care afforded the poor. Many of the residents suffered from malnutrition. Medical screening turned up chronic conditions that had never been treated. One physician who found a congenital heart condition in a nine-year-old Alabama boy learned that the child had seen a doctor back home, who told his mother to "stop worrying." Dr. Vinod Mody, a tropical disease specialist from India, treated a fifty-eight-year-old black Mississippi woman with a partially deformed bone structure resulting from two fractures of the arms that had never been treated. She also had rickets, with a rib cage so thin "that an easy blow with the hand could crack the bones." "I never would have thought this patient came from the United States," a shocked Dr. Mody told the *Washington Post*, "India, maybe. But not the United States." In addition to the problems they brought with them, the protesters had to contend with poor sanitation and the heavy rains, which became so bad that at one point women and children were temporarily evacuated to nearby churches.[17]

Throughout all of this, in an atmosphere charged with racial tension, the medical volunteers treated acute conditions such as upper respiratory infections, bronchitis, lacerations, and gastrointestinal disturbances. There were no epidemics inside the camp, and few cases required hospitalization. The doctors provided comprehensive physical examinations, and they immunized children against smallpox, diphtheria, polio, and typhoid. They also offered the residents programs in health education. MCHR's Arthur Franks speculated that people in Resurrection City were probably receiving better health care than the average resident of Washington.[18]

The high point of the Poor People's Campaign was Solidarity Day, a mass rally that drew approximately 75,000 people to the Lincoln Memorial to hear Abernathy and other movement activists speak, including Coretta Scott King, who received a rousing ovation. The rally took place on June 19, three days after the park permit had expired. After five weeks of encampment, most of the original residents of Resurrection City had left for home. A disproportionate number of the 500 or so who remained were young people from the inner cities. A week later a thousand police officers arrived at the gates of Resurrection City to clear them out. There was no physical resistance, but 115 protesters, ignoring the command to leave, were arrested while singing freedom songs. That afternoon National Park Service workers prepared to bulldoze the site.[19]

Of all the events of that turbulent spring of 1968, the Poor People's Campaign seems to have gotten lost in the shuffle. Internationally, student-led protests in Paris, Tokyo, West Berlin, and Mexico City led to violent confrontations with government authorities. In Czechoslovakia the Prague Spring rebellion was brutally crushed by Soviet tanks and troops. In the United States, by the time the PPC demonstrators arrived in Washington the country was already reeling from the assassination of Martin Luther King. And Bobby Kennedy was killed in June, while Resurrection City was in its early stages. By most accounts the Poor People's Campaign was a failure. Federal agencies did promise to increase the supply of free food and housing for the poor, but these were token gestures, as was the pledge by HEW to provide "adequate and essential health services to the poor." The War on Poverty was on its last legs. Less than a year later the administration of Richard Nixon would usher in a new era, one in which "benign neglect" was about the best that poor people and people of color could hope for from their government.

The response of health care professionals to the encampment at Resurrection City was admirable. Hundreds of doctors, nurses, and other volunteers provided twenty-four-hour coverage during the entire five weeks of the encampment. The members of the Washington MCHR chapter who spearheaded the medical effort worked closely with their black counterparts in the District. This cooperation did not last. With the nonviolent crusade of Dr. King fading into the background, Black Power militants symbolized by the Black Panther Party now held sway. The Medical Committee too was becoming more radical in keeping with the times, inspired in part by college students who were not just debating but taking action on a number of issues dividing the nation.[20]

Five days after King's assassination Grayson Kirk, the president of Columbia University, rose to speak at a campus memorial service commemorating the life and work of the slain leader. A "ruling-class liberal," Kirk was nearing retirement, hoping to serve out his remaining months in relative tranquility. But in the immediate aftermath of King's death he had watched the fire and smoke coming up from Harlem, and he was concerned about the relations between the exclusive, mostly white university and "the Negroes" in Harlem. In the middle of the service, a middle-class white undergraduate named Mark Rudd walked onto the stage, grabbed the microphone, and denounced the university for "honoring" King while disrespecting Harlem.

Speaking as the local president of the Students for a Democratic Society (SDS), the leading organization of the New Left, Rudd was not exaggerating. A study released in 1968 showed that since the beginning of the decade Columbia's expansion into Harlem had forced 7,500 residents out of their homes and the university was planning on pushing out 10,000 more. Most dramatically, Columbia had negotiated a lease with the city for more than two acres of public land to build a gymnasium in Morningside Park, overlooking Harlem, without consulting that community's leaders. Initially, Harlem residents were to be denied entrance to the gym. After protests, officials decided to build a separate entrance in the back for the local community, with their own little pool. This "Gym Crow" concession, as it came to be known, did not calm the waters, and the project became a potent symbol of Columbia's encroachment into the Harlem community. In addition, Rudd blasted the university for its complicity in the war in Vietnam, specifically its affiliation with the Institute for Defense Analysis, a consortium of universities doing research on military strategy for the Pentagon.[21]

For the next two weeks SDS held rallies on campus, culminating in the occupation of Hamilton Hall (which housed classrooms and the offices of the college dean) on April 23, 1968, by nearly three hundred people, including members of the Student Afro-American Society (SAS). The night of the takeover the two groups debated strategy. Most of the white students wanted to keep the building open for classes while the blacks wanted to shut it down. Early the next morning black leaders asked the whites to leave, and suggested that they take "[their] own building." And they did, breaking into Low Library and setting up shop in the office of President Kirk. Other takeovers followed. On Friday, with students occupying five buildings, President Kirk formally shut down the university and announced that work on the gymnasium had been suspended.[22]

At five A.M. on Wednesday morning, Dr. Richard Hauskenecht, a member of the faculty at Mount Sinai Hospital, received a call from the students who had just occupied Hamilton Hall, asking him to set up a first aid center there. A Medical Committee veteran who had worked in the South, Hauskenecht called other MCHR activists including Thomas Harper (a psychiatrist at Cornell Medical College), Al Moldovan, Hyman Gold, and June Finer, who had moved from Chicago and was teaching at New York Medical College. The group set up an aid station in Hamilton. Soon all the volunteers but one moved into the other occupied buildings. Finer remained in Hamilton, its only white resident. "I stayed in Hamilton constantly," she told journalist Roger Kahn. She handled minor injuries in the building, such as squashed fingers, sprained ankles, scalds, cuts, bruises—accidents that occur in any normal household. "I had alcohol, bandages, antiseptics, but no prescription drugs, no injectables, no syringes. I wasn't setting up a field hospital, but an aid station . . . After a few days in Hamilton I went to Fayerweather [Hall] for a while. Almost everyone there was white and liberal."[23]

Tensions escalated over the weekend, as attempts by an ad hoc faculty committee to work out a compromise failed. The five hundred students occupying the buildings insisted on amnesty, and Kirk refused to grant it. On Monday morning Finer responded to a call from Tom Harper, who needed more medical supplies in Low Library. She made two attempts to enter the building with the medicine, but was turned away by the Majority Coalition, a group of students (many were athletes) opposed to the occupation, which had surrounded the library to prevent the intruders from receiving reinforcements.[24]

Although the Columbia faculty divided over many issues relating to the takeover, a strong majority opposed bringing the police onto campus to remove the occupiers. By late that evening it was apparent that President Kirk had decided to do just that. The police action began around two thirty A.M. on Tuesday (the authorities wanted to be sure that Harlem was asleep) with the peaceful evacuation of Hamilton Hall, which had been occupied by black students for nearly a week. Administration officials were more concerned about Hamilton than with any of the other occupied buildings, and they persuaded several black faculty and community people, including Professor Kenneth Clark, to negotiate with the students. The last thing the Columbia administration wanted was for Harlem residents to wake up to the sight of black students being beaten up by white cops on TV. The students walked out of Hamilton voluntarily, through underground tunnels. Eighty-six of them were arrested. No one was injured.[25]

The police then moved on to Low Library, now with nightsticks flying, breaking through a protective cordon of faculty members in front of the building. Once inside, they came upon Tom Harper in President Kirk's office. Seeing Harper's white medical coat, and sensing that he was an authority figure, an officer asked, "Can you talk sense into these kids and get them to walk out?" Harper replied, "If I could, I wouldn't. And I can't. I'm only the medical aide. These young people make decisions on their own." Roger Kahn explains what happened next:

> Dr. Thomas Harper never saw the club that slit his scalp . . .
> Someone spun Harper. Someone else struck him from
> behind . . . a third policeman began to blackjack Harper. The
> doctor fell gradually, a look of surprise on his face . . . He sank
> to his knees. The police continued beating him. Blood stained
> his scalp. He made a guttural noise. Then he was down. Other
> policemen dragged him out of Grayson Kirk's office by his
> feet . . . There he was handcuffed. "My bag," Harper said. "I
> have to get my bag, so I can treat injuries . . ." "You don't need
> it, Doc," a plainclothesman said. "We'll take care of anyone
> who gets hurt."

The police cleared Low Library, breaking down the barricades, dragging students out, using their clubs against those who resisted (and in some cases against those who did not).[26]

Finer and David Goldman were in Fayerweather Hall. Before the police assault began they climbed out the window and stood outside with blankets and first aid supplies. About twenty-five faculty and students were sitting on the steps to the entrance of Fayerweather. Ordered to get out of the way, they refused, whereupon the police "rushed into the group, kicking, pushing, wrenching, and striking them," forcing their way into the building. "Some minutes later," Finer reported, "I saw four male students, handcuffed in pairs, being dragged down the stone steps, their heads banging on each one." Other students were also "pushed out of the building and dragged down the steps." Finer and Goldman made their way to the bottom of the steps and began giving first aid to people with scalp lacerations. Although wearing a white jacket and carrying a black bag, Finer was "pushed back over a hedge and knocked to the ground by the police." When she identified herself as a physician, an officer blocked her path, warning her to "keep out of the way, you'll just get hurt."[27]

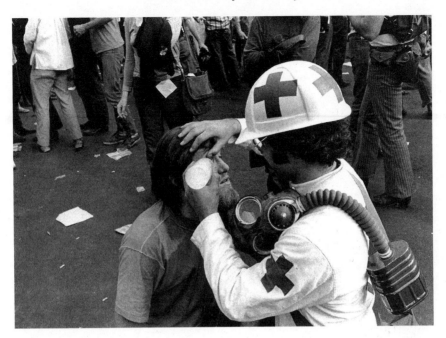

MCHR volunteer removes tear gas from the eye of a demonstrator. (Bill Wingell)

The same scene occurred at the other buildings. Anthropology professor Marvin Harris saw police pulling women students out by the hair, faculty members kicked in the groin, and "many students bleeding profusely from head wounds." Moving over to the mathematics building after Fayerweather had been cleared, Finer "saw five or six policemen's arms striking at someone on the ground. I heard him say 'I'll walk, I'll walk,' but they continued to strike him." Finer "personally gave first aid for some eight scalp wounds and about ten other injuries including those caused by beatings around the kidney area, groin kicks, wrenched arms, and scattered blows to trunk and limbs." Some students had to be carried off on tabletops put into use as stretchers.[28]

It took police about three hours to clear the buildings and the campus. With more than 100 students and a few police officers injured and 692 students arrested—129 of them women—it was the most violent confrontation on a college campus up to that time. In the end, the students won their basic demands. The university did not build a gymnasium in Morningside Park, and it dropped its affiliation with the Institute for Defense Analysis. President Kirk announced his retirement in August. Still, images of affluent students occupying the office of a university president and rifling through his files disgusted millions of Americans, feeding the growing backlash of working-class people against the children of privilege.[29]

College students heeded SDS leader Tom Hayden's call for "one, two, three many Columbias." The 1968–69 academic year witnessed an estimated 150 violent confrontations on campuses across the country, and wherever there were MCHR chapters, medical personnel were on the scene. As in Mississippi in 1964, their presence at times had a calming effect, but as the mood of the country became less tolerant and more divided, MCHR volunteers themselves increasingly fell victim to acts of violence. This was the case later in the summer in Mayor Daley's Chicago.

Back in October of 1967 when the Democrats selected Chicago as the site for their national convention, it appeared to be a logical choice. Illinois was a Democratic state, and controversial as he was, Chicago's mayor Richard Daley was a party loyalist who would roll out the red carpet for the thousands of delegates who, it was assumed, would nominate Lyndon Johnson to run for another term. But then came the Tet Offensive in Vietnam, an event that shifted American opinion against the war and made Johnson vulnerable to a challenge from within his party. Senator Eugene McCarthy of Minnesota ran as a peace candidate, and after he almost defeated the president in the New Hampshire primary, Johnson dramatically bowed out of the race. Senator Robert Kennedy threw his hat in the ring to challenge McCarthy and the sitting vice president, Hubert Humphrey, who now had the backing of Johnson and the party machinery. Then, in rapid succession came the assassinations of King and Kennedy, the uprising at Columbia University, and the debacle at Resurrection City. And to compound the Democrats' problems, thousands of angry and frustrated antiwar activists were promising to come to Chicago to disrupt their convention.

A coalition of groups under the umbrella of the National Mobilization Committee to End the War in Vietnam, or the MOBE, as it was called, spearheaded the protest effort. Most visible in this coalition was the Youth International Party, the Yippies. Led by Abbie Hoffman and Jerry Rubin, the Yippies saw themselves as the political arm of the counterculture. MOBE leader David Dellinger attempted to work with Chicago officials to obtain permits for protest marches, but found them uncooperative. Roger Wilkins, the head of the Justice Department's Community Relations Service, flew to Chicago to try to persuade Daley that the best way to avoid chaos was for the demonstration leaders and city officials to come to some sort of understanding. Daley was not persuaded. He curtly informed Wilkins that Chicago was an orderly city, and if there were to be trouble it would be caused by "outsiders," adding that his police could handle any problems. The Chicago police were known for their aggressive behavior, which was encouraged by the mayor. In the rioting in Chicago that followed Martin Luther King's death, Daley ordered his police to "shoot to kill arsonists and shoot to maim looters," and later that month police attacked a crowd of peaceful antiwar protesters, injuring twenty. Fear of the police kept many antiwar protesters away from Chicago. The expected tens of thousands of people did not materialize. In the end, only a couple of thousand came to Chicago to join forces with local dissidents. In all, an estimated five thousand protesters took to the streets during convention week (with maybe twice that number after a rally on Wednesday night). Dick Daley, on the other hand, put his twelve thousand police officers on twelve-hour shifts, with five thousand Illinois national guardsmen and six thousand federal troops at the ready.[30]

Leaders of MOBE had asked the Chicago chapter of the Medical Committee for Human Rights to provide medical presence during the convention. Over the past three years Chicago MCHR activists had been on the scene at a number of civil rights and antiwar demonstrations, but they sensed that this would be their biggest challenge. To comply with its stated policy that it would not assume the functions of public health organizations, the Medical Committee first contacted Chicago hospitals, the Board of Health, the mayor's office, and police and fire departments to learn what steps these agencies were taking to supply necessary medical care. Quentin Young recalls that "we started quite early, at least six months, to deal with the city authorities." Initial interviews were productive, but then "we'd come back once or twice later and have the door slammed. We knew that the Daley administration didn't want to have anything to do with us." Unlike in Washington, where local authorities recognized their responsibility to the residents of Resurrection City, Chicago officials had made it clear that "none of these agencies had any intention of providing medical or auxiliary services of any kind" to the demonstrators. MCHR would have to go it alone, or so it seemed at the time.[31]

Medical Committee activists, led by Young and Chicago co-chair Jane Kennedy (her antiwar arrest and jailing were still more than a year away), "put up a sign-up sheet, and maybe forty to fifty doctors, nurses, and medical students," many of them members of the Chicago Student Health

Organization, volunteered "to give three hours here, four hours there. That's what we started with." They solicited medical supplies from more than thirty private firms. The United Church Federation of Chicago, located near the Democratic convention headquarters at the Conrad Hilton Hotel, offered its offices as the central treatment and communications center. MCHR established an auxiliary center in a church near Lincoln Park where, it turned out, most of the violence would occur.[32]

The trouble began on Sunday night when five hundred police officers moved against a thousand demonstrators who refused to leave the park after an eleven P.M. curfew. By now some of the police, angered by the disrespectful, lewd remarks directed at them by the Yippies, were already over the edge. There were shouts of "Kill the commies" and "Let's get those bastards" from police officers as they charged into the crowd swinging their batons. They continued to beat the demonstrators after chasing them out of the park into the streets. Claude Lewis, a reporter for the *Philadelphia Bulletin*, took notes as the police clubbed a young woman to the sidewalk. Quickly sizing up the situation, an officer grabbed the reporter's notebook with one hand while clubbing him on the head with the other. Photographers covering the police action were singled out as targets that night. In all, the police assaulted ten reporters and photographers, representing such mainstream organizations as *Newsweek, Life,* and the Associated Press. The "battle of Lincoln Park" continued at curfew hour for the next three nights, with police attacking the demonstrators who were trying to get away. Reporters and volunteer medics were also among their victims.[33]

During the first night of violence local health care workers called the MCHR office offering their help. "It was a remarkable experience," Young recalls. "The whole house staff at Rush Hospital who were not on duty volunteered." The volunteers, easily identifiable in their medical attire, were also forcibly ejected from Lincoln Park each night, despite an earlier agreement with the city that medical workers would be regarded as "neutrals" and be given access to the wounded. In all, about four hundred volunteers—including fifty doctors, forty nurses or nursing students, and at least eighty-five medical students—participated, most of whom were from the Chicago area. Added to the "permanent" stations in Lincoln Park and the treatment center in the church nearby were ten part-time aid stations, some set up as the need arose.[34]

The medical effort was well organized. Teams, each consisting of a doctor or a nurse and three medical students, were dispatched throughout the area where daily demonstrations were taking place. Each team had a leader. Members were to remain together and stay on the periphery of any demonstration. In addition to basic first aid supplies, they carried plenty of bottles of water, for as the police escalated their responses the use of tear gas and mace became commonplace. The natural reaction of these victims was to run, with the possibility of people being trampled in a stampede. At this point the medical teams performed what they called "psychiatric first aid," chanting in unison "Walk! Walk," a technique that actually succeeded in getting people to slow their pace.[35]

The worst violence occurred on Wednesday night, as the convention delegates who were assembled in the Stockyards were defeating an antiwar resolution and nominating Hubert Humphrey for president. That afternoon, a mile away in Grant Park, across the street from the Hilton, the convention hotel, ten thousand people had gathered for the only demonstration of the week to be given a city permit. Now, in the evening, the crowd attempted to march from the Hilton to the convention site. Their first attempt, around six P.M., was halted by tear gas. Jane Kennedy was helping the victims when "I turned and there on Michigan Avenue was a Poor People's mule train slowly moving south." Ralph Abernathy had taken a small group of PPC veterans to Chicago to present their demands to the Democrats. His was the only protest group to be treated with civility by the Chicago police. An hour later, with the mule train out of sight, all hell broke loose. A British journalist on the scene observed the events from his vantage point outside the Hilton:

> Cohorts of police began to charge into the crowd from a street north of the Hilton. The kids screamed and were beaten to the ground by cops who had completely lost their cool. Some [demonstrators] tried to surrender by putting their hands on their heads. As they marched to the vans to be arrested they were rapped in the genitals by cops swinging billies. I saw one girl, surrounded by cops, screaming, "Please God, help me. Help me." . . . Some of the demonstrators were thrown against a window of the hotel and pushed through it. The cops were using mace indiscriminately . . . It was a sadistic romp.[36]

The medical volunteers followed in after the police charge, running to treat those downed by clubs or mace. As television cameras rolled, the crowd screamed at the police, "The whole world is watching! The whole world is watching!" Al Braverman, an MCHR physician and veteran of many campaigns, including Bogalusa, told a *New York Times* reporter that "I have never seen anything as bad as it is here. The injuries are incomparably worse than anything at the Pentagon last spring or at Columbia University or in the Southern civil rights marches."[37]

Braverman was one of nearly a dozen medical volunteers attacked by police during convention week. Tom Harper (who had sufficiently recovered from his beating at Columbia to volunteer in Chicago) observed one medical student who had been "set upon by several policemen, knocked to the ground, and repeatedly struck with nightsticks. He was treated at a local hospital for deep scalp lacerations, two broken fingers, and multiple contusions." "The police are hard to believe," said Braverman after he had been hit and pushed by a police officer. "When a friend said I was a doctor, the cop replied, 'I don't give a damn.'" Jane Kennedy, after reporting similar incidents, concluded that "the actions of the police toward MCHR were so variable that it appeared that each policeman made his own decision about how he would relate to us . . . many police were neutral to us. A few were helpful."[38]

The immediate response of reporters, delegates, and the American public to the conduct of the Chicago police and the mayor was one of shock and anger. An enduring image of the Chicago convention is the shot of an enraged Dick Daley, shouting back at Senator Abraham Ribicoff, who from the podium was condemning "Gestapo tactics on the streets of Chicago." Daley's voice was drowned out in the bedlam, but TV viewers clearly saw him mouthing the words, "Fuck you, you Jew son of a bitch." Less than twenty-four hours later, however, a remarkable shift in public opinion began to occur.[39]

On the final night of the convention, TV newscaster Walter Cronkite, who had been a vocal critic of the Chicago police actions, invited the mayor into his CBS booth, listening without comment as Daley smeared the organizers of the protests as Communists and claimed that the presence of the medical teams was evidence of the violent intent of the demonstrators. The mayor then got an endorsement from the Democratic nominee himself. Talking with CBS's Roger Mudd before he left Chicago, Hubert Humphrey said, "I think the blame ought to be put where it belongs. I think we ought to quit pretending that Mayor Daley did anything wrong. He didn't . . . I know what caused these demonstrations. They were planned, premeditated by certain people in this country that feel that all they have to do is riot and they'll get their way." After castigating the demonstrators for their "obscenity," "profanity," and "filth," Humphrey concluded, "Is it any wonder police had to take action?" Within a very short time representatives of the national media, so critical of the conduct of the police at the time, were singing a different tune. The *Washington Post* conceded that "of course" police officers would be expected to be annoyed by the sight of men in beards. As Daley and his aides continued their counterattack against the demonstrators while exonerating the police of wrongdoing, Medical Committee leaders found themselves in the middle of a controversy over what really did happen on the streets of Chicago that week in August.[40]

Less than two weeks after the convention the mayor issued his official report, *The Strategy of Confrontation,* a document that demonized the demonstrators. "The overwhelming majority" of those arrested were "adult troublemakers who came to Chicago for the avowed purpose of a hostile confrontation with law enforcement." Weapons employed against the police by the "revolutionaries" and "terrorists" included "rocks, bricks, two-by-fours . . . cellophane bags of human excrement, cans of urine . . . Molotov cocktails." While some demonstrators fought back against the police outside the Hilton Hotel (most of the police injuries occurred that night), there is no mention of a Molotov cocktail ever being thrown. Most remarkably, the official report does not include "guns" in the arsenal of the "terrorists." One of the most interesting facts to come out of convention week is that no one was killed. There was no gunplay. Unlike earlier in the year when the ghetto exploded after King's death, the Chicago police had no "shoot to kill" or "shoot to maim" orders for dealing with this mainly white, middle-class group of troublemakers. Kent State was still more than a year away.[41]

The Daley report's section on casualties produced the astonishing statistic that Chicago hospitals treated only "approximately 60" demonstrators that week, while 198 police officers suffered some injury. For the casual reader, it appeared that more than three times as many police had been injured as demonstrators. But twenty of the police injuries were self-inflicted (tear gas) and seventy others were insignificant ("laceration to the tip of left finger, "abrasion to thumb," "split fingernail"). The number of hand injuries reported by the police led Chicago columnist Mike Royko to suggest that a lot of the demonstrators must have been going around smashing the officers' knuckles with their faces![42]

Four days after *The Strategy of Confrontation* appeared, the Chicago MCHR held a press conference and issued its own report, titled *The Strategy of Contusion.* The Medical Committee had written records on 425

protesters treated at the "stationary medical centers." Of these, 112 suffered from head, face, or neck wounds, 83 had injuries to the body or below the neck, and more than 80 were treated for the effects of tear gas
and mace. Mobile medical teams, unable to keep records, reported treating an additional 200 to 300 people for medical conditions and providing first aid for tear gas and mace to another 400 to 600 demonstrators.
The MCHR report projected about a thousand casualties, with both
hard and empirical evidence to back it up. Mayor Daley's people did not
consult the Medical Committee in preparing their report, but Daniel
Walker, a Chicago lawyer did. *Rights in Conflict*, more commonly known
as the *Walker Report*, was based on the work of 212 investigators and
nearly 3,500 eyewitness accounts. While the *Walker Report* cited examples
of abuse and provocation by the demonstrators, it also found evidence
of "unrestrained and indiscriminate police violence," which led to "the
presence of what only can be called a police riot." The report contained
and upheld the evidence submitted by MCHR. The British journalists
who wrote *American Melodrama* concluded that "the treatment figures
supplied by the Medical Committee for Human Rights . . . knocked
the whole Daley thesis lopsided. There could hardly have been a
more fitting demonstration of the indestructible quality of the Big
Lie."[43]

In the following weeks, however, MCHR found itself on the defensive as the fallout from the convention continued. In September a federal
grand jury in Chicago subpoenaed MCHR for the records of the people
it treated or referred for treatment during the convention, claiming it
needed these files to pursue "possible violations resulting from police activity." The Medical Committee responded that the records were privileged information, and it would release them only with the permission of
the patients. The U.S. attorney countered that he would subpoena the
records with or without the consent forms. At this time there were rumors
that various governmental investigative bodies, including the House
Un-American Activities Committee (HUAC), were planning hearings to
"look into the crossing of state lines to foment riots." Any records handed
over to one federal agency could well be passed onto another, and MCHR
feared that harassment of patients and the medical volunteers was "a clear
and present danger." Forced to turn over its records, MCHR did so "under protest." The records were of little use to the grand jury, and there is
no information that the patients suffered harassment or intimidation.

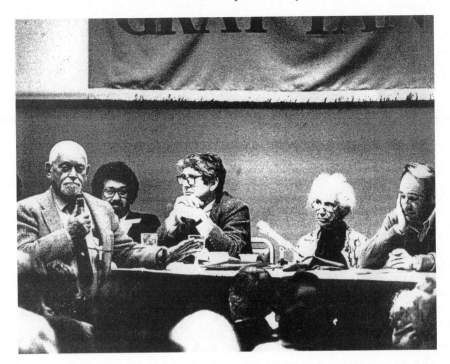

Quentin Young (center). (Institute of Social Medicine and Community Health)

Nonetheless, the subpoena had a "chilling effect" on MCHR, and the suspicion that there was a larger agenda was confirmed when Quentin Young was served a subpoena to testify before the House Un-American Activities Committee.[44]

By the summer of 1968, Young, the most visible person in the Medical Committee, had been politically active in Chicago for three decades. He was born in Hyde Park in 1923, the child of Jewish immigrants. Although his family was not political, at an early age Quentin got caught up in the left-wing scene that flourished in and around the University of Chicago. He joined about 150 other teenagers in a Marxist study group, and became a member of the radical American Student Union. (In 1939, the sixteen-year-old activist wrote ASU president Joseph Lash, warning him that local Communists were attacking Lash over the latter's opposition to the Hitler-Stalin Pact and the Soviet invasion of Lithuania.) Young interrupted his education at the University of Chicago in 1943 to enlist as a private in the Army Medical Department.[45]

After the war he enrolled in medical school at Northwestern, and by the early 1950s he had established a private practice in the racially mixed neighborhood of Hyde Park.*[46]

A committed antiracist, Young was a founding member of the Committee to End Racial Discrimination in Chicago Medical Institutions. Throughout the 1950s he continued to publicly identify with leftist organizations. "I had five children and had to tell them not to talk to people about their parents and what they did," he recalled. A Mississippi volunteer during the summer of 1964, he became the driving force behind the Chicago MCHR. When the New York office collapsed in 1966, Young was responsible for the organization's relocation to Chicago ("We won the booby prize!"), and during his tenure as national chairman in 1967–68, MCHR got back on its feet. His public career as a radical physician in the campaign for social justice, together with his leadership of the MCHR medical presence team at the Democratic convention, had landed him in the HUAC witness chair in the fall of 1968. Young saw the hand of the mayor behind the subpoena. "The Daley machine wanted to hurt me and the Medical Committee for Human Rights because of our activities during the convention week."[47]

According to subcommittee chair Richard Ichord, a Missouri Democrat, the HUAC hearing was to "determine the extent of Communist and subversive participation in the Chicago disturbances." Also summoned to testify were Yippie leaders Abbie Hoffman and Jerry Rubin, along with David Dellinger, Tom Hayden, and Rennie Davis of the National Mobilization Committee. (They would later be tried as part of the infamous "Chicago Seven" conspiracy.) While Rubin and Hoffman did their best to turn the hearings into a circus, Young avoided histrionics, choosing to use this public forum to defend the work of MCHR volunteers during the convention and to attack the conduct of the Chicago police. The Chicago physician did not fit the stereotype of the sixties radical. He wore conservative business suits and plain black-rimmed glasses, and his youthful appearance (one reporter wrote that "the 45-year-old doctor looks 30") belied his long history as an activist. The committee members didn't know quite what to make of him.

---

*Young was unique among MCHR leaders, most of whom made their living by teaching in prestigious medical schools or were "more careerist outside of private practice." Conceding that "left-wing physicians were critical of private practice," Young nonetheless saw an upside. "You are very close to your patients, you are community based, and . . . it gives you economic freedom to say what you want to say." Although he made good money as a self-employed physician, Young had long been an advocate of national health insurance and group medical practice.

HUAC staff counsel Chester Smith cut to the chase. He asked Young if he were a member of MCHR. He then established that the witness was a practicing physician in Chicago. Question number three: "Dr. Young, are you a member of the Communist Party?" That Young declined to answer the question did not surprise committee members, but what startled them was his citation of the First Amendment rather than the Fifth in his defense. Young's decision to base his refusal on his constitutional right to free speech rather than to plead the Fifth, which protected him against self-incrimination, placed him at risk. Back in 1947 members of the Hollywood Ten, who had cited the First Amendment in their testimony before HUAC, went to jail for contempt of Congress. Young was aware, however, that by 1968 HUAC was in decline, and that it was unlikely he would do jail time. But by taking this position he had changed the nature of the inquisition. If the committee members expected him to take the Fifth or walk out of the hearing or become unruly, they were mistaken. For the remainder of that day and the next Young more than held his own as committee members attempted time and again to gain information about his political affiliations and his relationship to the organizers of the convention demonstrations.[48]

At one point committee counsel Smith asserted that HUAC "has received information that you have been a member of the Communist Party, specifically a member of the Doctor's Club of the Party on the North Side of Chicago, a club that was called the Bethune Club. Would you affirm or deny this information?" Young's response that "I am sorely tempted to answer those ridiculous charges" ended with his taking the First. When he was asked, "Did you serve as a member of the governing council of the Medical Committee for Human Rights pursuant to a plan or directive of the Communist Party?" Young's answer was a flat no. Had he taken the Fifth, he would not have been able to answer this question without answering all the others. Attempting to link Young to MOBE leaders, the committee counsel cited as evidence his check for one thousand dollars to rent an office for the MOBE in Chicago. Young replied that this was a personal loan to MOBE leader Rennie Davis, and that Davis paid it back within forty-eight hours. And so it went for the rest of the afternoon.[49]

The next morning the hearing resumed with Young on the offensive. He read a letter of support from the Student American Medical Association, a mainstream organization comprised of thousands of medical students. (During the two days of hearings the more militant Student Health Organizations circulated a petition signed by 1,500 medical students and 700 allied health professional students praising Young and denouncing "the continuing existence of HUAC and its harassment of Dr. Young and other American citizens.") He was also able to read into the record a letter from Washington, D.C., police captain Michael F. Molesky, thanking the Medical Committee for saving the life of the soldier in his precinct who had suffered a heart attack during the riots after King's death. Young contrasted the cooperation MCHR had received from the D.C. authorities in April and May with the hostility the organization faced from the Daley administration, which had refused to work with MCHR and yet had no plan of its own to deal with health care issues outside the convention center. Ichord even let Young read MCHR's *The Strategy of Contusion*, its rebuttal of the Daley report, into the record. Although from time to time committee members came back with questions about Young's alleged Communist proclivities, their hearts were not in it. In the end, they didn't know what to do with Quentin Young, so they let him go. HUAC's attempt to link the Medical Committee with the Communist Party and with the more radical factions at the convention had failed, and Young became something of a hero in the New Left for his testimony.[50]

On the West Coast, MCHR activists became involved in several highly publicized actions, for the Bay Area had been a hotbed of protest since the free speech movement hit Berkeley in late 1964. The San Francisco chapter was led by Philip Shapiro, a respected psychiatrist. He had been working closely with Huey Newton and Eldridge Cleaver of the Black Panthers to provide better health care for residents of inner-city Oakland, and he was active in prison reform issues. Shapiro organized meetings, speeches, and charity events to rally public opinion against American foreign policy in Southeast Asia, and he was involved in the effort to rebuild the Bach Mai hospital in Vietnam, which had been destroyed in a B-29 bombing raid. Under his leadership, MCHR expanded its activities in the Bay Area.[51]

Among Shapiro's recruits was Dick Fine, a Cornell Medical School graduate who had moved to California to do his internship and residency. When violence broke out at San Francisco State University after students went on strike, Fine was in charge of medical presence on campus. "Every day at twelve o'clock we would come to San Francisco State for the riot," he recalls. MCHR was also present when efforts by local activists to create a "People's Park" on a University of California parking lot turned ugly. After demonstrators threw rocks and bottles at the police, the officers responded with gunfire, wounding thirty of them. Medical Committee volunteers also came to the aid of the group of American Indians who had occupied the abandoned prison on Alcatraz Island in San Francisco Bay.[52]

The takeover on Alcatraz began on the night of November 20, 1969, when seventy-two Indians clandestinely boarded boats in Sausalito, crossed the bay, and climbed ashore on "The Rock." For the next eighteen months they held the island, insisting that the federal government turn it over to them, "the Indians of all tribes." They planned to establish an educational center for Native American Studies and a Spiritual Center, along with a training school and a museum. The new Nixon administration decided against using force to evict the intruders from this federal property, as the audacious takeover had drawn widespread attention, much of it favorable. Most of the early occupants were college students, but after they went back to school, families moved into the abandoned prison buildings and set up their own community government.

From the outset, health care was a problem. The prison, closed in 1963, badly needed repairs. Sanitary facilities were terrible, and soon after the occupation the government cut off electrical power to the island. An Indian leader, Anthony Garcia, set up a temporary health clinic, while emergency cases were evacuated by helicopter to the mainland. There were no physicians on the island, and as days passed into weeks it became clear that a professional medical presence was essential. The Medical Committee stepped in to fill the void.[53]

The Bureau of Caucasian Affairs (a pun on the federal government's Bureau of Indian Affairs) asked the San Francisco MCHR to assist in running the island clinic. One of the doctors who spent time on the island was Larry Brilliant. Editor of the short-lived, irreverent MCHR counterculture journal, *The Body Politic,* the twenty-five-year-old Brilliant received his M.D. degree from Wayne State University and had moved west to do his internship at the Pacific Medical Center. He delivered the first baby born on Alcatraz, assisted by two midwives affiliated with MCHR, Elly Bare and Linda Brow. Other medical volunteers who made regular visits to the island included Count Gibson, who had just become the chair of Community Medicine at Stanford. Dick Fine made a weekly trip to bring medical supplies to the island on the "official" ferryboat and remained to treat patients for minor injuries, colds, and pneumonia as well as victims of physical assault.[54]

By early spring of 1970 local media coverage was beginning to wane. The Alcatraz community consisted of about a hundred residents, a disparate group of young idealists, community people and families, and "street punks and winos" from the mainland. Drugs and alcohol became a problem, and acts of violence were common. In its final days, Alcatraz took on the personality of Resurrection City, with leaders unable to lead, a "security force" of young militants threatening and beating up people, the federal government refusing demands, and, finally, a dwindling number of residents staying because they had no place to go. On June 11, 1971, a Coast Guard force came onto the island and evicted the remaining fifteen residents, who left peacefully.[55]

While the occupiers had failed to acquire Alcatraz for the Indian people, they had raised awareness over the plight of Native Americans and the failed government policies of Indian relocation and assimilation. The taking of the island was also prophetic. "Alcatraz!" became a rallying cry among Native American militants, and in the five years after the seizure of the island there were more than sixty occupations of government land and buildings. The leading force of behind this new wave of activism was the American Indian Movement (AIM), formed in July of 1968 by 250 Indians representing several organizations. AIM saw itself as the cutting edge of the civil rights movement for Native Americans. Its leaders, Russell Means, Dennis Banks, and Clyde Bellencourt, were veterans of the streets with prison records, and they admired the style and militancy of the Black Panthers. AIM first drew national attention in November of 1972 when it led a group of Indians on the Trail of Broken Promises, a movement similar to the Poor People's Campaign. Three months later the group shocked the country when it occupied a historic battleground called Wounded Knee.[56]

Wounded Knee, of course, was the scene of the massacre of more than two hundred starving Sioux Indians in the winter of 1890. Led by Chief Big Foot, the Sioux were on their way to surrender when they were mowed down by the U.S. Cavalry. The occupation of the village of Wounded Knee nearly three quarters of a century later by Oglala Sioux and AIM militants is too complex a story to be examined here except in its broadest detail. The Pine Ridge reservation in South Dakota was one of the poorest regions of the country. The tribal chairman was alleged to be both corrupt and brutal, but all efforts by local people to get the Bureau of Indian Affairs to remove him had failed. When the desperate leaders of the Oglala Sioux Civil Rights Organization called on AIM to join them,

Means, Bellencourt, and Banks, an Oglala Sioux born on the reservation, were quick to respond. With the blessings of the tribal chiefs and medicine men, AIM led a convoy to Wounded Knee on February 27, 1973. The militants took over the town, obtaining guns, ammunition, and food by raiding the local trading post. Their demands included the firing of the corrupt chief and a meeting with Secretary of State Henry Kissinger. (Under the terms of an 1868 treaty, they claimed that the Sioux were an independent nation.) Aware of the symbolism involved—one Nixon official warned that "we don't want another Wounded Knee at Wounded Knee"—the federal government decided against forced eviction and laid siege instead. For weeks on end the town was the site of sporadic gunfire coming from both sides, peace talks, and clandestine movement in and out of the city.[57]

The Medical Committee for Human Rights offered to send personnel and supplies, and began raising funds to support the occupation. Dick Fine and other Alcatraz veterans volunteered, as did a number of staff members from Lincoln Hospital in the Bronx. All doctors and nurses were under the supervision of medicine man Leonard Crow Dog, who taught the white volunteers how to use natural medicines and to "say the proper prayers before treating a patient." The medics found the inhabitants "without sanitation, good food, pure water, or electricity. They sleep in cramped quarters. Respiratory and diarrheal diseases are epidemic." They also treated gunshot wounds inflicted by the government marshals firing from a distance. On one occasion an MCHR volunteer nurse reported that "M-16 bullets whizzed through the hospital all night." Throughout April the government tightened the siege. Denied access, volunteers smuggled in supplies on their backs at night by sneaking past guards at the perimeter. Over the next month more than three hundred people were arrested for attempting to bring provisions into Wounded Knee.[58]

Dr. James Waller arrived in Pine Ridge in late April, and kept a diary of his time there. A medical school classmate of Fitzhugh Mullan, Waller was currently on the staff of Lincoln Hospital, part of a "collective" in the pediatric department. (See chapter 9.) In Pine Ridge, Waller spent his time assembling the packs of medicine to be taken in to Wounded Knee each night. Inspired by the spirituality of the Indians, he wrote movingly about taking part in a sweat lodge ceremony led by medicine man Henry Crow Dog. Still, he was restless because "there is a war going on and we are in the rear lines." On May 3, Waller wrote that Pine Ridge "has all the qualities of a bad Fellini movie. Enemies sit cordially together. Blue jump-suited marshals parade around with feathers in their hair. Bearded CBS newsmen lounge in the grass looking like the FBI . . . People wait in silence for something to happen."[59]

Less than a week later it was all over. No longer able to obtain food and supplies, the remaining occupiers put down their weapons. After holding the village for seventy-one days, they left Wounded Knee. Many of them were arrested and put on trial. Two Indians had died from federal gunfire during the siege. There were no fatalities among the federal forces. The medical volunteers returned to their jobs or schools. They had come to Wounded Knee to provide medical care and to bear witness. No doubt some were there because that was where the action was. They were "tripping," eager to regale their colleagues with stories from the front. ("Medics who were at Wounded Knee are available for speaking engagements," stated an MCHR fund-raising letter.) But most medical volunteers came out of a genuine commitment to social justice, and, like Jim Waller, were moved by the examples of courage and spirituality they encountered among the Oglala Sioux.[60]

Whatever its merits as a tactic or program, medical presence had once again given MCHR visibility and popularity. The work of the Washington, New York, Chicago, and San Francisco affiliates during the chaotic protests of the late 1960s attracted new members, with chapters forming across the country. Seemingly on the brink of collapse in the spring of 1966, the Medical Committee had staged a remarkable recovery. It had also received a shot in the arm from a rowdy band of young health care students and professionals, whose bold behavior made their elders appear tame in comparison.

CHAPTER 9

The Young Turks

We were the New Left in medicine.
Subjective, principled, angry, often arrogant,
we felt no ties with the past.

—Fitzhugh Mullan

The 117th convention of the American Medical Association met in San Francisco ten days after the assassination of Robert Kennedy and three thousand miles from Resurrection City. On a pleasant Sunday afternoon in June of 1968 more than a thousand physicians and their wives assembled in the huge grand ballroom of the plush Fairmount Hotel to watch the color guard complete its routine and to view a film extolling the glories of San Francisco. They were just settling in for the opening round of speeches when suddenly two young men, one black and the other white, strode down the aisle through a phalanx of uniformed guards and onto the podium, where the speaker of the AMA House of Delegates was warning his audience of pickets outside the hotel. The white intruder, Peter Schnall, who had worked with MCHR in Selma and was now a fourth-year medical student at Stanford, grabbed the microphone and began reading a statement from the MCHR executive board. He was met with catcalls, boos, and cries of "Shut up" and "Throw him out." Then the microphones went dead.[1]

Things quieted down some as Schnall continued to read, now shouting at the audience. His message was that the American health care system

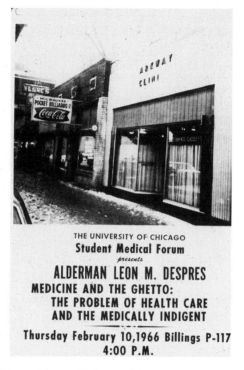

The Student Medical Forum, Chicago Student Health Organization. (Fitzhugh Mullan donation)

was failing, due to a systematic pattern of racial and economic discrimination and an "archaic, poorly delivered and inadequate health program." The AMA was "the culprit," in part because it "has kept medical care a privilege rather than a right" for poor people. Schnall went on to charge that "the AMA has refused to cleanse its ranks of open racial discrimination" by its refusal to force local affiliates in the South to admit black physicians in to their organizations.

After Schnall finished, Jimmy Rogers read his statement in a voice so quiet he could not be heard at all. A Berkeley social worker who represented the Poor People's Campaign, Rogers asked "why the American know-how that can move a wounded marine from the jungles of Vietnam to the finest medical care in minutes cannot and does not do the same for a sick child in the Mississippi Delta or on an Indian reservation? We come to ask why this rich nation with the most advanced medical knowledge in the world can develop artificial organs yet cannot provide inoculations against disease to many of its poorest children?" Rogers then read a list of ten demands put forth earlier by Ralph Abernathy in Resurrection City. They included priority health care for the poor, expansion of Medicare to cover all the indigent, AMA support for maternal health clinics in poverty areas, and training poor people for careers in the health care professions. At the end of Rogers's remarks, Schnall shouted angrily, "Did you hear the representative of the poor?" When the audience roared "No!" Schnall shot back, "This is the whole trouble. You never listen to the poor. Until you hear them, I don't believe you people have the right to call yourselves physicians or humanists."[2]

The protest was not unexpected. The previous day Dr. Donald Goldmacher of the San Francisco MCHR chapter told a reporter from the *San Francisco Chronicle* that MCHR and PPC representatives "will attempt to invade" the opening session of the conference because the AMA had denied their request to speak. Anticipating this action, the AMA decided not to arrest any protesters, fearing that MCHR physicians inside the hall might hold a sit-in on the stage. Outside, nearly a hundred picketers, including Black Panther activists Bobby Seale and Eldridge and Kathleen Cleaver, marched and carried signs denouncing the AMA. The MCHR demonstrators were encouraged by the protest, which received prominent coverage in the major newspapers. Their actions may also have had an impact on a dramatic change in MCHR policy.[3]

Prior to the convention the Massachusetts Medical Society had submitted a resolution to the committee on amendments requiring the judicial council of the AMA to expel any medical society that excluded physicians on racial or religious grounds. Earlier in the year, AMA president Milford O. Rouse had claimed that such action was unnecessary because "we cannot find a single state medical association where any discrimination exists. Neither does it exist on the level of the county societies." The National Medical Association countered that upward of 450 southern black doctors were denied local society membership and related hospital privileges. Not surprisingly, the committee on amendments recommended that no action be taken on the Massachusetts resolution.[4]

The day following the MCHR protest Dr. Urban Eversole of Boston stood up to warn the delegates that "this is a matter of such vital concern that it must be faced, without equivocation, and the report of the reference committee fails to do this." Then Howard A. Nelson, a Greenwood physician, stunned the audience by stating that Mississippi's two-man delegation supported the resolution, claiming (with a straight face) that "we have never discriminated against anyone in Mississippi on race, creed, or ethnic grounds." Following a round of applause, the house of delegates overruled the committee recommendation (to take no action) and endorsed the resolution, directing that it be placed on the agenda at its December meeting in Miami for final approval. There, by a vote of 170 to 69, more than the needed two-thirds majority, the delegates voted to expel any "constituent society found repeatedly guilty of barring physicians from membership."[5]

Why the "sudden" AMA turnaround after years of refusing to deal with discrimination in its ranks? Pressure had been building within the mainstream medical community for some time. Four months before the San Francisco convention an editorial in the prestigious *New England Journal of Medicine* demanded that the AMA take action against its racist affiliates. Moreover, by the late 1960s the AMA had been suffering from internal discord and declining membership and needed to improve its image within the medical community as well as with the general public. The most persuasive explanation for the about-face is that southern hospitals now *had* to award privileges to local black doctors or face the loss of millions of dollars in Medicare and Medicaid funds for violating Title VI of the 1964 Civil Rights Act. Knowing the game was up, the southern medical societies did not strenuously object to the AMA resolution. Still, the Medical Committee deserves its share of credit. For five years it had publicized the AMA's failure to take a stand, and in San Francisco it forced the AMA's hand by dramatizing the issue of racial discrimination to a nation still mourning the loss of Martin Luther King. (Forty years later, in July of 2008, the AMA officially apologized for its "past history of racial inequality toward African American physicians.")[6]

By the late 1960s the Medical Committee for Human Rights had completed its evolution from a national organization providing medical presence to southern civil rights workers to a loose federation of chapters working largely independently of the national office. In the spring of 1967, Quentin Young had been elected national chairman, replacing David French. T. G. G. "George" Wilson, a Philadelphia physician and biochemist, succeeded Young the following year, and Paul Lowinger, a Detroit psychiatrist and antiwar activist, took over in 1969. Eli Messinger, a New York psychiatrist and Marxist scholar, won election in 1970. It is safe to say that each of them would have welcomed a stronger national office during his tenure, but the local chapters enjoyed their autonomy and were not about to give it up. As Walter Lear put it in a letter to Messinger, "It is clear to me that the real strength of MCHR is in the chapters and that the chapters are not particularly interested in a large national office with power over the chapters." For Lear, the national office should function as a clearinghouse, maintaining communication with the chapters, conducting fund-raising campaigns, and recruiting new members.[7]

Even in its diminished state, the national office played an important role as medical watchdog, educator, and vocal critic of the war in Vietnam. Its publications, most notably the periodical *Health Rights News*, reached thousands of people interested in the delivery—and politics—of health care. To operate on this scale required money, but without a strong national program, fund-raising proved difficult.

The largest single source of revenue for MCHR was membership dues. Of the annual $15 fee, half went to the national office, the other half to the chapter. During its civil rights phase, MCHR could count on generous donations from individuals and from events attended by celebrities. By 1969 this source of revenue had all but dried up. That year the national office collected dues from fewer than one thousand members in sixteen chapters, and its total income was $16,836. Office expenses for that year accounted for all but $600 of that total, and *Health Rights News* production cost another $9,500. For the year, the national office ran a deficit of $12,000. It could not pay its part-time staff members their total salaries. The "national office" headquarters was in George Wilson's basement in Philadelphia.[8]

Another problem was that of the changing demographics of the Medical Committee's membership. Many of the physicians who had founded MCHR during Freedom Summer were now gone, replaced by younger men and women from diverse backgrounds, many of whom saw health care reform as just one phase of the larger revolutionary struggle. Staff member Alan Venable noted this development in October of 1970. "You're probably aware of some of the hassles MCHR is going through right now," he wrote to Patricia Lievow, "including a large shift in emphasis away from doctors and towards nurses, hospital technicians and other 'middle level' type people." That same year MCHR activist Larry Brilliant noted "the astounding fact that nearly 2/3 of MCHR members are women, a fact not reflected in the emphasis of *Health Rights News*." Whether the latter figure is "fact" is impossible to prove, given that the national office compiled no membership lists. It is clear that MCHR's traditional leadership—established male physicians—was under attack from feminists and health care students who identified with the New Left. Among the most interesting of these insurgents were members of the Student Health Organizations (SHO).[9]

SHO activists saw themselves as the radical vanguard of the medical profession. They dressed informally in the style of sixties militants, questioned the wisdom of their elders, and believed that ordinary people should have a major say in the health care decisions now being made for them. SHO evolved from the Student Medical Conference, which was founded in 1965 and comprised of medical, nursing, and dental students from ten schools in the Los Angeles area. The first multidisciplinary health student organization in the country, the SMC published its own newspaper, *Borborygmi* (the medical term for stomach rumbles), which dealt with issues of concern to health students such as school curriculum, elitism in the profession, and health care delivery (or lack of it) in poor communities.[10]

The SMC's founder was Bill Bronston, a senior medical student at USC. The child of Russian Jewish immigrant parents, Bronston grew up in California, where his father had become a successful Hollywood producer (*El Cid*, *55 Days in Peking*). Bill was raised in the lap of Beverly Hills luxury, graduating from Hollywood High School and enrolling at UCLA, where he majored in U.S. history, taking science courses on the side because "I always wanted to be a doctor." The Cuban missile crisis occurred during his first year of medical school, leaving Bronston outraged and frustrated because "we were literally days away from global war—and I was incapable of doing anything constructive." He wrote an angry letter to President John F. Kennedy and posted it on the student bulletin board, which made him for a time something of a pariah among his patriotic peers. But Bronston had begun his commitment to political activism. He started reading Marx and Mao and leftist journals such as *Ramparts*, made an unsuccessful run for president of the medical school student body on a platform of student power, and then founded the Medical School Forum, which brought well-known activists like Michael Harrington and Benjamin Spock to address broader questions of health and society that were ignored in the formal curriculum.[11]

With encouragement from the medical school dean, Roger Egeberg, the Student Medical Conference began to take on health care projects in poor communities. One group working with Head Start initiated an audiovisual screening project for twelve hundred youngsters. During the summer of 1965, five students received funding to work with MCHR in Mississippi, while eleven volunteers, most of them nursing students serving without pay, lived and worked with poor immigrants in the San Joaquin Valley. They established a pattern of testing, screening, and community involvement that became "a model for future involvement of health-science students in the deplorable conditions of California's rural poor."[12]

This outpouring of activism in Southern California convinced Bronston to reach out to health care students across the country. The time appeared ripe for a national movement to fill the void for progressive health care students that had existed since the Association of Internes and Medical Students (AIMS) had been red-baited out of existence two decades earlier. Flamboyant and energetic, Bronston began calling around, talking to the secretaries of medical school deans, asking them to identify their "very outspoken and rascalian and activist students." He then contacted the students to arrange a meeting. "I told them, 'I'll bring you our underground newspaper. I'll show you how we are organizing all the schools in the region. I'll show you how we're doing the seminar series.'" On weekends Bronston would jump on a plane (he was then married to a flight attendant who worked for TWA, so he could travel for free) and head out for Baltimore, Cleveland, Denver, Chicago ("Fitz Mullan and I were already friends"), San Francisco, and other cities, meeting with groups of fifteen or twenty students. Organizing them "was so easy it was ridiculous. Within six months we had this national network."[13]

One of Bronston's early recruits was Michael "Mick" McGarvey, a fellow USC med student who had become radicalized while attending Reed College. McGarvey remembers Bronston as "a charismatic, powerful personality, and a good organizer." When they would recruit on other campuses, "We were a one-two team. He would go in and polarize a group, and I would pull them back together to figure out how to get them from A to B." In the fall of 1965, sixty-five students from twenty-five schools of medicine, dentistry, nursing, and social work met in Chicago to form the Student Health Organizations (named after the World Health Organization). From the outset SHO was a loose federation of autonomous chapters—the plural in the name was there for a reason—but the students cooperated closely on a number of summer community health service projects.[14]

McGarvey had developed contacts in the Office of Economic Opportunity (OEO), particularly with program officer Joseph English, who arranged for a hundred-thousand-dollar demonstration grant for a summer project in 1966. Ninety health care students from forty institutions came to California to work in multidisciplinary groups in poverty areas of nine counties. They were joined by fifteen local community workers, who received the same stipend as the students. The project was to provide health services, "stimulate community action for social change," and "educate the students about the problems involving health care for the poor." It was similar to the type of work done in Mississippi by Phyllis Cunningham and Josephine Disparti, who had served as mentors for medical volunteers like Mullan in the summer of 1965. The California project won acclaim, and the OEO funded more ambitious programs the following year in Chicago and New York as well as California. The student participants returned to their campuses full of enthusiasm, and new Student Health Organizations sprang up across the country, with many publishing their own newspapers.[15]

The second national SHO convention, held in New York, drew 350 representatives from seventy-five schools. These delegates called for sweeping curriculum reforms, including adding full departments of community medicine and allowing medical students to have direct contact with patients early in their training. They chose *Encounter*, a magazine that came out of the 1966 summer program, as the official SHO publication, and wrote proposals to fund more projects in other cities. By 1968 there were nine summer projects in inner cities and impoverished rural areas throughout the nation involving more than six hundred students at a cost of more than a million dollars in federal poverty funds.[16]

Older Medical Committee members did not know what to make of this upstart organization. They were impressed with the students' energy and dedication, and hoped they would "graduate" into MCHR chapters after they finished their medical training. Tom Levin wrote that "the kids are as smart as whips, flexible, and responsible. We have a lot more to learn from them than they can from us." On the other hand, this new generation had little respect for authority, and some veteran MCHR physicians found the brash behavior of the students off-putting. As for the SHO leaders, they respected activists like Young and Holloman, but they did not want to be swallowed up by the older organization. (At the beginning of the decade, SNCC activists had experienced the same kinds of feelings toward Martin Luther King and the SCLC.) Believing that MCHR presented a threat to the fledgling group's autonomy ("they were doctors, we were students"), Bronston warned delegates at an SHO conference in early 1967 that "any contact with MCHR would result in the collapse of SHO." MCHR was a "stodgy" organization plagued by "bureaucracy" and "infighting over ideological matters," and SHO, with its action agenda, should keep its distance.[17]

Bronston's remarks at the SHO conference attracted the attention of MCHR leaders, with chairman Young inviting Bronston and McGarvey to participate in a Student Activities Seminar at the national convention in April. There SHO presented MCHR with an "action mandate" calling for its chapters to support SHO groups and their projects. The Medical Committee should also "seize every opportunity to express its dissent, ideas, and programs in the lay and professional press." Young stressed the importance of establishing a liaison between the two organizations, and as chairman he took this responsibility upon himself. He wrote to Bronston and McGarvey that the "most important development at the just completed convention . . . was the drawing much closer together of our two organizations," and that the two of them had "played the paramount role." When a concerned MCHR member asked whether MCHR would "have any advisory rights" if SHO "started off in the wrong direction at times," Young replied that "I have found the SHO youngsters to have a fierce sense of independence which they jealously guard," and that "the only remedy for this youthful malady seems to be good personal and organizational experiences with individual 'adults' in their environment." The two groups, he felt, "are now in a period of testing and collaboration" that "offers a real hope for the future." Shortly thereafter SHO leaders Bronston and Lambert King were added to the MCHR executive committee.[18]

In several of the 1967 and 1968 SHO projects, volunteers had to face troubling questions of race and class. Mullan and King were the directors of an ambitious program centered in Chicago's inner-city slums, where they supervised a staff of 125 health science students and 75 high school interns working at forty-one sites. From the outset, the white students met with mixed reactions from blacks. In the Robert Taylor Homes, the largest public housing project in the world, SHO students were welcomed by the women of the Taylor Residents Health Committee, who were excited by the prospect of a health clinic in the project. In the summer of 1968, eight SHO students began work at Taylor, assisted by six local black youths serving as interns. The Taylor project got off to a bad start when word got out that the SHO students' summer stipend was eight hundred dollars while the inner-city interns received only six hundred dollars, a situation that "caused dissension [and] perpetuated the professional-community dichotomy." Too often the white students did not permit the interns to do meaningful work. At one site in Chicago the health-science students "had the interns preoccupied with painting walls and washing floors."

Overall, SHO found that "the 'interns' were extremely critical of the health-science students and their approach to the ghetto or ghetto problems." The white volunteers also fell victim to the rising tide of black nationalism that had intensified after the assassination of Dr. King. At the Taylor project, black youths ordered all whites to leave their community. When the white volunteers refused, the young blacks threatened them with bodily harm. At the end of the summer, the volunteers wrote a self-critical report that highlighted their ignorance of and inattention to the residents of Taylor. One student sadly concluded that "I don't think we should have been there in the first place."[19]

Experiences in summer projects in other major cities were much the same as in Chicago, causing SHO leaders to question their priorities. "We're at a point where we have to change," said King. "The projects have been very effective in meeting the educational needs of the students and in exposing community health issues, but they didn't help the communities in any significant way. So now we are going through a period of reassessment." That summer six students worked with Ralph Nader's group investigating environmental pollution and the operation of the Food and Drug Administration. And the Philadelphia SHO hit upon a creative and confrontational approach to deal with one of the most serious health care problems facing the black community.[20]

Addressing the National Medical Association on August 14, 1968, President Lyndon Johnson asked his audience to "Consider this fact: among white citizens one American in 670 becomes a doctor, but among Negroes one in 670? No. Among Negroes it is one in 5,000 . . . That is a tragedy, a complete absolute indictment of our entire educational system." The president said that the country must recruit "more talented Negro students for the medical professions and assist more institutions to educate more Negro doctors, Negro dentists, Negro nurses, and Negro technicians. We must persuade American universities to stretch and expand their resources to give special attention to training Negroes to take their rightful place in the health profession." Three weeks later a group calling itself the Committee on Black Admissions of the Philadelphia Student Health Organizations (CBA) delivered a letter to the deans of the six local medical schools demanding that one third of the students admitted in 1969 be black, a figure commensurate with the African American population of the city. (Of the 2,795 students in the six Philadelphia schools, only 27—less than 1 percent—were black.) The letter stated that "since the black citizens of Philadelphia, as ward and clinic patients, serve as an important source of medical instruction for the Philadelphia schools of medicine it is reasonable that these schools make a special effort to offer educational opportunities to Philadelphia residents who are black." It concluded by asking for a meeting with the six deans the following week.[21]

One of the organizers of the CBA was Mick McGarvey, who had moved to Washington to work with the Public Health Service and commuted up to Philadelphia for the meeting with the deans. He recalls that "it was hilarious. It was one of the funniest meetings I had ever attended. One of the deans was so angry he couldn't even speak." The students had anticipated the questions the deans might ask. CBA members would help conduct a national recruitment campaign to get qualified students. They would approach foundations for funds to defray the cost of a medical education for students who needed financial aid. They would develop a network of local black families to be a support group for the students. And they would institute a summer program to provide remedial work for those students who needed intensive study in the sciences before entering medical school. "We did all those things," McGarvey modestly concluded. And while the Philadelphia medical schools never approached the CBA goal of 33 percent, the number of blacks admitted increased in the following years. The CBA continued to be a positive force in the recruiting drive, joined by the Philadelphia chapter of MCHR, which secured a grant of ten thousand dollars in 1970 to set up a summer program for "disadvantaged students in the Philadelphia area health schools."[22]

Medical schools across the country now took steps to improve their woeful record in black student admissions. By 1970, fifty-four schools had initiated special programs to recruit minorities, and many included financial and academic assistance to the entering students. During the 1971–72 academic year, 2,056 black students were enrolled in medical schools, 4.7 percent of the total, almost double that of 1968–69. Recruitment of minority students intensified in major universities across the country during the late 1960s and 1970s. Health care activists deserve credit for pressuring medical and nursing schools to take affirmative action.[23]

By 1968 SHO had chapters in forty states. Membership may have run as high as three thousand, about three fifths of whom were medical students. It remained a loose federation of local groups, with no national officers. While best known for its summer projects, SHO chapters were active on a number of fronts, including issues relating to school curriculum. Some members wanted SHO to take a public stand on pressing concerns, such as national health insurance and the Vietnam War, and to establish a central office run by a full-time executive. All this came to a head at the third national SHO conference, held in Detroit at the end of February in 1968. That assembly proved to be a turning point for the student organization.[24]

Nearly six hundred students from more than one hundred schools had registered for the conference. A thousand people attended the opening session, which featured a talk by Benjamin Spock and a keynote address by SHO cofounder Fitzhugh Mullan. Perhaps the nation's best-known critic of the war, Spock focused his remarks on the need for a national health plan that covered all Americans, and he drew much applause when he attacked the AMA. Mullan argued that for SHO to be nationally effective it must have a national presence. His call for the assembly to endorse his proposal to create a central executive office was heatedly debated and eventually defeated. (The SHO members' distrust of a strong central office had its counterpart in MCHR.) The resulting compromise was the establishment of a National Service Center, to be overseen by a Coordination Council. For Mullan, SHO's refusal to "put together a national organization with staying power" resulted from "centrifugal tendencies within SHO" and an "enormous paranoia" that the national office "would be infiltrated immediately" by hostile government forces.[25]

Failure to establish a strong national office was a factor in SHO's decline, but the question of whether the organization should take a stand on the war proved equally as damaging. McGarvey put it bluntly. "SHO self-destructed on the breakwater of the Vietnam War." The issue was the same one that had split the Medical Committee in 1966. Practically all the SHO students opposed the war, but, like their MCHR counterparts, they did not see antiwar activity as a proper function for a medical organization. Some were concerned that taking a public stand would undercut the organization's primary program, the summer projects, which were dependent on government money. Needlessly antagonizing the Johnson administration was not good politics. A number of the delegates didn't even want Dr. Spock to speak. Sensing the tension, Spock tried to calm the waters by stating that SHO might "restrict its usefulness by becoming solely another anti-war group," but this drew an angry response from Bill Bronston, who insisted that SHO speak out against the war, as MCHR had done a year earlier. The debate raged on and was not "resolved" until the final session when the assembly passed a weak resolution that supported "the right of individuals in SHO to dissent and resist service in the armed forces."[26]

Divided over questions of the war and the need for a strong national organization, SHO went into decline. It maintained an office in Chicago for a time, funded by the Carnegie Corporation. The organization had no summer projects in 1969, and by the following year SHO as a national confederation had ceased to function. During its relatively short existence, the Student Health Organizations had empowered students in the medical community to bring about curricular reforms in their schools and had lobbied successfully for the recruitment of more minority students to the health care professions. Its summer projects called attention to the nation's failure to provide anything resembling adequate health care for the poor. One of the lasting legacies of SHO was its impact on the Student American Medical Association, which had been under the thumb of the "parent" AMA. "We had a lot of students who were active in SAMA," Mullan recalls, and in 1969 SAMA chapters operated thirty-two summer projects, which followed the SHO model. Eventually SAMA changed its name to the American Medical Student Association so that it would not be identified with the AMA. According to Mullan, "a lot of the energy, the vision we had in SHO got embedded in SAMA and lives on today in AMSA, which generation after generation keeps picking leaders who would have been comfortable with SHO."[27]

After graduating from medical school many SHO activists did their internships in inner-city public hospitals, where most patients were poor blacks and Hispanics. Fitz Mullan chose Jacobi Hospital in the northeast Bronx, affiliated with Albert Einstein College of Medicine. Like the other interns, he spent a hundred hours a week in the hospital, working a six-day week, on call every other night. The hospital encompassed his life. Later, Mullan recalled that "we made no home visits, worked with no community organizations, visited no local practitioners, and generally maintained a kind of medical school isolation despite the fact that we were a city hospital." The hospital "lacked any sense of community base or any vehicle for community involvement." Administrators at Jacobi were responsible only to the City Department of Hospitals and to the sponsoring medical school. Mullan and other SHO veterans had embraced the idea of "participatory democracy" popularized by the Students for a Democratic Society, and this meant that those served by the hospitals—the patients—should have a major say in the decisions made by these institutions.

Throughout his internship, Mullan struggled with his inability to work in the surrounding community (as he had done in Holmes County in Mississippi), and with the hospital's unwillingness to permit any citizen involvement in its operation. During his second-year residency in pediatrics he worked with Marty Stein, a SHO veteran from Berkeley. Both wondered where their experiences at Jacobi were leading them. "Weren't we becoming an indistinguishable part of the system?" They knew that other SHO alumni were working in isolation in hospitals across the country, where their recommendations for institutional reform were easily dismissed. During one conversation Stein hit upon the idea of creating a critical mass of like-minded interns and residents who would work together at the same hospital. Through sheer force of numbers they could create an environment more hospitable to their ideas. Barbara Blase, a fellow resident, joined their discussions, as did Charlotte Fein and David Stead, who were residents at Lincoln Hospital, and an Einstein student, Peter Rothstein. The group began to develop recruitment strategies to staff such a program.[28]

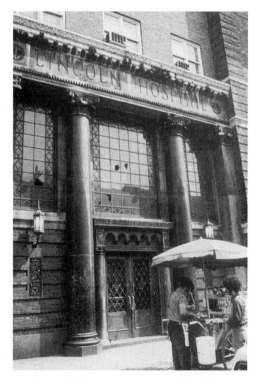

Front entrance to Lincoln Hospital, Bronx, New York, 1972. (Fitzhugh Mullan donation)

First they had to select a hospital. Jacobi was too big, and as a referral center it did not serve a specific neighborhood. They settled on Lincoln, a small, ancient hospital with 350 beds in the South Bronx. Built as a nursing home for runaway slaves in 1839, this dilapidated structure had been condemned as early as 1950 for its "substandard physical conditions." The *New York Times* called Lincoln "a medical disaster area." For as long as anyone could remember, local residents had referred to it as "the butcher shop." Back in 1967 the city announced plans for a new nine-hundred-bed hospital, but three years had passed without even a groundbreaking. In the meantime the area's 350,000 residents, 80 percent Puerto Rican and 20 percent black, had to rely on a medical facility that seemed right out of Charles Dickens. For Mullan and his friends, all of whom had spent time at Lincoln, the hospital had everything they wanted: "a small medical staff, a real community base, a medical school affiliation necessary for the training program and, additionally, a chronic problem of understaffing."[29]

The base of their operations would be the Pediatric Department, then staffed almost entirely by physicians from the Philippines and Korea. Department chief Arnold Einhorn was a native of Belgium who at age seventeen had been a member of the French resistance. He graduated from medical school in Paris and immigrated to the United States in 1954 to do his internship and residency. A dedicated and competent physician, Einhorn had been at Lincoln since 1958. When Mullan and others met him and promised to recruit a staff of American interns and residents from leading medical schools, Einhorn was ecstatic. "I have worked here at Lincoln for many years in the hope of improving medical care for the poor. Finally there seems to be someone else who agrees with me . . . Where do we begin?" With approval from Einhorn and other administrators, the young doctors used their SHO network to attract an impressive team of eighteen interns, five first-year residents, and six second-year residents. Included in the group were Jim Waller, Mullan's friend from medical school, and MCHR activists Henry Kahn and Peter Schnall, who with his wife, Susan, had moved to New York from California. All the recruits were white, a third of them were women, and a majority were Jewish. The Lincoln Collective, as it came to be called, developed a political program centered on community involvement in the work of the hospital. All agreed that decisions would be made by the group, not by individuals. Some members lived communally and shared expenses.[30]

For years patients had been critical of the services provided at Lincoln.

In June of 1970, a month before the new interns and residents began their work, a group of local people calling themselves Think Lincoln came into the hospital and set up a complaint table stocked with pamphlets discussing hospital abuses, patients' rights, and the need for community control. Then, in a dramatic move on July 14, 150 members of the Young Lords, a Puerto Rican group that patterned itself after the Black Panthers, occupied the Nurses' Residence for twelve hours. They left only after presenting hospital officials with a list of demands that included a door-to-door preventive medicine program, a day care center for the children of parents and workers, and the creation of a board of community members and hospital workers to operate the hospital. Lincoln administrators responded by setting up a day care center. The Lincoln Collective, in place for only two weeks, endorsed both the demands and the takeover. Most of the permanent staff physicians at Lincoln were uncomfortable with this kind of activism.[31]

Initially, Einhorn seemed to accept the idea of "community involvement," but it soon became apparent that he did not take kindly to input from the likes of the Young Lords or, for that matter, the Lincoln Collective. In the fall the collective presented Einhorn with a position paper calling for creation of a community-hospital board that would control hiring, firing, and budget decisions. Another proposal asked that the Pediatric Department formally associate with the Young Lords and the Black Panthers. Einhorn rejected both petitions, adding that he did not think the Young Lords had "legitimate constituencies" in the South Bronx. For a dozen years Einhorn's word had been law in his department, and the mostly foreign-born interns and residents had not challenged his authority. They appreciated his dedication and the stability he represented. Now all that was being threatened by community agitators and the New Left activists who had joined his house staff.[32]

On July 28, only four weeks after the arrival of the new doctors and nurses, twelve physicians (eleven Filipinos and one Korean) asked to be relieved of their jobs in pediatrics, claiming "harassment and intimidation" by the Young Lords and other community people, who questioned their competence and even referred to them as "foreign mercenaries." Einhorn defended the physicians in an interview with the *New York Times*, adding that "I'm probably on my way out too. I can't continue to operate under these conditions." This possibility pleased members of the Lincoln Collective, for Einhorn was standing in the way of their reforms. Administrators at Einstein Medical College, the sponsoring institution, had been aware of the growing turmoil at Lincoln, but they admired the idealism of the Collective members and were delighted that such bright young people had chosen to work in a ghetto environment. Replacing Einhorn might restore harmony to the department.[33]

During the fall of 1970 a forty-one-year-old pediatrician from Puerto Rico named Helen Rodriguez applied for a position at Lincoln. Her credentials and personality impressed both Einstein administrators and members of the Collective. "She felt like one of us," observed one of the doctors. The plan was that after a brief period on the Lincoln staff, Dr. Rodriguez would take over as chief of pediatrics, while Einhorn would be reassigned to another position within the Einstein system. Although he had previously requested a transfer, Einhorn now had second thoughts, believing that he was being forced out. In the end, he insisted that Dean Labe Scheinberg at Einstein issue a statement that he was "being replaced for political reasons," and that "the department finds it essential at this time to have a director of a different ethnic background."[34]

When news of the specifics of the agreement leaked out, the Jewish community in New York was outraged. Recently, a controversy had erupted in the Ocean Hill-Brownsville district over community control of schools that culminated in the firing of several Jewish principals. Now it appeared that Puerto Ricans and blacks were out to get a competent and dedicated Jewish physician. The Jewish Defense League responded by staging a sit-in at Dean Scheinberg's office and issuing a series of press releases. The *New York Times* lauded Einhorn as "an underground fighter against the Nazis in World War II." The *Times* editorial correctly called attention to Einhorn's dispute with "a staff of junior physicians dominated by radicals," but then mistakenly concluded that "he was removed simply because he was not of Puerto Rican origin." The Anti-Defamation League of B'nai B'rith weighed in, citing the Lincoln example in an attack on four "politically oriented [medical] groups committed to radical change." The guilty organizations were the Student Health Organizations, the Medical Committee for Human Rights, Physicians for Social Responsibility, and the Health Policy Advisory Center (Health-PAC), a left-wing think tank in New York. Six months later, after an investigation, the New York Human Relations Commission concluded that Einhorn had not been the victim of ethnic discrimination, but was let go because Einstein officials "felt that a rebellious pediatric staff and community unrest had produced a complex political and administrative situation which . . . was adversely affecting the pediatrics program at the hospital."[35]

As a result of the Einhorn controversy, the Lincoln Collective received a lot of mostly negative publicity. (Victor Sidel, one of the nation's leading health care reformers and head of the Division of Social Medicine at Montefiore Hospital, resigned his membership in MCHR over the refusal of the organization to repudiate intemperate remarks made by several Lincoln physicians identifying themselves as MCHR.) The charges of anti-Semitism stunned the Collective, for most of them were Jewish, as was the administration at Einstein Medical College. Had Einhorn backed their program they would not have sought his removal. But after it became apparent that he did not support their agenda, the Collective did demand that Einhorn be replaced, and they did play the ethnic card in advancing Dr. Rodriguez's candidacy. The immediate impact of Einhorn's departure on the Collective was an increased workload, because the foreign medical graduates—comprising about one quarter of the house staff—left with Einhorn and they were not replaced.[36]

All this happened during the first six months of the Collective's existence. For the next year and a half the members met regularly to discuss practical problems and political theory. They read selections from Mao's *The Little Red Book* and examined the changes in health care brought about in the Chinese countryside by the Communists. They engaged in criticism and self-criticism. (Several Collective members later joined the Revolutionary Union, the forerunner of the Revolutionary Communist Party.) Women raised issues of male chauvinism within the Collective and on the hospital floor. Efforts to establish rapport with the clerical and nursing staffs were largely unsuccessful, in part because many of the people working at Lincoln were uncomfortable with the politics and lifestyle of the Collective. Ironically, the group that fervently preached egalitarianism was coming across as elitist, a problem that confronted New Left activists elsewhere.[37]

The Collective had its successes. Mullan helped organize the Pediatric Parents Association, a group of community people who had a direct interest in the hospital. At their first meeting Mullan served cookies and soft drinks to about twenty parents. (The congenial, down-home atmosphere reminded him of Holmes County and the Mississippi Freedom Democratic Party.) At future meetings the parents listened to lectures and toured a section of the Pediatric Department, where they interviewed the people working there. They took on a political role by supporting the staff's efforts to block budget cuts and, most important, they selected representatives to participate in the selection of new interns and residents. The

Collective also took over operation of the Community Medical Corps, a door-to-door health screening program in the South Bronx started by two medical students from Einstein in the late 1960s. It continued to support the Young Lords and other militant community organizations. But its failure to develop its own political program led to increasing disillusionment and alienation among those who had come to Lincoln to revolutionize the practice and delivery of health care. In July of 1972 a new "class" of house staff arrived at Lincoln, "with many members leaving the Collective for other areas of work." The Collective continued through the mid-1970s, but by then the Pediatric Department was looking much the same as it had in 1969, with foreign-born medical graduates once again the majority of the house staff. "Collectivism, community control, and worker democracy" were no longer issues.[38]

What is most interesting about the Lincoln Collective is not that it ultimately failed but that it came to be in the first place. The audacity of a handful of medical graduates moving into a hospital department, in effect taking it over and then planning and operating with a freedom unknown in other teaching hospitals, is in itself remarkable. Like their counterparts in SDS, the members of the Collective engaged in endless debates about culture and politics, but they also worked long hours in a run-down hospital and faced life-and-death issues every day. Looking back on that experience, Mullan observed that although "we did not achieve the sweeping changes in medical care that we had hoped for when we first came together . . . we made an honest stand for what we thought was right and worked hard in support of it." Ultimately, the failure of government at all levels to adequately fund public hospitals, together with the leaden bureaucracy that administered these institutions, doomed experiments like the Lincoln Collective. Frustrated by their inability to have any lasting impact in hospitals that operated in the ghetto, some young health care activists turned their backs on establishment medicine and searched for new ways to deliver health care to the urban poor.[39]

The free community clinic, a storefront operation providing basic medical services in economically deprived neighborhoods, took hold in the late 1960s. By 1971 more than 150 such clinics were operating across the country, most but not all in urban areas. MCHR and SHO activists helped organize and staff many of these centers, with doctors, dentists, nurses, and students volunteering their time to treat anyone who walked in needing

medical assistance. The three most common types of clinics were the so-
called hippie clinics that were aimed at young people and dealing primarily
with drug problems, those clinics initiated by community organizations,
and clinics opened by groups with a radical political agenda, like the Black
Panthers.[40]

The HEAD clinic (Health Emergency Aid Dispensary) in the New
Orleans French Quarter served a young, mostly itinerant clientele. Initiated
by the New Orleans MCHR in late 1969 and governed by a local board,
HEAD included a pharmacy and a complete emergency laboratory staffed
by volunteers. Open four days a week, it had a twenty-four-hour hotline
that referred patients to other sources of assistance when the clinic was
closed. HEAD filled a need unmet by local health providers. "We haven't
seen one person yet who could have afforded a private doctor," reported
MCHR chair Dr. Jeoff Gordon, "and most of them can't get into Charity
Hospital except in emergency cases because they haven't lived in New Orleans six months to meet the residency requirement." Moreover, he said,

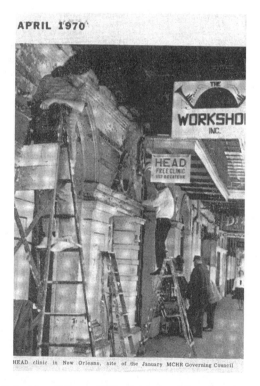

The HEAD free clinic, New Orleans, 1970. (Institute of Social Medicine and Community
Health)

"People with drug-related problems stay away from hospitals because of the risks of arrest and the unsympathetic reception they get there."[41]

June Finer was the prime mover in establishing the Judson Mobile Health Unit, a fifty-foot trailer parked in the heart of New York's Lower East Side. "We're here to give health care to any East Village kid who needs it," said Finer. "We don't ask questions and we don't make judgments." Serving mostly impoverished blacks and Hispanics, the Mobile Health Unit offered free treatment for a range of ailments, from rat bites and cuts to venereal disease and bad drug trips. The clinic provided immunizations, pregnancy diagnosis, and counseling and referral for legal, welfare, and housing problems, as well as a remedial reading program, informal day care, and a youth "rap group" for neighborhood kids. There was also a political component to the clinic. Community organizer Paul Ramos noted that most of the health problems they encountered stemmed from the oppressive poverty in the East Village slums. "Part of our job is to make people politically aware of why they are sick: overcrowding in their houses, miserable garbage pickup, a poor health system, and welfare which doesn't give them enough money to live on." Finer believed that it was the efforts of community organizers like Ramos and the Job Corps workers assigned to the clinic that made it an example of "guerrilla medicine." "Without them," she said, "the unit would have been just another straight health clinic, a dull, moderate success. The generation we're trying to reach is a revolutionary generation."[42]

Young people who had left home to experience life in the streets found medical help in places like the Haight-Ashbury clinic in San Francisco, the Corner Drug Store in Gainesville, Florida, and the Heads Up Center in Washington, D.C. Perhaps a majority of the clinics throughout the country were "straight," initiated by community people simply wanting to provide some health care services to a deprived population. But a number of clinics were operated by militant organizations with a radical agenda. The best known of these groups was the Black Panthers.

Founded in Oakland, California, in 1966 by Huey Newton and Bobby Seale, the Black Panther Party for Self-Defense established a foothold in major cities across the country. Preaching a blend of black nationalism and Marxism, the Panthers were intimidating in their black leather jackets and berets and their public display of weapons. The FBI and local law enforcement agencies identified the Panthers as a primary target in 1969, a year when an estimated twenty-eight Panthers were killed by police, with hundreds of others imprisoned. The most shocking case was the killing of

Panther leader Fred Hampton by Chicago police, who raided an apartment where he was sleeping and shot him down in cold blood. The Black Panthers had also been organizing inner-city communities, offering free breakfasts for schoolchildren, educational programs, and free health clinics. White liberals and radicals were attracted to this side of the Panther profile.[43]

MCHR members embraced the Panthers' cause and rallied to their defense. On December 12, 1969, the Medical Committee called a press conference in New York, where an "outraged" Don Goldmacher charged that it had "become abundantly clear that genocide is being practiced against the Black Panther Party in the United States." Condemning "the tactics of early morning raids and of shooting people in their sleep," MCHR demanded the immediate release of "all Black Panthers now in jail in violation of their constitutional rights" and a congressional investigation of the FBI and its tactics. The statement ended with a warning that "if the Panthers are destroyed, we are all guilty and will surely suffer the consequences—the loss of civil liberties for all." MCHR's identification with the Panthers may appear to be another example of "radical chic" (the disparaging term the writer Tom Wolfe applied to white liberals who unquestionably accepted the Panther agenda). But unlike most whites, MCHR members had been volunteering in a number of clinics established by the Black Panthers. At the time of his death, Fred Hampton had been working with the Medical Committee to set up a free health clinic on the West Side of Chicago. MCHR activists, then, felt a direct kinship to the members of a group the government was attempting to destroy.[44]

The Medical Committee helped the Panthers open clinics in several areas, including Los Angeles, New Haven, and the San Francisco Bay Area. MCHR volunteers assisted black community activists in obtaining medical equipment and drugs for the clinics, and arranged for laboratory tests at local hospitals. Relations between the black street activists and the mostly white middle-class health professionals were not always harmonious. Ann Garland, an African American nurse and an officer in the Philadelphia MCHR, reported that a Panther clinic official "threw out a nurse who was not black." Garland promised to bring a semblance of order to the clinic, which "is one big mess! Everything remains unorganized; lists of doctors, etc., have all been lost." She also observed that "in its anxiety to please, MCHR has neglected to speak up with constructive criticism of the Black Panther effort." George Wilson agreed, warning that "we should be careful to avoid 'reverse paternalism' by letting the Panthers do it all alone, when they obviously need professional expertise."[45]

One of the most successful Panther clinics was the People's Free Medical Care Center in Chicago, inspired by Fred Hampton. Its opening had been delayed because of his death, and the center's director, nineteen-year-old Ronald "Doc" Satchell, had himself been shot five times in that police attack on Panther headquarters. The center was "bright, warmly decorated and well-equipped without frills as an efficient out-patient service," thanks to the work of local black carpenters, who donated their services. The Chicago MCHR had assessed each member five dollars to support the center, and supervised the schedules of the more than 150 nurses, technicians, physicians, and health science students who volunteered to work in the evenings and on Sundays. Quentin Young recalls that Satchell demanded professionalism in appearance as well as service. Seeing Dr. Young make his rounds wearing white coat and tie, Satchell instructed the young medical volunteers to get rid of their Levi's and sneakers and come to work professionally attired.[46]

The medical establishment's reaction to the free clinics was mixed. In Chicago the Board of Health invoked a thirty-one-year-old ordinance and charged that four clinics did not meet official standards and thus were operating illegally. The offending clinics just happened to be the ones operated by the Black Panthers, the Young Lords (Puerto Rican), the Young Patriots (Appalachian whites), and the Latin American Defense Organization—all militant ethnic groups. The cases were thrown out after a judge ruled that the definition of a clinic was "so vague and so indefinite as to be completely unenforceable." On the other hand, many local medical societies and hospitals welcomed the clinics, a development that MCHR reformer Tom Bodenheimer found problematic. In a 1972 article, the California physician wrote that "in the five years since the first free clinic opened, the free clinic movement has gained the support and blessing of the health establishment—drug companies, medical schools, even the Nixon administration." Bodenheimer concluded that the "general effect of most free clinics is to perpetuate and assist establishment health care institutions to continue in their anti-patient policies." The hospitals were using the free clinics as "an escape valve—the free clinics see patients these establishment institutions don't want to deal with." And while there were exceptions, "the day-to-day work of most free clinics is no challenge to the health care structure." Bodenheimer was not recommending that the free clinics close their doors, but that they "use the energy present in free clinics as a springboard to challenge local health care institutions." The free clinic movement could become "a powerful force creating change in the health care system." It did not succeed in doing so.[47]

Quentin Young, a clinic supporter, saw them as "a symbolic attempt to address the problems of health care in the deprived community of poor blacks and whites." Yet he believed "they could never do this in a comprehensive way." The clinics served only a tiny fraction of the millions of people deprived of decent medical care. By 1970, Young and other MCHR leaders were putting together an ambitious "comprehensive" reform program that would become the centerpiece of a National Health Crusade. Five years earlier, working quietly and largely without fanfare, a small group of MCHR physicians had initiated a pathbreaking, successful, and permanent innovation in the field of health care for the poor, one that could serve as a foundation for the national organization's proposed overhaul of the American health care system.

CHAPTER 10

Health Care Is a Human Right

If we believe that men have any personal rights at
all as human beings, they have an absolute moral
right to such measure of good health as society,
and society alone, is able to give them.

—Aristotle

The comprehensive community health center movement was the
most significant and enduring achievement in the field of health
care to come out of the civil rights years. Discussions held by Jack
Geiger, Count Gibson, Bob Smith, and other MCHR activists in Mississippi in the fall of 1964 led to the Office of Economic Opportunity's funding of two centers, one in the Columbia Point section of Boston and the
other in a rural southern community. Tufts University was the administrative agent for the centers, with Count Gibson in charge of Columbia
Point and Jack Geiger responsible for the southern operation. (See pages
81–83.) After visiting several communities, the site chosen was Mound
Bayou, Mississippi, a historically black town made famous by the patron-
age of Booker T. Washington early in the twentieth century.[1]

Mound Bayou is in Bolivar County in the heart of the Mississippi
Delta, one hundred miles south of Memphis and twenty miles east of the
Mississippi River. The town had two private, fraternally sponsored hospitals, and although they were run-down and badly in need of funds, they
would benefit from the presence of the health center while providing beds

and care for center patients needing hospitalization. Bolivar was the third-poorest county in the nation, with an unemployment rate over 50 percent. Cotton had been king, but now sharecroppers had been replaced by machines. Without jobs, blacks had little or no access to health care. Medicare had just passed Congress; Mississippi would not join the Medicaid program until 1971. The few public health facilities in the county were inadequate and unwelcoming. Most blacks had never seen a doctor. In such an environment, where one had to choose between food, rent, and medicine, good health was almost impossible.[2]

Geiger and his colleagues, recognizing that basic medical services alone would not address the underlying causes of poverty, envisioned the health center as a primary agent of social change, affecting all aspects of the lives of the population it served. Its mission was to implement "social, economic and human rights in concrete ways by providing health care, but also by addressing the social determinants of health through employment, environmental interventions, housing repair and development, a massive self-help

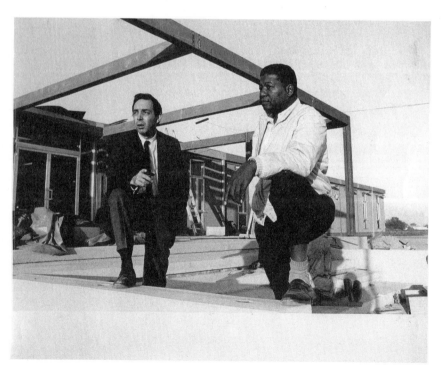

H. Jack Geiger and John Hatch at construction site of the Tufts-Delta Health Center, 1966. (H. Jack Geiger donation)

nutrition program, community organization for economic and political empowerment, and—above all—the provision of educational opportunity."[3]

Taking their cue from the civil rights movement, the Tufts team saw community organization as key to the success of their health centers. Gibson recruited Jo Disparti, who had organized the neighborhood health committees in Holmes County, to work at Columbia Point. Going door-to-door in the housing project, Disparti spread the word about the new center, identifying people to work there and to serve on the advisory board. Another seasoned organizer was John Hatch, a veteran African American activist. Hatch was born and raised in the rural South. After a three-year stint in the army he enrolled in Knoxville College and graduated in 1957 with a degree in sociology. After receiving his master's degree in social work from Atlanta University, Hatch moved to Boston and spent three years as senior community organizer for the South End Planning Council before becoming the assistant director of the Boston Housing Authority's Division of Tenant and Community Relations.[4]

As the first comprehensive community health center, Columbia Point received national attention. A visit in 1967 so impressed Senator Edward Kennedy—the Senate's champion of health care—that he secured a $51 million appropriation to the OEO budget to start up new health centers. But it was Mound Bayou that would command the most interest, in part because it was the first rural health center, and also because many Americans were familiar with the Mississippi Delta, both as a battleground in the civil rights movement and as one of the most poverty-stricken regions in the country. As soon as the Columbia Point center was on a sure footing, Disparti and Hatch headed south to begin organizing black communities in North Bolivar County.[5]

In Mound Bayou, Hatch tried to win over those people "most likely to be threatened by the proposed project." That group included medical practitioners who feared new competition, the traditional elites who had controlled Mound Bayou political and economic life for decades, and black power militants opposed to a "white" institution invading a historically black and proud community. Efforts at pacification were generally successful. According to Hatch, "our accessibility and willingness to talk probably defused several potentially explosive situations." The next step was to meet with the county residents to gather data on their problems and needs and to prepare them for the opening of the center. Hatch and a team of volunteers made house calls, then met with small groups, and finally held large community meetings that led to the formation of health associations.[6]

The Tufts-Delta Health Center, as it was formally called, finally opened its doors in November of 1967, offering free clinical health services in a remodeled parsonage. The original clinical team consisted of three doctors who came down from Tufts, five registered nurses led by Disparti, and a social worker. Geiger recruited Bob Smith and Aaron Shirley, who for a year spent two days a week in Mound Bayou, in addition to maintaining their practices in Jackson. Smith took flying lessons so that he could shorten his commute, and Shirley left Jackson at six A.M. and returned in the evening. (Shirley applied what he learned in Mound Bayou when he opened the Jackson-Hinds Comprehensive Health Center in 1970.) Within two years Geiger, the director, and his associate director John Hatch had assembled a staff of ten doctors, ten nurses, two trained midwives, plus twenty-three other professionals, including social workers, clinical technicians, a psychologist, a nutritionist, and a pharmacist. A majority of this professional staff was black and recruited from the North. During its first two years the center treated more than eight thousand patients. By 1970 thirty-two medical, nursing, and graduate students were doing their internships at the center, which also recruited personnel from the National Health Service Corps, created by Congress in 1970 to attract badly needed doctors and nurses to rural and impoverished areas.[7]

In the Mississippi Delta, a patient's basic needs went far beyond the diagnosis and treatment of illness. As one resident put it, "I've been sick sometime, always broke, sometimes hungry, and never lived in a decent house. I do believe that one begets the other." Thanks to mechanization and the government's cotton crop reduction program, demand for plantation seasonal labor had fallen by more than 75 percent between 1965 and 1967. And for the thousands of black families now without any income, the implementation of the highly touted federal food stamp program came as a cruel blow. Food stamps were to replace the commodities program, which had distributed free staples like flour, powdered milk, and eggs. The major problem with the original food stamp program was that recipients had to pay hard cash to get them. It cost a family of six twelve dollars a month for stamps, even if it had no income at all.[8]

The result was predictable. In the spring of 1967, six distinguished physicians made a tour of the Delta and were shocked by what they encountered. "In child after child" they saw "thin arms, sunken eyes, lethargic behavior [and] swollen bellies . . . homes with children who are lucky to eat one meal a day." They found children who were "fed communally— that is, by neighbors who give scraps of food to children whose own parents have nothing to give them." The panel's conclusion was grim. "We do not want to quibble over words, but 'malnutrition' is not quite what we found . . . They are suffering from hunger and disease and directly or indirectly they are dying from them—which is exactly what 'starvation' means." At the Mound Bayou health center Geiger began writing prescriptions for food. When some government bureaucrat objected to this unorthodox procedure, the physician responded, "The last time we looked in the book, the specific therapy for malnutrition was food."[9]

Prescribing food for hungry patients was a stopgap measure, and Hatch came up with the idea of a cooperative farm, where people could use their agricultural skills to grow vegetables instead of cotton. During 1968 five hundred families too poor to afford food stamps cultivated 158 acres, trading their labor for shares in the harvest. Within a short time the North Bolivar Farm Cooperative had expanded to five hundred acres, with a thousand families growing hundreds of tons of vegetables annually.[10]

The food cooperative was but one example of what made the Tufts-Delta Health Center program unique, both for its time and for ours. Where the traditional public health center dispensed pills and shots, at Mound Bayou the staff attacked the root causes of poor health and deprivation. The team of physicians touring the Delta in 1967 had found "homes without running water, without electricity, without screens, where children drink contaminated water and live with germ-bearing mosquitoes and flies everywhere around." Sanitation expert Andy James headed an environmental team at Mound Bayou that dug protected wells and built sanitary privies, put screens in windows and fumigated houses to control if not eliminate the rats and mosquitoes and other disease carriers. Helen Barnes, an obstetrician-gynecologist, directed family planning and nurse-midwifery programs, including early child care, which led to a dramatic decrease in infant mortality. The center also sponsored nutritional and social programs for senior citizens living in isolated areas, and it initiated a bus transportation system to bring people from rural communities to the clinic for treatment.[11]

The involvement and direct participation of the residents of northern Bolivar County was crucial to the center's success. Hatch had laid the groundwork by organizing the first of ten local community health associations even before the center opened. Each association would select its own officers and initiate programs, with elected delegates from each association comprising the membership of the North Bolivar County Health Council. This larger group developed programs for the entire area and had direct representation on the center's board of directors. (In 1972, the health council took over as the owner and operator of the center.) Direct participation in the decisions that affected them empowered Bolivar blacks.[12]

Perhaps the most enduring—and inspirational—aspect of the health center was its educational program. At night the doctors, nurses, and social workers taught GED high school equivalency courses. An arrangement with Mary Holmes Junior College allowed the students to get college credit for advanced courses taught by the center staff. Local people got training for such center jobs as secretaries, medical assistants, librarians, technicians, and sanitarians. Staff members used their northern contacts to place Bolivar County blacks at leading universities and professional schools. By the fall of 1970—three years after the center's opening—five local blacks were enrolled in medical schools at Tufts and the University of Wisconsin, seven were in nursing schools, three were pursuing advanced degrees in social work, four in environmental health, and one each in clinical psychology, pharmacy, and elementary education. An additional seventeen students were enrolled in undergraduate programs at colleges and universities across the country. By 1975, the health center educational program had produced seven physicians, five Ph.D.s in clinical sciences, two environmental engineers, six social workers, numerous nurses, and the first ten black registered sanitarians in Mississippi history.[13]

Of all the success stories, that of L. C. Dorsey stands out. A high school dropout who married a sharecropper, Dorsey had six children in ten years, and she brought them to the health center as soon as it opened. Dorsey liked what she saw, applied for a job, and Hatch hired her as a training associate. She helped him organize the farm cooperative and became its director in 1968. She also took advantage of the educational program, and in 1971 she enrolled at the State University of New York at Stony Brook, where she received her master's degree in social work. Dorsey returned to Mississippi to work in the criminal justice field, and then went on to earn her doctorate in public health at Howard University. In 1988 she came back to Bolivar County—as director of the Delta Health Center. She replaced Willie Lucas, another local success story. Lucas had been teaching high school chemistry in Mound Bayou when the center first opened. He told Geiger he had always wanted to be a doctor, but lacked the means to do so. Lucas recalls that Geiger "set up an interview with me at Tufts. He flew me up to Boston, and two or three weeks later I was in." After receiving his M.D. degree Lucas came back to the center as a physician, then later became its medical director. After Dorsey took over, Lucas stayed in the state to open his own practice in Greenville.[14]

The Tufts-Delta Health Center also served as a model for physicians who were eager to start up their own centers. The OEO initially gave enthusiastic support to these innovative programs. Unlike in many politically charged poverty projects, where those in charge were found guilty of mismanagement or worse, the health centers were corruption free and operated by professionals affiliated with medical schools or hospitals. Most important, they were providing free health care to thousands of impoverished citizens. The Community Action Program of OEO funded eight neighborhood health centers in 1966 and 1967, and a hundred more between 1967 and 1971 in inner cities and in isolated rural areas like Mound Bayou. The Department of Health, Education, and Welfare also got into the act, funding another fifty centers as demonstration projects.[15]

While Geiger and Gibson were MCHR members, the Medical Committee did not become directly involved in the burgeoning community health center movement. For reasons largely bureaucratic, OEO could not fund an MCHR-sponsored health center. (Most of the early centers were awarded to medical schools.) There were, however, opportunities for MCHR chapters to receive poverty funds to initiate projects. Geiger and Gibson envisioned opening "neighborhood health action centers" in northern inner cities. MCHR chapters could play a major role establishing and overseeing these centers, which would be primarily health education and advocacy agencies with a permanent staff. The two physicians met with federal officials in the middle of 1965 and reported back to the executive committee that OEO was "inviting program proposals and suggestions from MCHR." Under a proposed arrangement, OEO would fund the project through a local Community Action Program (CAP), which in turn would subcontract the program to an MCHR chapter. There was some discussion, but little enthusiasm for this idea. Some members feared cooptation by OEO, and others expressed doubts "as to whether we could really supply enough professional staff on the local level."[16]

That said, the Medical Committee deserves much of the credit for creating the climate that made the health center movement possible. Without its Freedom Summer presence in Mississippi, the Mileston clinic as a model, and the Greenville meeting attended by a half-dozen MCHR activists, it is questionable whether the community health center concept would have emerged as it did and when it did. And while MCHR itself did not commit its resources to this program, members like Des Callan and Mike Holloman went on to found and direct community health centers of their own.[17]

By the early 1970s, the federal government's enthusiasm for health centers was waning. During the Nixon years the program was transferred to HEW, while funding was reduced for the Medicare and Medicaid programs. At Columbia Point, the local health council assumed direct management of the center in 1972. The Delta Health Center, now under local control, persevered, although beset by political infighting and funding cuts that forced a cutback in social programming. Nationally the community health centers survived the 1970s and expanded their coverage in the decades that followed.[18]

Health care reformers recognized that community health centers were no substitute for a national health program, and when a movement got under way in the late 1960s to provide government-funded universal national health insurance, a lively debate ensued. Not surprisingly MCHR activists were ready to jump into the fray with their own proposals.

The United States was the only industrial country without a national health program covering all its citizens. Back in 1883, Chancellor Otto Von Bismarck sponsored the Sickness and Insurance Act, a law providing medical coverage for German workers and their families. Other European countries followed suit, with the National Health Service in Great Britain the most ambitious in scope. In America, Progressive Era reformers talked of providing insurance for workers, but it was not until the mid-1920s that the United States began to give serious attention to the problem. Then a physician named Ray Lyman Wilbur chaired a blue ribbon Committee on the Cost of Medical Care (CCMC), an independent group of fifteen economists, physicians, and public health specialists. Over the next five years, the CCMC issued twenty-seven research papers "providing the most detailed information yet assembled on medical care in America." Its final report, published in 1932 in the midst of the Great Depression, advocated group practice and group payment for medical care, and called for voluntary, not compulsory, health insurance. No fire-breathing radical, Wilbur had been president of Stanford University, Herbert Hoover's secretary of the interior, and a past president of the AMA. But his ideas met with almost unanimous opposition from mainstream physicians, who denounced the plan as "socialism and communism" and as "an incitement to revolution."[19]

The furor over the CCMC report helped persuade the administration of Franklin D. Roosevelt to delete a national health insurance component from its Social Security bill. Just to be sure, early in 1935 the AMA called a special meeting of its House of Delegates to condemn compulsory health insurance, agreeing to consider voluntary programs only if they were under the control of the AMA and its state affiliates. During World War II a group of liberal senators tried unsuccessfully to amend the Social Security act to include health coverage. FDR had indicated he would push for national health insurance once the war had ended, and his successor, Harry S Truman, took up the challenge. Truman's federal security administrator, Oscar Ewing, declared that the United States "must provide that all people shall have access to such health and medical services as they require, through a system of insurance covering the entire population." The program would be financed by up to a 4 percent increase in the Social Security tax on payrolls, and administered by the states, with the federal government acting only as the collecting and disbursing agent. Truman insisted his bill was not "socialized medicine." Patients could choose their doctors, and physicians would be free to join the plan or not.[20]

Once again, critics of government-sponsored health insurance came out in force. The AMA assessed each member twenty-five dollars to employ a public relations firm to organize a campaign to defeat the bill. The Cold War had just begun to heat up, and AMA lobbyists wasted no time in linking national health insurance to the menace of international communism. One pamphlet read: "Would socialized medicine lead to socialization of other phases of American life? . . . Lenin thought so." Senator Robert A. Taft, "Mr. Republican," declared, "I consider [this bill] the most socialistic measure this Congress ever had before it." Although it debated the proposal several times during the Truman years, Congress never made a serious effort to pass a comprehensive health insurance law.[21]

Given that polls always showed a majority of Americans supporting national health insurance, why did efforts to enact it always fail? In his influential book *The Social Transformation of American Medicine*, Paul Starr argues that while America is thought to be a less ideological society than Europe, the debate over health insurance was intensely ideological here (but not there). Moreover, although a majority of Americans said they wanted national health insurance, they were uncertain as to what kind, and the AMA and its lobbyists were able to exploit this uncertainty to undercut public support. (This pattern repeated in the 1990s. The "Harry and Louise" television advertising campaign, for example, effectively raised doubts about the Clinton administration's health care program.) Finally, Starr notes that there "was a gross imbalance in resources—partly material, partly social, partly symbolic." The AMA spent $2.5 million in 1950 to defeat the Truman plan, while the leading advocacy group, the Committee for the Nation's Health, could muster only $36,000. The pharmaceutical companies and insurance corporations also poured their resources into the AMA-led campaign. Class divisions were important, with poor and working-class people supporting the legislation, while wealthier individuals (who were satisfied with the care they received) and powerful federations like the National Association of Manufacturers and the U.S. Chamber of Commerce opposed it. Add to this the postwar "red scare," with its fear and loathing of all things socialistic, and the defeat of the Truman health care program was not just predictable, it was inevitable.[22]

Fifteen years later, Lyndon Johnson thwarted another attack by the AMA and its allies, persuading Congress to provide health insurance for people sixty-five and older under Medicare and for indigent people under Medicaid. Why this partial victory in the struggle for national health insurance after a half century of failure? Inspired by the civil rights movement and moved by revelations of widespread poverty (chronicled in Michael Harrington's bestselling *The Other America*), voters in 1964 elected representatives to Congress who, over the next two years, enacted sweeping progressive legislation as part of President Johnson's Great Society initiative. The only other significant period of liberal reform had occurred in 1935–1936, when overwhelming New Deal majorities had pushed through Social Security and labor and banking-reform laws. In each instance reformers had little time to savor their success, as backlash set in, with conservatives in Congress determined to turn the clock back. Ironically, it was in the midst of the revolt against the Great Society agenda that support for some form of national health insurance surfaced again, this time from the right as well as the left.

Undoubtedly, Medicare and Medicaid were providing better care for millions of senior citizens and poor people. The problem was—and still is—that millions of working people under age sixty-five had no coverage, and health care costs were skyrocketing. Here are a few quick statistics: The growth rate in the cost of medical services rose from 3.2 percent per year in the years before Medicare to 7.9 percent annually after passage of the law. Per capita health expenditures, which had increased from $142 to $198 between 1960 and 1965, shot up to $336 by 1970. Most patients did not feel the crunch immediately, because medical expenses paid by third parties—private insurance and government programs—went up from 45 to 67 percent between 1960 and 1975. Government's share of the health expenses during that period rose at a rate of 20.8 percent, from $10.8 billion to $27.8 billion.[23]

The greater number of Americans covered, along with expensive new medical technology, increased health care costs. However, the Medicare program also had structural flaws that contributed to the taxpayer's burden while enriching the providers. For example, Medicare did not impose a fee rate on doctors; instead, it paid them according to their "customary" fees. Younger doctors, with no track record, billed at unprecedented levels, and they were paid. Older doctors then followed suit, with the result being rampant inflation. Under a fee-for-service payment system, the more services provided, the more fees, and both doctors and hospitals exploited the system. According to Starr, studies revealed that not only were Americans having unnecessary operations, as many as one fifth of the patients in hospitals did not need to be there. By the late sixties each city had its example of physicians and health care institutions like nursing homes "making small fortunes off government programs through inflated reimbursements or outright fraud." By 1968, three years after the enactment of Medicare, the situation had become so serious that reformers began to look for a health care plan that would provide better coverage without bankrupting the federal treasury.[24]

Walter Reuther, head of the United Auto Workers, put out the call for a comprehensive national health insurance program in an address to the American Public Health Association in November of 1968. The labor leader noted the paradox that while "we are the richest nation [and] have the highest level of medical competence, America ranks 21st among the nations of the world in life expectancy for males and 12th for females," and 16th in the rate of infant mortality. With an estimated eighty million Americans lacking adequate health care, nearly 40 percent of the population, Reuther maintained that instead of a health care system "what we have, in fact, is a disorganized, disjoined, obsolete nonsystem of health care." He then announced the formation of a Committee of 100 for National Health Insurance to lobby for a comprehensive program. Members included medical school deans, black activists Whitney Young, Coretta Scott King, and Ralph Abernathy, senators Ted Kennedy and John Sherman Cooper, and public intellectuals like economist John Kenneth Galbraith. MCHR activists Mike Holloman, David French, Jack Geiger, and George Wilson were members of Reuther's group, as were SHO leaders

Fitzhugh Mullan and Lambert King. The subsequent national discussion over health care led to a number of specific proposals submitted by Senator Kennedy, the AMA, the Nixon administration—and the Medical Committee for Human Rights.[25]

MCHR entered the health care debate in late 1967 with a full-page ad in the *New York Times* attacking the AMA and its president, Dr. Milford O. Rouse. The Bible-thumping, sixty-four-year-old Sunday school teacher from Dallas was a former director of the right-wing Life Line Foundation, the brainchild of Texas billionaire H. L. Hunt. Rouse had used his inaugural speech at the 1967 AMA convention to warn delegates that "the system of medicine . . . is now threatened . . . by those who advocate central government planning and coercion in the field of medicine." Angry about increased government intervention (he did not mention Medicare specifically), price and wage fixing, attacks on the drug industry, and an "emphasis on a nonprofit approach to medicine," Rouse found particularly alarming "the concept of health care as a right rather than a privilege." In the *Times* advertisement, under the banner headline "WE CHALLENGE THE A.M.A.," MCHR declared that "HEALTH IS A HUMAN RIGHT, basic, universal and non-partisan, which all movements for human progress must encompass," and, without getting into specifics, called for "prepaid, comprehensive health care for all."[26]

The Medical Committee sensed that the once all-powerful AMA was vulnerable, for it had been taking negative positions on important health programs. The group had spent millions of dollars opposing the popular Medicare bill, and its president denounced the highly regarded comprehensive community health centers as "unnecessary and wasteful." Following the U.S. surgeon general's warning of links between smoking and cancer in 1964, the AMA accepted a $10 million research grant from six tobacco companies and publicly condemned the government proposal to place a health warning label on cigarette packages. Opposition to programs that were winning high ratings from the general public was costing the AMA support among physicians as well, with membership declining significantly in the late 1960s. By taking on the AMA in the "newspaper of record," MCHR was sending a signal that it wanted to be included in the national debate over the direction of health care in this country.[27]

The *Times* advertisement marked the beginning of a campaign by Quentin Young and other activists to revitalize MCHR's national office, which had been little more than a clearinghouse for the local chapters. By 1970 the organization was beginning to reassert itself. The demise of the

Student Health Organizations intensified recruitment efforts in medical schools and public hospitals to attract interns, residents, and nurses. Membership increased to about six thousand, while the number of chapters rose to thirty-one. A hardworking and successful fund-raiser, Young got grants from the United Auto Workers and the New York Foundation, and a donation from artist Georgia O'Keeffe. The singer James Taylor wrote a check for ten thousand dollars. Luke Wilson gave MCHR one hundred shares of Woodward and Lothrop stock. And veteran members of the organization renewed their financial support now that the organization was once again showing signs of life.[28]

The 1971 national convention in Philadelphia had as its theme "The Consumer and Health Care." The gathering drew substantial numbers of women, blacks, nonprofessional health workers, and consumers, whose demands for representation resulted in an expanded national governing council that reflected this diversity. (See chapter 11.) The delegates agreed that the Medical Committee should have a strong national office, one that could develop its own programs in conjunction with the chapter affiliates. Two years after his first term ended, Young was again elected chairman, and at his urging the national office moved from Philadelphia to Chicago, (where he lived) with the addition of two full-time staff members. Frank Goldsmith, who had worked for the UAW, became the national organizer, and Patricia Murchie the executive secretary. Finally, with momentum building across the country for medical reform, convention delegates pledged to "fight the makers of our present health care catastrophe and to bring the issues to the health care consumer." The following month the executive council announced the beginning of a National Health Crusade to promote a comprehensive health care program that was more far-reaching than the proposals being debated in the U.S. Congress.[29]

Shortly after taking office, and with Medicare on his mind, Richard Nixon warned that "we face a massive crisis" in the area of health care. "Unless action is taken within the next two or three years," the president predicted, "we will have a breakdown in the medical system." From the vantage point of the twenty-first century, it is somewhat astonishing to see that not only was health care reform a significant issue during Nixon's first term, but that there existed a widely held assumption that passage of some kind of national health insurance program was likely. Of the many proposals, the AMA produced the most conservative. Called "Medicredit," it provided for tax credits for people voluntarily purchasing private insurance. Those who paid federal income tax under three hundred dollars would receive free coverage, those with higher incomes would receive tax credits to pay for part of their private health insurance, and Medicaid would remain for those who paid no taxes and Medicare for those sixty-five and over. The AMA plan, then, would use federal tax dollars to subsidize private health insurance. It would be voluntary and coverage would be limited, with significant out-of-pocket expenses for most people. Medicredit left the medical establishment intact, with no cost controls or new administrative apparatus. Although conservative, this plan was "a quantum leap ideologically and medical-socially for the AMA."[30]

Nixon's major concern was to keep the rapidly increasing medical costs under control. At the heart of his plan was the creation of health maintenance organizations. Individuals or families would enroll in HMOs, paying a fixed amount for an itemized list of health care services. The HMOs would compete with one another for customers, and ideally through competition and bargaining they would use the free market to bring down the cost of medical care. The idea of prepaid group practice (as opposed to fee-for-service) had long been denounced by conservatives. Now, as Paul Starr wryly observed, it seemed as though "the socialized medicine of one era had become the corporate reform of the next." Nixon began funding HMO start-ups even before legislation passed Congress. In 1971, thirty HMOs were in operation and the administration's goal was to have seventeen hundred HMOs by 1976, enrolling forty million Americans.[31]

The health maintenance organizations pleased neither the AMA nor liberals, who were particularly uncomfortable with the idea that HMOs set up as for-profit corporations could make more money by rationing medical services. In addition, the Nixon plan called on employers to provide some health benefits. The millions of Americans who could not afford health insurance would fall under Nixon's Family Health Insurance Program (FHIP), which was more complicated than Medicredit but similar in that tax revenues would be used to buy private health insurance policies for low-income people. Benefits for those who were voluntarily enrolled in FHIP were limited, allowing only eight doctor visits a year, thirty days of hospital care, and no payments for drugs or dental care. Nixon's proposal to help finance his plan by cutting funding for Medicare also drew fire from health care activists, who noted that the president's plan would still leave from twenty to forty million Americans uninsured.[32]

Several proposals, including those by New Yorkers Nelson Rockefeller and Jacob Javits, were more generous than the AMA or Nixon plans, but by 1971 the one garnering the most popular support was the bill introduced by Senator Edward Kennedy and representatives Martha Griffiths and James Gorman. Supported by the Committee for National Health Insurance and by major labor unions, the proposed Health Security Act (more commonly known as the Kennedy bill) offered free, comprehensive health care to all Americans. Services included unlimited hospital, physician, optometrist, and podiatrist care; home health care; X-rays and laboratory tests; and limited nursing home care, drug prescriptions, psychiatric, and dental care. The patient would pay no insurance premiums or incur out-of-pocket expenses. The system would be financed nationally through a new Health Security Trust Fund, with half the money coming from general tax revenue. The other half would be raised by social security payroll taxes on employers and to a lesser extent on employees. Patients would choose their own physicians. A Health Security Board would control all medical costs, establish a national budget, allocate funds to different regions of the country, and require private hospitals and physicians to operate within the regional budget. Nonprofit prepaid HMOs would be encouraged, but fee-for-service payments could still be made to independent physicians. If enacted, the Kennedy bill would replace all public and private health plans. Insurance companies like Blue Cross could still exist, but at best would play a minor role as a fiscal intermediary if so requested by doctors.[33]

In the midst of the spring 1971 debate in Congress and in the media over the merits of the various health insurance proposals, the Medical Committee for Human Rights, believing it could play a unique role, launched its campaign to educate the American public. In early June the national office distributed a leaflet with the headline AWAKE AMERICANS!! THE NATIONAL HEALTH CRUSADE IS COMING YOUR WAY. MCHR members in all chapters were to engage in "leafleting, canvassing door-to-door, polling/petitioning their neighbors and friends to bring pressure for quality health care on a national scale." The campaign was launched at a national press conference on June 15, and volunteers spent the day distributing the first leaflet—"it is of high quality and of great organizational use"—at schools, shopping centers, hospitals, and other public locations. This pattern was to be repeated throughout the summer, with new leaflets and additional press conferences.[34]

The Medical Committee took the position that all the proposed health care measures were unacceptable. The AMA and Nixon plans both left millions of Americans uninsured, and held patients with insurance responsible for out-of-pocket payments up front that many could not afford. There were no effective controls in place. Drug companies, hospitals, and insurance companies would operate as they had before, only with an influx of federal dollars to swell their profits. As one MCHR spokesman put it, "the ruling class is figuring out how to give the people a little national health insurance, while giving itself a lot of profits."

At first glance, it appeared that MCHR should endorse the Kennedy bill. It covered the entire population, it was "free," and there would be a national Health Security Board to oversee the allocation of funds to health care providers. Young called the Kennedy bill "far and away the best one offered." And yet MCHR opposed this liberal proposal as well, in large part because of its regressive funding system. For the health care radicals, what this country needed was not national health insurance but a national health service.[35]

The architect and major publicist of the MCHR plan was a young physician named Thomas Bodenheimer. A 1965 graduate of Harvard Medical School, Bodenheimer served as a physician in the Peace Corps in Costa Rica before returning to get his master's degree in public health at Berkeley. In 1971, while doing his residency at San Francisco State Hospital, Bodenheimer wrote extensively about the competing health insurance proposals. With two other San Francisco health care workers he wrote and edited a 128-page book (in inexpensive magazine format) called *Billions for Band-Aids*, a series of essays that attacked the Nixon and Kennedy plans, the HMOs (referred to as "Profit Maintenance Organizations"), drug manufacturers, and insurance companies. The book concluded with the *MCHR Position Paper on National Health Care*.[36]

Bodenheimer recalls that "it probably took me a day to write the [MCHR] national health care program." It provided complete, comprehensive, and preventive health care for all Americans, with no charges for any services. To pay for this expansion in coverage, Congress would enact a new progressive tax on total wealth. This plan would end profit-making in health care. All health care workers, including physicians, would be salaried employees of the government. The new system would eliminate health insurance companies and private drug manufacturers. (A federal nonprofit corporation would develop, produce, and distribute all drugs and medical supplies.) All schooling for health care students would be free, with steps taken to increase the number of health care workers on all levels. Racial minorities and women would be represented "in proportion to their numbers in the general population."

Finally, all health care institutions would be run by consumers (patients) and by "those who work in the institution." These boards were to be both institutional and regional, with consumers always in the majority. They would set policy, hire all employees, and allocate the budget, which would be determined by a regional consumer-worker board. Just what role, if any, federal government agencies and Congress would play in the administration of these institutions was not spelled out. Bodenheimer later summed up the MCHR plan as "single payer plus national health service. But it wasn't the British National Health Service. It was a community-worker controlled national health service."[37]

At the heart of the MCHR plan to restructure health care in America were the neighborhood community health centers, with the Tufts-Delta Health Center in Mound Bayou and urban health centers serving as models. Every designated community (up to 25,000 in the cities, fewer people in rural areas) would have a health center. It would provide a wide range of treatment for all citizens, not just the poor, including preventive, educational, social, and rehabilitative services, as well as transportation, child care, and home visits. Each community health center would be connected to a general hospital for hospitalization or specialized treatment, with that hospital in turn linked with regional specialty hospitals to handle difficult medical problems. "Every doctor in the country should be working in these kinds of institutions," declared Bodenheimer. "This will distribute the doctors to where they should be, and organize medical care in a rational kind of way." MCHR planners were influenced by the experiences of European countries, including the British National Health Service, and by health care delivery systems in the third world, particularly those in China and Cuba.[38]

The MCHR analysis of the shortcomings in the health care "nonsystem" has special resonance: we are facing the same problems today. By 2008 an estimated forty-seven million people, more than 18 percent of the nonelderly population, had no health insurance, Medicare and Medicaid costs were continuing to rise dramatically, and pharmaceutical manufacturers and insurance companies remained free to run their institutions in such a manner as to guarantee high prices and profits, with exorbitant salaries for their CEOs. The MCHR national health service proposal promised to eliminate capitalism in the health care world: no more private drug manufacturers, insurance companies, private hospitals, or physicians setting their own fees. Aside from the lack of details, the major drawback to the MCHR health care plan was that it had absolutely no chance of being enacted by Congress. Such an audacious reform was impossible in the

1970s, and in the decades that followed. Caught up in the revolutionary spirit of the times, the radical MCHR activists had simply lost touch with reality. With the mainstream liberal community united behind the Kennedy bill, only a few political leaders (including California congressman Ron Dellums) took the MCHR plan seriously. The AMA simply refused to speak on the same platform with MCHR, maintaining that it would only debate participants representing proposals "that have been introduced into Congress or proposals of which introduction into Congress seems imminent." (Later, both the architect of the MCHR national health service proposal and the organization's chairman had second thoughts about the course of action MCHR took during the earlier debate over health care. Tom Bodenheimer now believes that "we made this horrible mistake of saying, 'The Kennedy bill is a piece of crap.' We should have supported the Kennedy bill." Quentin Young concurs. The Physicians for a National Health Program, of which he was a cofounder, advocates a program for national health insurance that is closely modeled after the Kennedy bill.)[39]

Without a viable product to market, the National Health Crusade never really got off the ground. Despite the exhortations of the national office staff in Chicago, the individual chapters largely ignored it. Just the idea of distributing leaflets at shopping centers and department stores was off-putting to a number of MCHR members. Others resented the public relations effort, which smacked of Madison Avenue. (One communication urged members to distribute the leaflets "as soon as possible so your friends and neighbors can Sign Up for quality health care!") And finally, for those chapters that did take the National Health Crusade seriously, the question remained: Once we educate and mobilize people in our communities, what are we going to ask them to do? The Medical Committee did not want people to lobby their congressional representatives, because it opposed all the bills under consideration, including the Kennedy bill. Not only was the MCHR proposal not "legislatively viable," it was not even up for consideration. (In 1974 Representative Dellums introduced a bill similar to the MCHR plan, but nothing came of his efforts.) MCHR representatives did testify later in the year at the House Ways and Means Committee hearings on health legislation, and sent fifty thousand copies of a letter supporting its program from congressional representative Shirley Chisholm of New York, but by the end of 1971 the National Health Crusade had succeeded mainly as a means of recruiting new members and attracting media attention. Critics inside MCHR believed, perhaps unfairly, that this was the goal of the leadership all along. "Instead of asking what MCHR could do for a national health care plan, MCHR instead asked what a national health care plan could do for it."[40]

If the National Health Crusade was a failure, so were the efforts to achieve any kind of national insurance legislation during 1972. Although the AMA's influence had weakened somewhat, it still had powerful allies in the drug and insurance industries, both of which would have been adversely affected had the Kennedy bill become law. Since there was no consensus on a single program, opponents were able to employ the tried-and-true tactics of divide and conquer. In 1971 numerous political observers had predicted that health care would be a major issue, if not *the* major issue in the 1972 presidential campaign. It didn't turn out that way. The Vietnam War and how to end it became a central issue, and President Nixon's surprise trip to China captured and diverted the nation's attention. In the end, there was no grassroots campaign to demand that Congress take action. Health care first became an issue when leaders in the government and in the medical community became alarmed over increasing costs. Once they decided to defer action on the matter to an unspecified future date, there was no consumer movement in place to demand that they take action. It would be another twenty years before health care again became a major national issue, and then the administration of Bill Clinton would find the enemies of national health insurance still too powerful to overcome. During the first decade of the twenty-first century the health care system was once again high on the political agenda, particularly among Democrats. But still fearing the charge of "socialized medicine," party leaders refused to endorse a comprehensive, single-payer program.

Many inside MCHR had hoped that the campaign for a national health care system would do what the civil rights movement had done earlier: provide the organization with a single programmatic focus that would attract the loyalty and dedication of an enthusiastic member base. That did not happen. The Medical Committee had achieved renewed vitality as the public debate over health care intensified. Once again it was a player. But when universal health care subsided as a pressing public issue, MCHR had no other national program around which to rally its increasingly diverse constituency, so it turned once again to organizing on the local level. This time, however, activists formed task forces designed to coordinate common activities throughout the country.

*   *   *

The most ambitious of these groups was the task force on occupational health. Even though conditions in the workplace caused fifteen thousand deaths and more than a million illnesses and injuries in a typical year, the medical profession had neglected the field of occupational health, virtually excluding the subject from the medical school curriculum. MCHR accelerated its work in this area after passage of the Occupational Safety and Health Act of 1970 (OSHA). First proposed by Lyndon Johnson in his last State of the Union address and signed into law by a reluctant Richard Nixon, OSHA established an enforcement agency to investigate working conditions in plants and businesses and require offenders to comply with standards set by the federal government. The problem was that the officials whose job it was to carry out the law were extremely reluctant to do so. Two MCHR physicians, Phyllis Cullen of Denver and Donald Whorton from Washington, hit upon the idea of holding a series of conferences involving health care professionals, labor leaders and rank-and-file members, and environmentalists. Their purpose was to generate interest and activity in occupational health and to talk with workers about the hazards they faced in the workplace from dust, gas, noise, radiation, solvents, and heat.[41]

The first conference was a successful collaboration involving the Medical Committee, the University of Illinois Medical School, and the United Auto Workers. Held in Chicago in early 1972, the meeting attracted health care activists and union members. The workers talked about their jobs and the risks they faced, while the doctors discussed the causes and elimination of workplace hazards. Speakers also pointed out the need for agitation to get OSHA to do its job. MCHR participants, always conscious of their status as members of an elite profession, enjoyed this event, where "burly, close-shaven steel mill workers [were] seen mixing amiably with shaggy, bearded medical students." A reporter noted that "the disparate members of the audience seemed to have forgotten their usual animosities in behalf of a common cause."[42]

Encouraged by the response in Chicago, Cullen and Whorton took their show on the road, holding conferences in communities where a dominant industry created widespread health hazards. Thus, in Houston, sessions focused on problems of workers in the oil industry, a meeting in Kentucky dealt with black lung disease in coal miners, and the conference in Durham concerned brown lung disease among cotton mill workers. Occupational health became such a popular program that the task force was able to employ a full-time staff member, Don Berman, who had worked on health issues with the Teamsters in St. Louis. Soon it was publishing a newsletter and churning out booklets and pamphlets that described health care problems in language that nonspecialists could understand.[43]

But problems in communication and logistics developed between the staff of the task force and the national MCHR office, and funding difficulties arose in late 1972. Dan Berman informed members that although labor unions had initially been enthusiastic about cooperating with MCHR, they had contributed only three thousand dollars, far less than the task force needed to survive as a national operation. In some cities MCHR radicals alienated local labor leaders by making direct appeals to union members that included disparaging remarks about the conservative nature of the union leadership. All this led Berman to conclude that it "was unlikely that the unions will be funding the project."[44]

The occupational health project was only one of several MCHR task forces designed to coordinate common activities throughout the country. Big city chapters campaigned to eliminate lead poisoning by lobbying Congress to pass laws outlawing lead in paint, publicizing the problem in their area, and screening children for the disease. Affiliates in Philadelphia, Boston, Detroit, Chicago, and Seattle worked with African American health organizations to screen blacks for sickle cell disease, which had only recently come to the nation's attention.[45]

One of MCHR's most popular causes was prison reform. After the riot at the state penitentiary in Attica, New York, in September of 1971, where a police assault resulted in the deaths of twenty-nine inmates and ten hostages, MCHR intensified efforts to develop a "National Prison Health Program" to "upgrade health services and conditions" in penal institutions. Prisoners should be entitled to health care as a right, enjoying the same constitutional guarantee as their access to legal services. MCHR also wanted to end "the selective use of prison medicine as a form of punishment," which meant that responsibility for medical care had to be taken from prison authorities to an independent health team. MCHR chapters instituted prison programs in eighteen cities. The projects did not achieve their lofty goals, but they did help raise public awareness about conditions in the prisons.[46]

Other groups formed to support women's health issues, including the right to an abortion. (MCHR began its agitation several years before *Roe v. Wade*.) By the early 1970s there were strong women's health movements in most cities where MCHR was operating, and the organization's primary function was to assist these groups. Boston MCHR formed an Abortion

Counseling Committee to help women desiring to terminate their pregnancies. This program led to the opening of women's clinics in Somerville, Jamaica Plain, and Cambridge. Medical Committee activists also participated in the Boston women's collective, which wrote *Our Bodies, Our Selves,* the guide to women's health that sold two hundred thousand copies in its first two years, millions thereafter, and over the next three decades was translated into seventeen languages.[47]

Task forces lobbied to liberalize drug laws, and to defend the rights of patients, including mental patients. Bill Bronston and other volunteers from New York were active in the campaign against Willowbrook State Hospital, where the medical staff infected mentally retarded children with hepatitis so that they might gauge the effects of gamma globulin in combating the disease. (MCHR members were among those staging protests at the 1972 convention of the American College of Physicians, which was presenting an award to Dr. Saul Krugman, the physician in charge of the hepatitis research project.) After a long lobbying campaign by Walter Lear, MCHR took a stand in support of gay rights at its 1972 convention, condemning the widely held view in the medical profession that homosexuality was a mental disorder.[48]

The Medical Committee continued its work in occupational health projects, in prisons, and in other programs (such as sickle cell and lead poisoning) through the mid-seventies, but after 1972 these were largely independent efforts, with little support from the national MCHR. For in addition to their internal problems, the task forces were affected by the steps taken at the 1971 national convention to broaden MCHR's constituency. That meeting in Philadelphia proved to be among the most important in the Medical Committee's history, setting the stage for its long and painful final act.

CHAPTER II

Years of Decline

A lthough MCHR had attracted young health professionals since its founding, established male physicians had always constituted its leadership. In the late sixties, as older members dropped out for a variety of reasons, more medical students, nurses, interns, and residents came in. As an organization of the New Left, the Medical Committee had to respond to the women and minorities who had always been underrepresented in the organization's membership and who were now seeking a substantial share of the leadership positions. Women led the charge in Philadelphia, presenting a list of demands that a few years earlier would have been dismissed out of hand by their male elders.

The "Statement of the Women's Caucus" asserted that "men have a vested interest in our old form of leadership. Because of the understanding growing from our oppression as women, we have a unique perspective and responsibility in creation of new forms of organization and leadership." Here, women in MCHR were reflecting the concerns already expressed by their counterparts in SNCC and SDS. That organizations founded on egalitarian principles assigned second-class status to members based solely on physical characteristics was a sad fact in virtually all leftist groups, and it was particularly pervasive in medical organizations, where the male physician had long stood as a symbol of power and entitlement.

The caucus nominated women to fill three of the four national offices, and called for the expansion of MCHR's governing body, the National Executive Council (NEC), to include women from each region. The caucus made it clear that "nominees for the Women's Slate have agreed to run as a unit. They all will serve, or none will serve." These women were making it clear they would not accept token representation. The Third World Caucus followed suit, demanding that one fourth of all officers be people of color and that MCHR employ a full-time organizer to recruit blacks and other minorities. Despite some grumbling in the ranks that members "should work their way up and serve on the basis of ability, not sex or color," the convention endorsed both caucus reports. Three of the four national officers were women (Quentin Young, now in his late forties, was elected chair), and of the new twenty-six-member NEC, sixteen were women and six were black—none of whom was a physician. Only six doctors served on the new board. The Medical Committee had determined to eliminate sexism and racism from its ranks. The result, according to one critic, "was an elaborate structure that was to prove as unwieldy and dysfunctional as it was superficially democratic." On the other hand, MCHR stood alone among medical organizations in its commitment to its women and African American members.[1]

A number of the women and blacks attending the national convention were political activists from outside the field of health care. They demanded that the "elitist" MCHR expand its constituency to include them and the people they claimed to represent. In response, the organization's leaders agreed to transform MCHR into a mass organization "incorporating all strata of health workers and of consumers as well." A Health-PAC report later observed that

> *MCHR* was to be the radical health vehicle of both the doctor and the dishwasher, the medical student and the ward clerk, the administrator and the consumer, the privileged and the poor, the Third World and the white, the man and the woman. In short, there was no one who was not part of MCHR's newly defined constituency. MCHR would no longer simply serve the vanguard—MCHR would *be* the vanguard by shedding its skin and wishing itself a new one.

The decisions made in Philadelphia did, for a time, inject new life into MCHR. With Young at the helm raising money from foundations, labor unions, and wealthy individuals, MCHR's coffers swelled. The Chicago office became something of a propaganda mill, churning out leaflets, broadsides, and two internal newsletters. *Health Rights News*, which had suspended publication for lack of funds, now appeared monthly, with a new upbeat tone celebrating the organization's rapid expansion.[2]

The campaign for new members had produced results. In 1970, MCHR figures showed 6,000 members in twenty-six chapters. A year later the journal *Science* reported that MCHR claimed "some 20,000 members in 40 local chapters across the country," and in 1972 Young told reporters that the number of chapters had risen to seventy-four. The Medical Committee had experienced substantial growth in 1971 and in the early part of 1972, but the numbers are both debatable and misleading. In a report prepared for the NEC meeting in August of 1971, staff member Frank Goldsmith revealed that the claim that MCHR had "an active membership of approximately 6,000 to 7,000" was not verifiable because "there has not been a national dues billing for 18 months and national contact with local membership drives has been next to nil." When dues notices went out in the fall of 1971 they netted only 950 paid responses. Chapter growth figures were even more suspect. In his organizational report for that year Goldsmith listed fifty-three cities with chapters, but forty-one of these had fewer than ten members. After boasting of the formation of the fifty-third chapter, Goldsmith was forced to admit that it consisted of three people—who had not even met one another![3]

The national office's public relations campaign celebrating expansion masked an internal conflict with a number of the older chapters in cities like Boston, Los Angeles, and New York. Members there chafed at the bureaucratic, top-down operation of Young and his staff, of which the National Health Crusade was a prime example. Minor matters of miscommunication escalated into name-calling. When the officers in Chicago determined that the New York chapter was withholding that portion of its members' dues designated for the national office, executive secretary Pat Murchie wrote a blistering letter accusing New York of "hostile and uncomradly [sic] activity," and demanded "in a comradly way for you to pay your rebates." If they did not, she threatened, "none of the New York people will receive *Health Rights News* or the national mailings." When it turned out that New York had in fact paid its dues, Young wrote a sheepish apology, but the damage had been done. In late 1971, when the Los Angeles chapter was experiencing an "internal struggle," its NEC representative, Helena van Raan, accused Goldsmith of taking sides, disregarding her warning that the national office should stay out. Many in the big-city chapters also resented the decision to recruit consumers into MCHR. Since 1964 they had operated as an organization of professionals, and while most saw the need to attract more midlevel health care workers, they took pride in their identity as a medical organization. The national office responded with a report that evaluated chapters by a list of criteria including sexism, racism, and professional dominance, and, not surprisingly, the older chapters were found guilty on each count. If a local chapter was reluctant to recruit consumers, this was prima facie evidence of sexism or racism.[4]

A fascinating example of the latter occurred when the Medical Committee sent a delegation to the People's Republic of China. The practice of medicine in socialist countries had long been of interest to MCHR members, and several had visited Cuba, the Soviet Union, and Eastern Europe. Travel to "Red China" had always been illegal, but a thaw in relations made it possible for educational groups to tour the country at the invitation of the Chinese government. When MCHR learned that it could send a delegation, members expressed keen interest in the trip. Chairperson Young declared that "only members (for at least six months and current dues paid)" would be eligible. The national office chose a selection committee exclusively from the Chicago area. There were the usual problems of miscommunication, but the real trouble began when an independent group with no previous ties to the New York chapter started an MCHR branch at Columbia Presbyterian Medical Center. They then nominated Dr. Calvin H. Sinnette, clinical professor of pediatrics at Columbia, to be a New York representative on the China delegation.

The black scholar seemed an ideal candidate. His extensive writing on disease in African countries, as well as his serving as Malcolm X's personal physician, would be of interest to his Chinese hosts. The problem was that Sinnette had never been active in MCHR, was not even a member, and had made it clear that he would not speak to groups on behalf of the Medical Committee when he returned. Noting that Sinnette did not meet the national office guidelines, the New York chapter declined to recommend him. But the selection committee in Chicago chose Sinnette anyway, claiming he had the endorsement of the Third World Caucus. New York vehemently objected to the arbitrary selection process. Former MCHR chair Eli Messinger wanted to be part of the delegation—"I thought I deserved to go"—and when he was not selected he took it as "a big personal affront." In defense of Sinnette's selection, Third World Caucus representatives Ann Garland (also MCHR treasurer) and Gwen Smith wrote an angry letter labeling the New Yorkers' protests "an example of the illusions brought on by typical ego-tripping of so-called intellectuals . . . Isn't it time Third World people decide their own destiny?" they asked. "Is this too much for 'white radicals' to stand? Make up your mind, New

York, as to whether or not you are racists." Garland and Smith concluded that "it is blatantly apparent to us third worlders that New York does not want a black doctor on the trip to China."[5]

In late June, Walter Lear led the delegation of sixteen people on a tour of health facilities and services in China. In addition to Sinnette, the group included MCHR officers Ann Garland and Kay Fitts and executive secretary Pat Murchie. What had promised to be a feather in MCHR's cap (Richard Nixon did not make the trip until later in the year) resulted only in increasing the acrimony between the older chapters and the national office led by Young, Goldsmith, and Murchie. Before the year was out Murchie and Goldsmith would be gone, and Young would relinquish his dominant role in the organization.[6]

If there was a defining moment in the decline of the Medical Committee for Human Rights it was Quentin Young's decision shortly after his reelection as national chair in April of 1972 to become chief of medicine at Cook County Hospital. Some in the Chicago office were dismayed at Young's action, correctly assuming that the prospects for maintaining a strong national presence were slim without his day-to-day leadership. A founding member of the Medical Committee, Young had been a stabilizing force in an organization increasingly beset by sectarian infighting. He was its major fund-raiser, using his vast personal contacts (and his own money) to put MCHR back on a sound footing. Perhaps the failure of the

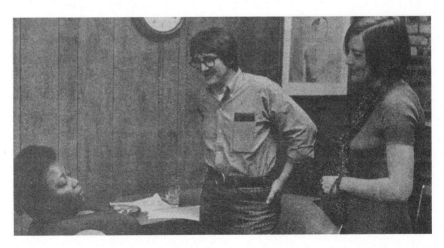

Ann Garland, Quentin Young, and Felicia Hance, Chicago MCHR office, 1972. (Institute of Social Medicine and Community Health)

National Health Crusade to catch hold, as well as the increasingly nasty exchanges between the chapter presidents and Goldsmith, influenced Young's decision to take the Cook County job. Whatever the reason, his reduced commitment to MCHR was felt immediately, both in staff morale and in the pocketbook.

During 1971 and the first part of 1972, MCHR raised and spent a lot of money—$160,000 by one estimate—and the proposed budget for the fiscal year beginning June 1, 1972, was a whopping $306,000. But with Young no longer available to raise funds (and with the McGovern presidential campaign of 1972 soaking up a lot of liberal money), the Medical Committee found itself once again without financial resources. Publication of *Health Rights News* was suspended for most of 1972. Owed back pay and denied a thousand-dollar cost of living raise, both Murchie and Goldsmith quit. When *Health Rights News* finally published an issue that December, the news was somber: "Our operating funds are nearly nonexistent; we have no national full-time staff; we have little communication on projects and chapter activities." Not only was the national office in limbo, the Chicago chapter, consumed by factional infighting, "is essentially nonfunctional." MCHR would survive as an organization, but it was greatly weakened, and it now had to beat back takeover attempts by Marxist factions.[7]

There had always been Communists in the Medical Committee. Several of the founders had joined the Communist Party U.S.A. during its "popular front" period in the 1930s, and a few were still active members when MCHR formed in 1964. While there were arguments among individuals representing competing Marxist groups, the Communist Party made no effort to take over MCHR, either then or later. Party members were enthusiastic supporters of MCHR's southern civil rights initiatives, but so were non-Communists. Even the FBI did not see the Communist Party as a threat in MCHR, as the Bureau's COINTELPRO files show. (It is ironic that while it was determined to ferret out Communists in every mainstream civil rights organization, the FBI pretty much left card-carrying party members in MCHR alone. Perhaps the aura surrounding the medical profession protected them.)

The role of alleged Communists in the Medical Committee became an organizational issue in the early 1970s. MCHR members Ronda Kotelchuck and Howard Levy wrote a critical article in the *Health/PAC*

Bulletin, charging that a "national office faction" that included Young, Goldsmith, and Murchie, among others, contained "open or reputed members of the Communist Party." Moreover, the national office "could depend on support from groups and or individuals in New York and the South that had long been associated with the Party." The authors claimed that "many aspects of the national office leadership were reminiscent of the Old Left, including its united-front approach to constituency . . . its bureaucratic style . . . and its centralist orientation." Levy and Kotelchuck did not name names, but their message was clear. They sent an early draft to Young, who replied that while he acknowledged their effort "to avoid the cesspool of redbaiting in your formulation," they had in fact done just that. He further took them to task for "characterizing individuals or groups with the labels that at once legitimize cannibalism within our movement and genocide by the common enemy." Young implored the writers to avoid the Communist issue, but they printed the allegations anyway. Peter Orris, who was then a member of the National Executive Committee— and the Communist Party—later stated that while there was some truth to the assessment, Kotelchuck and Levy exaggerated their claims. He believes he was the only Communist Party member in the leadership at that time, and when the article "makes it sound like there are serious revolutionaries sitting there planning a line, figuring out what will go where and how, and all these things, that's wrong!"[8]

From 1972 to 1975, MCHR carried out the policies and program agreed to at the 1971 convention, including broadening its constituency to include "consumers." The campaign for a National Health Service remained the major national effort, but among the rank and file there was little enthusiasm to do the educational and lobbying work to promote this radical alternative. Antiwar momentum subsided after the January 1973 cease-fire agreement between the United States and North Vietnam, and the reelection of Richard Nixon had dispirited progressives everywhere. With few resources and no effective national program, the Medical Committee went into decline. The number of chapters fell drastically, while most existing chapters reported only five or ten active members at most. All this made MCHR vulnerable to infiltration and takeover by the growing number of left sectarian factions and political parties.[9]

The Medical Committee for Human Rights was the only remaining organization of the New Left with both a national presence and a proud history, which made it appealing to revolutionary groups grounded in Marxist principles. The first of these was the Progressive Labor Party (PL).

Formed in 1961 by members of the Communist Party who had become disenchanted with the Soviet Union (which in their eyes had become revisionist and reformist), PL proclaimed the working class as the vanguard of the Communist revolution and attacked other leftist groups for their popular front mentality, which was demonstrated by their willingness to form coalitions with more conservative organizations. In the mid-sixties, PL members joined the Students for a Democratic Society, a move that ultimately split SDS into separate organizations.

With active members in the health professions in New England, PL decided to move into the small Boston chapter of MCHR in 1973. At the NEC meeting in June, Rena Leib complained that PL people were organizing in health care institutions in Boston under the MCHR name. The local chapter failed to call a regional meeting for fear of its being taken over by PL activists. (When that meeting did take place in October, a "nasty session," the Boston delegation did succeed in blocking the NEC nomination of a PL member from New York.) San Francisco activist Dick Fine recalled that "the PL group was just a nightmare. There was this constant struggle around ideology rather than practice. It drove us nuts." Eventually PL members were excluded from the San Francisco MCHR's meetings. The New York and Washington, D.C., chapters also came under PL attack. Quentin Young observed that MCHR was particularly vulnerable because it was "a wide open organization." The threat from PL subsided the following year, as many members left that organization over internal ideological disputes.[10]

Increasingly, MCHR was caught up in political controversies that overshadowed programmatic concerns. At the fall 1973 NEC meeting, Rena Leib questioned a national office decision to put a "member of the C.P." on the staff, to which Peter Orris responded, "Why should this fact have any influence?" Susan Schnall, now secretary of the NEC, said she wanted to know where a person's loyalty would lie if there were a conflict between a party decision and an MCHR position. Orris believed it wrong to single out Communist Party membership—as opposed to membership in other groups—because "that didn't recognize anticommunism in this country and what was going on." In the end, the candidate persuaded the group that there was no conflict of interest, and he was hired.[11]

At the 1974 national convention in Pittsburgh, which elected New Haven activist Art Mazur as national chair, organizers tried to push aside internal political concerns, with little success. Attendance was disappointing. Of the three hundred registrants nearly half were from the area, and most were medical students, nurses, and social workers. Physicians were conspicuous by their absence, as were "representatives from black and Spanish-speaking peoples." The major session, on national health insurance, attracted a small crowd. A key panelist, Victor Sidel, did not show. Another, Herbert Denenberg, the former Pennsylvania insurance commissioner then running for the U.S. Senate, angered the audience by affirming his opposition to both abortion and gun control and by defending capital punishment. No one even discussed the MCHR plan for a national health service. The most significant event was not on the program. A group of Communist physicians and students, unhappy with what they perceived as the authoritarian style of the national leaders and inspired by the example of Mao Zedong, formed the Anti-Imperialist Caucus and set out to make their voices heard.[12]

The group was influenced by the Revolutionary Union (RU), founded by activist Bob Avakian in the late 1960s. The RU called for the "overthrow of the imperialists by the working class, the replacement of capitalism and all exploitation with socialism, under the role of the working class, which will advance society to communism." Inside MCHR the Anti-Imperialist Caucus—which soon changed its name to the Activist Caucus to appear less dogmatic—opposed practically every program that the Medical Committee had championed. As revolutionaries they ridiculed the campaign to legislate a national health service because such efforts "create the illusion that the rotten health care system can be reformed, or that socialized medicine . . . can be achieved under capitalism." The free clinics "could only put a few band-aids on a leaky ship and create the illusion it could be patched up." The move to recruit consumers into MCHR and to promote "special constituencies—women, blacks, old, young" were doomed because "they ignored the class nature of society."[13]

The Activist Caucus planned to lead MCHR in a new direction by narrowing its constituency. "Our main task will be to organize health professionals and students in all aspects of their contradictions with the ruling class, and especially to take up the social issues of the day that prevent us from delivering good health care." That idea appealed to a number of non-Communist members uncomfortable with MCHR's "big tent" approach to constituency, who wanted to focus on problems facing health care workers and institutions. The Activist Caucus promised that by "building the struggle of health care professionals against the ruling class and linking it to the working class struggle, MCHR will flourish and become the fighting organization of health professionals."[14]

Naturally the national office did not take kindly to this insurgency, and held fast to the direction it charted in 1971. The Pittsburgh chapter had assumed responsibility for housing the national office after the 1973 convention. There was now little contact with local chapters, and by early 1975 the Medical Committee was facing yet another "crisis." Pittsburgh informed the national executive committee that "there was no money to continue our present operation," and that without additional resources the chapter could no longer be home to the national office. Two months later MCHR held its eleventh annual convention in Freeport, Illinois. The old guard was still in charge, and elected Susan Schnall as the Medical Committee's first woman chairperson. After her court-martial by the navy in 1968 Schnall moved to New York, where she participated in the Lincoln Collective, and later became an administrator in the Department of Community Relations in the city's Health and Hospitals Corporation.[15]

The Freeport Convention was poorly attended and contentious. About a third of the 150 delegates were from the Activist Caucus, who used the conference to push their agenda, which included the demand that MCHR limit its constituency to health professionals and students. Quentin Young was there, and told a reporter that "MCHR never really solved its constituency problem, whether it was to be a professional group . . . or a consumer group." (Later that year, Young privately admitted that the decision to broaden the constituency to include consumers had been a mistake.) Noting MCHR's "sharp decline" in recent years, Young expressed regret "at the degree of disintegration" of the national office, but his duties at Cook County Hospital kept him from giving much time to the organization. *American Medical* published a story on the convention under the headline "Apathy a Major Problem for MCHR," which was "a shadow of its former self."[16]

The Activist Caucus, however, was anything but apathetic. Although the insurgents lost the elections for national office, they dominated the plenary session at the end of the convention. When they attempted to pass resolutions, Schnall rejected the motions, declaring the absence of a quorum ("I became an expert on Robert's Rules of Order!"). Schnall recalls this as a time when it became "difficult to maintain an independent political analysis without joining one of the parties. I had differences with all of them. We needed an independent American left." Over the next several months the Activist Caucus held several national meetings on its own. Hoping to forestall a takeover of the national executive committee, Schnall and other independents joined forces with more doctrinaire members of the board, but to no avail. By early 1976 the Activist Caucus, firmly allied with the Revolutionary Union, had taken over almost half of the remaining MCHR chapters—and now controlled the NEC.[17]

Faced with this show of force, staff member Jim Ferlo and other members of the Pittsburgh chapter called for "the dissolution of the MCHR national organization." Noting that "MCHR has dwindled down into a loosely organized bunch of activists across the country," they deplored the Revolutionary Union's "organized 'invasion' into MCHR, at a time when there is such weak organization and weak political structure." As one member put it, "We are allowing vultures to pick over the carcass of an organization we are all proud of." Later, in the spring of 1976, Schnall and four members of the New York chapter wrote a position paper attacking the Activist Caucus for "camouflaging their intention to stifle every concept which does not agree with their particular analysis," and for "operating on democratic centralist practices which are inappropriate and mortally harmful to a mass organization." They concluded that "we cannot in good conscience attend this national convention," and called upon "those health workers and consumers who agree with us" to join them in a boycott.[18]

When the 1976 convention met in Cincinnati, an Activist Caucus stronghold, Schnall and the other national officers were conspicuously absent. ("We didn't have the numbers, we didn't have the organization, we didn't have the will," reflected Schnall.) Of the fewer than one hundred delegates, the majority supported the Activist Caucus, which elected their own people to the most important offices. For the next year and a half, backed by the new Revolutionary Communist Party (RCP), the Caucus dominated national MCHR. The death of Mao in 1976, however, had led to a split in the RCP, which coincided with the last hurrah of the Medical Committee for Human Rights.[19]

RCP founder Bob Avakian and the majority of the party's leaders believed that the post-Maoist Chinese Communist Party was revisionist, moving the nation toward capitalism. A substantial minority in the RCP, however, remained loyal to the new Chinese government, and broke away from the RCP to found a group with the unwieldy name Revolutionary Workers Headquarters (RWH). The schism, charges, and countercharges all played out in MCHR as well, and culminated in heated disagreement over how to respond to the Bakke case, which had become a cause célèbre among civil rights activists.

In both 1973 and 1974, Allan Bakke, a thirty-four-year-old white engineer, was denied admission to the medical school at the University of

California at Davis. He sued the University of California Board of Regents, claiming he was rejected because of his race, because minority students less qualified than he had been admitted. (The UC–Davis Medical School had set aside up to sixteen of its one hundred admissions for students with "disadvantaged" backgrounds.) A lower court ruled that Bakke was indeed a victim of discrimination, and on appeal the State Supreme Court went further, declaring the special admissions program at UC–Davis unconstitutional. When the Board of Regents appealed to the U.S. Supreme Court, there ensued a national debate over what legal scholars were calling the most important school case since *Brown v. Board of Education.*[20]

By the time the Supreme Court began hearing the case on October 12, 1977, a number of civil rights groups had been mobilizing public opinion against Bakke. The largest, the National Committee to Overturn the Bakke Decision (NCOBD), called on "all those people who oppose racism" to join with them. The National Executive Committee of MCHR, still dominated by members of the Revolutionary Communist Party, stated that "the Bakke case is a political attack to drive minorities down and crush their aspirations." It went on to claim that the California court's decision "is an attempt by the rulers of this country to dump their economic crisis on the backs of minorities." While the NCOBD declared that racism was the dominant force behind the drive to eliminate affirmative action programs for minorities, the MCHR board contended that this was just another manifestation of a decaying capitalist system. Indeed, the MCHR statement on Bakke never mentioned the words "race" or "racism."[21]

All the organizations maintained that the Supreme Court should rule against Bakke, but disagreements arose over questions of ideology and turf. MCHR chose Peter Moyer, a New York physician, to head its Bakke task force, and he attended a number of meetings called by the NCOBD. Moyer later acknowledged that "we were sectarian. We didn't listen to what others had to say. We refused to unite with Blacks and other minorities in their fight against racism unless they agreed—from the start—with our understanding that racism flowed from capitalism . . . We found we had become isolated from the masses and hadn't built the struggle." National MCHR had done nothing to link up with other Bakke opponents, including the National Medical Association and the American Student Medical Association. This isolation led Moyer and other New Yorkers, including Harold Osborne and Sheila Ditchik, to demand a revaluation of MCHR policy, and they helped organize a conference of "professional people from all over the country" to be held at Howard University in November of 1977. Its purpose was to unite Bakke opponents under one banner. That meeting was harmonious, and the participants agreed to organize a massive public protest in Washington.[22]

The Revolutionary Communist Party faction denounced the Howard Conference and the MCHR members who helped put it together. The party's newspaper, *Revolution*, lectured the black leadership of the NCOBD. "They make racism the central question, rather than correctly understanding national oppression . . . and the source of the Bakke attack—U.S. capitalism and its crisis." The editorial advocated "one united movement against Bakke, but only if the unity is guided by a correct political line." The flap over whether to join the NCOBD-led coalition exposed the internal struggle over the direction of MCHR. RCP members still held most national offices, but many East Coast chapter members had joined the Revolutionary Workers Headquarters faction. New members drawn into the organization by the Bakke action were both confused and impatient over the factional infighting.[23]

All this came to a head when, after the MCHR Bakke task force endorsed the demonstration, Moyer and others proposed that the Medical Committee form and march under the banner of a "Health Professionals Contingent" (similar to the coalition Walter Lear had put together for the March on Washington fifteen years earlier). When the National Executive Committee endorsed the proposal by a 12–7 vote, RCP members strenuously objected. They would not walk side by side with health care workers who did not espouse the correct political line. The march itself, held in mid-April, was well attended, with nearly fifteen thousand people demonstrating in Washington against Bakke. About twenty-five MCHR activists fell in line with members of other groups, including the presidents of the black Student National Medical Association and the largely white American Medical Student Association. Nearly a dozen MCHR demonstrators marched with the Revolutionary Communist Youth Brigade under the banner "Oppose Imperialism, the Source of All Oppression." The U.S. Supreme Court was not impressed, and later in the summer of 1978 ordered that Bakke be admitted to the UC–Davis Medical School. It also declared that the university's quota system, which reserved places for minorities, was unconstitutional. The court did rule that plans to promote diversity that included race or ethnic background among other criteria for admission were acceptable, a partial victory for the anti-Bakke forces.[24]

The controversy over the Bakke case marked the end of RCP domination of MCHR. At the fifteenth national convention, held in Philadelphia, the election of officers "reflected a victory for the RWH," whose candidates won three out of the five major offices, including chairperson and vice-chairperson. The new editorial board of *MCHR News,* the most recent house organ, changed course. Under the patient guidance of Walter Lear, who almost alone had hung in with his organization through thick and thin, the periodical shifted its focus to coverage of local projects, avoiding strident rhetoric about "imperialism" and "capitalism's crisis." The Medical Committee again reached out to other progressive medical organizations, and "coalition" was no longer a forbidden word. The RCP faction, now a minority, became more strident. It reinvented itself as the Norman Bethune Caucus (named for a Canadian doctor who served with Mao in the early days of the Chinese Revolution), once again touting "anti-imperialism" as the basis for unity in all MCHR work. The Bethune Caucus toed the Revolutionary Communist Party line, now including support for the revolutionaries in Iran who had overthrown the Shah. Internally, the Bethune caucus disrupted meetings by forcing ideological discussions and ignoring the will of the majority. On June 30, 1979, the National Executive Committee expelled the Norman Bethune Caucus from MCHR.[25]

Freed from sectarian wrangling, MCHR once again vowed to "build a broad-based united organization of health care activists." But it was too late. The election of Ronald Reagan did not mark the end of MCHR, but it did symbolize the changes that had been taking place in the American electorate. There was little enthusiasm for organizations dedicated to reforming the health care system, let alone bringing about a social revolution. At the opening session of the 1980 MCHR convention, two questions dominated discussion. "Can we continue? How?" A year later, a fund-raising letter announced that "we are slowly rebuilding from the effects of sectarian infighting and apathy, [but] we need your help." MCHR limped along into the early 1980s, with periodic, sparsely attended meetings at homes in a few major cities. When it finally vanished from the political landscape, few would be aware of, let alone mourn, its passing.[26]

Coda

In many respects Dr. James Michael Waller personified the idealism and commitment of the second wave of MCHR activists. Born in Chicago in 1942, Jim Waller grew up in a Jewish family, and his maternal grandfather was a Chicago physician who fought anti-Semitism in the medical profession in the 1920s. Jim became a member of the nation's first chapter of the Students for a Democratic Society (SDS) at the University of Michigan, where he majored in English. He went on to the University of Chicago Medical School, where he became friends with Fitzhugh Mullan. In his memoir of that era, Mullan recalls that Waller was the only student in his class to sport a beard, and he refused to shave it off despite threats by members of the medical faculty. Soon "Save Waller's Beard" became a rallying cry among the students, and their nonconformist colleague kept his whiskers. During the 1968 Democratic convention Waller was in the streets as part of the MCHR-led medical team that provided emergency medical care to the antiwar demonstrators beaten by the police.[1]

Waller's chosen field was pediatrics, and along with Mullan he chose to do his residency at Lincoln Hospital in the Bronx. A fellow member of the Lincoln Collective, Mike Dooley, praised Waller for his "thoroughness and warmth . . . his high standards of medicine and his empathy for the troubles of his patients." Waller spent four years at Lincoln in the early 1970s, and it was during that time that he helped supply the medical clinic for the Oglala Sioux at Wounded Knee. He also visited Cuba and came away impressed with that nation's attempt to provide free health care for every citizen. And he fell in love with Jean Sharpe, also a pediatrician. When in 1974 Waller was awarded a postdoctoral fellowship by Duke University in pediatric infectious diseases, she came with him.[2]

At Duke, Waller became close friends with two young activist physicians, Mike Nathan and Paul Bermanzohn. As an undergraduate, Nathan had led protests for union recognition for Duke service workers, who were paid eighty-five cents an hour. The child of Holocaust survivors, Bermanzohn was raised in the Bronx, and moved to the South to enroll at Duke Medical School. Classmates at Duke, Nathan and Bermanzohn organized the Durham-Chapel Hill chapter of the Medical Committee for Human Rights in 1973, which Waller and Sharpe joined once they got settled in North Carolina. Waller became active in the Carolina Brown Lung Association, and along with Bermanzohn worked in a local screening project for cotton mill workers. Politically, Waller had been moving further to the left. He joined the Durham Organizing Committee, a Marxist group, and became interested in the Workers Viewpoint Organization (WVO), a Maoist faction that was part of the New Communist Movement of the 1970s. It was about this time that the Revolutionary Communist Party took over the national MCHR and the Durham-Chapel Hill chapter disbanded in protest, claiming, among other things, that the RCP "was neither revolutionary nor communist."[3]

The Workers Viewpoint Organization was a small group operating in about twenty cities. It actively recruited minority members, believing that working people of color suffered from national as well as class oppression. Although the WVO had become alienated from the Communist Party of the United States, it embraced the discarded CP belief that blacks in the South constituted an oppressed nation with the right to self-determination, even secession from the United States. In North Carolina, the WVO was comprised of two major groups: white radicals from the Durham Organizing Committee, and black activists in Greensboro who had formed the Bolshevik Organizing Committee. Their leader, Nelson Johnson, had played a prominent role in the civil rights movement in Greensboro in the 1960s. Waller joined a WVO-sponsored study group, and learned from reading Marx, Lenin, and Mao that revolutionaries should "go to the proletariat," abandoning their professions to take jobs in factories and organize the workers. Waller resigned from Duke in the summer of 1976 to work on the assembly line at the Cone Mills plant at Haw River. Paul Bermanzohn also left the medical profession to work in a factory. Mike Nathan continued to practice medicine and was the head pediatrician at the Lincoln Community Health Center in inner-city Durham.

Waller's new ideological commitment precipitated a breakup with Jean Sharpe. He wrote to his sister that "I love Jean more than I have ever loved another. But she is not a communist, nor does she intend to become a communist." At a WVO meeting in late 1976 Waller met Signe Burke Goldstein, a divorced mother of two with a Ph.D. in philosophy from Columbia. She had quit her teaching position in North Carolina to work at a Cone plant in Greensboro, a city about an hour east of Chapel Hill and Durham. In early 1978 the two married and moved to Greensboro.

Waller threw himself into the task of organizing black and white workers at the Cone plant, and in June of 1978 led them out on strike. It failed, but the union grew and Waller was elected vice president of the local. Then Cone fired him, allegedly because he had not recorded on his job application that he was a physician. That fall, Waller attended the first convention of the Trade Union Educational League (TUEL), a national union created by the WVO to unite workers across lines of race, nationality, and occupation. In the spring of 1979 he was elected TUEL's president. Attempts to organize workers in the North Carolina cotton mills had been threatened by a revived Ku Klux Klan, which militantly opposed the formation of interracial unions.

Waller, Nelson Johnson, and other local leaders decided to oppose the Klan actively, in public, both as an act of conscience and as a means of gathering support for their organizing efforts. The first confrontation between the WVO and the Klan occurred in the small Carolina town of China Grove on July 8, 1979. The Klan had announced a public showing at the town hall of D. W. Griffith's racist film, *Birth of a Nation,* which glorified the KKK. About fifty WVO activists, including Waller, Nathan, and Bermanzohn, joined local blacks in downtown China Grove to face about fifteen armed white men (one in full Klan regalia, another wearing the uniform of a Nazi storm trooper). Several armed WVO members started moving against the smaller Klan group, which retreated to the porch of the town hall. The local police then moved in and persuaded the Klansmen to go inside the building. The anti-Klan activists celebrated the victory by burning a Confederate flag, while their humiliated adversaries peered out from inside the town hall. Flushed with success, the WVO planned a larger "death to the Klan" march in Greensboro the first week in November. The Greensboro rally was to mark the inaugural appearance of the Communist Workers Party, formed by the WVO that fall, with its most active contingent in North Carolina.

Buoyed by their success at literally backing down the Klan at China Grove, Waller, Johnson, and other activists launched a publicity campaign, mocking the Klan and its members with flyers labeling them "nothing but a bunch of racist cowards," and challenging them to "attend our November 3rd rally in Greensboro." The poster advertising the event showed a picture of the marchers at China Grove, with a smaller shot of the burning of the Confederate flag, all under the banner "DEATH TO THE KLAN." Mike Nathan was horrified at the level of Klan-baiting, convinced that "what the WVO was calling boldness was something more akin to insanity." Nonetheless he would attend the November 3 rally, which was to begin in the black Morningside neighborhood in Greensboro. Police granted a permit for the rally and march, but specified that the activists could not carry arms. Waller and his comrades assumed, mistakenly as it turned out, that the police would be on the scene to keep order.

But the television cameras were there that morning. Demonstrators sang freedom songs while the event's organizers prepared about a hundred people, black and white, for a march across town. Then a caravan of nine cars carrying some three dozen Klansmen and neo-Nazis drove slowly into the black housing project, a Confederate flag atop the lead vehicle. Several of the demonstrators hit the passing cars with their picket sticks. Then someone from one of the cars fired a pistol shot in the air and a scuffle broke out, while Klansmen in two rear vehicles up the street methodically began unloading an arsenal of shotguns, pistols, and a semiautomatic rifle. Moving to the front, they took aim and opened fire. Eighty-eight seconds later four demonstrators lay dead and eleven wounded. Dr. Paul Bermanzohn was shot in the head and arm while trying to protect his friend Cesar Cauce, who was trying to fend off a Klansman's attack. Bermanzohn would survive; Cauce, a Cuban-born labor organizer with a degree in history from Duke, did not. Bill Sampson, a graduate of Harvard Divinity School, was killed by a gunshot wound to the heart. Sandi Smith, the only black person and woman murdered that day, had been president of the student body at Bennett College. Dr. Mike Nathan was shot squarely in the face and died later in the hospital. After struggling with an attacker, Dr. Jim Waller ran for cover and died where he fell from gunshot wounds in the back.

The Klansmen were brought to trial twice and found not guilty by state and federal juries, despite TV footage that showed one defendant pumping bullets into a demonstrator already on the ground. The accused claimed self-defense. That all the victims were card-carrying Communists did little to elicit sympathy from the juries. Three months after the Greensboro Massacre, as it was now being called, seven thousand demonstrators from all over the country marched in Greensboro to protest Klan terror. Prominent in a delegation of health care professionals from New York were representatives of the Medical Committee for Human Rights. As it had at southern civil rights marches in the 1960s, MCHR provided medical presence, staffing first aid stations and two mobile vans along the parade route. Later in the year the Communist Workers Party distributed a pamphlet paying tribute to its members in the medical profession who had been killed or wounded in Greensboro. The pamphlet's title was *Being a Doctor Is Not Enough.*[4]

The tragedy of Greensboro aside, it is difficult to work up much sympathy, let alone enthusiasm, for the radicals who claimed to represent the vanguard of the health care movement in the late 1970s, a time when the term "politically correct" was employed without irony, when people met in somebody's basement to work up the proper slogans with which to reach the masses. The cadre of the Revolutionary Union who plotted the takeover of the Medical Committee seems far removed from the idealistic commitment of the doctors and nurses who went to Mississippi in the summer of 1964. And yet the figure of Jim Waller comes back to haunt us: the nonconforming medical student who fought to save his beard, transformed into the Communist revolutionary gunned down at the barricades by Ku Klux Klansmen. Like most health care activists, Waller had seen racial discrimination and economic injustice firsthand, at its most elemental level—in the teaching hospitals of inner-city ghettos. The determination to change that environment, together with the belief that society as a whole could be transformed, linked Waller and his comrades to the older founders of the Medical Committee for Human Rights. Proceeding from the assumption that health care is a right, not a privilege, they all came to see that "being a doctor is not enough." These professionals had to become political, to take to the streets if necessary to awaken Americans to the inequities inherent in the health care system. As Des Callan put it, "To get good health care, you've got to make noise, got to make trouble, got to speak out."[5]

The Medical Committee for Human Rights has left its mark on American society. From Greenwood to Greensboro, MCHR provided aid, comfort, and a degree of security to activists demonstrating in the streets against racism and war. The organization's work in the South did make a difference in the lives of civil rights workers, particularly those suffering from burnout and in need of counseling or a change of scene. MCHR doctors and nurses in Mississippi and Alabama also gave hope to thousands of community people denied health care. Although they were an overwhelmingly white group of professionals, the Medical Committee embraced the local perspective of black southerners, breaking through barriers of class and race to work with even the most militant African American activists and organizations.

In addition, MCHR helped bring about permanent improvements in the availability and delivery of health care. Its five-year campaign against the AMA facilitated the desegregation of state and local medical societies in the South, and the subsequent awarding of hospital privileges to hundreds of black physicians. It played a major role in desegregating southern hospitals and other health facilities. MCHR stimulated consumer participation in health affairs, and successfully pressured medical schools to add programs in family and community medicine and to admit more black and female students. Medical Committee lobbyists directly influenced passage of health care legislation and implementation of federal programs. It was in the creation of the model for the comprehensive community health

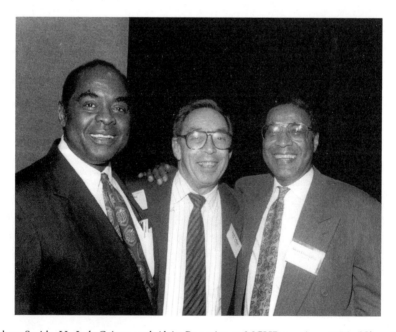

Robert Smith, H. Jack Geiger, and Alvin Poussaint at MCHR reunion, 1995. (Charmian Redding)

center that MCHR activists made their most important contribution to the well-being of impoverished Americans. By 2009 nearly 1,300 centers were providing primary care for more than sixteen million Americans at 7,354 sites in urban and rural medically underserved communities across the nation.[6]

The Medical Committee provided a model for organizations that succeeded it, like Physicians for Human Rights, Partners in Health, Remote Area Medicine, and Physicians for a National Health Insurance Program. However, its most enduring legacy has been the continuing social activism of its former members. Tom Bodenheimer has observed that "we tried to do something then, but if there's anything lasting, it's us. It's the alumni of MCHR trying to keep the flame alive, not in the name of MCHR anymore, but with the same principles."[7]

The MCHR Legacy

Former MCHR chair Mike Holloman became the first black president of the New York City Health and Hospital Corporation. He taught at the University of North Carolina School of Public Health, and was a staff member of the Health Subcommittee of the House Ways and Means Committee. Holloman practiced medicine in Harlem for more than a half century, and for twenty years he was medical director of the William F. Ryan Community Health Center. His was an early voice warning of the threat of AIDS in the black community, and he continued to agitate for national health insurance. "Unless we take the profit motive out of it and provide health care for all of our citizens, we are always going to have somebody who's left out," he told an interviewer, "because there are so many people on whom there is no profit to be made." Until he suffered a debilitating stroke in 1996, Holloman made a weekly visit to an armory to provide medical care for the homeless people sheltered there. He also continued to make house calls, noting that he and his patients were growing old together. Mike Holloman died in 2002.[1]

From 1968 to 1970 Des Callan was the medical director and then executive director of the Northeast Neighborhood Association (NENA) Health Center. Situated on New York's Lower East Side, this was the first community planned and sponsored center to receive federal funding. In the early 1970s Callan wrote extensively about health issues for the Health Policy Advisory Center (Health-PAC), and in 1975 he moved to rural New York, where he opened a family practice in Hillsdale. Later, he taught community medicine at Baystate Medical Center in Massachusetts. He remained a fervent supporter of the health center model, including

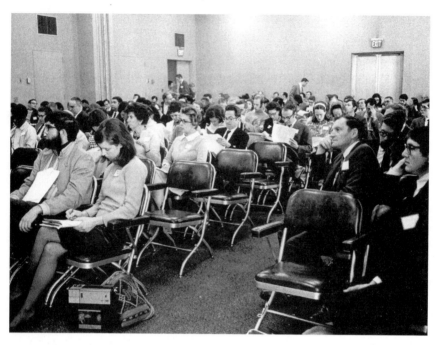

MCHR conference, Chicago, 1966. (Charmian Redding)

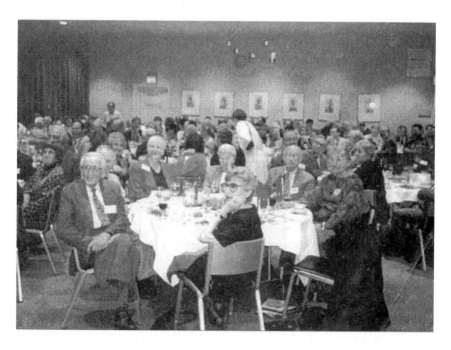

MCHR reunion, New York, 1995. (Institute of Social Medicine and Community Health)

community governance and control, but believed they should serve a broad spectrum of patients from different income groups. "There should not be poverty programs in health," he said in an interview shortly before his death in 2002, "because invariably poverty medicine becomes poor medicine." In 2006 the Desmond Callan Community Health Center opened its doors in Orange, Massachusetts.[2]

Tom Levin maintained his individual and group therapy practice in New York. He became the United Nations liaison for the World Association for Psycho-Social Rehabilitation, a group dedicated to the protection of the rights of the medically ill. In 1995 the Group Psychotherapy Foundation presented him with its first Humanitarian Award "for a lifelong contribution to social change and the advancement of society through the use of small groups." Levin died on the Fourth of July, 2008.

Al Moldovan has carried on his family practice in Spanish Harlem for more than four decades, and in his spare time he has assembled one of the most important Judaica collections in the world. Les Falk joined the faculty at Meharry Medical College in 1967, where he served as chair of the Department of Family and Community Medicine, teaching hundreds of African American medical students. He was the founder and first director of the Matthew Walker Community Health Center, in Nashville. Upon his retirement in 1987, Falk moved to Vermont, where he wrote a memoir, *My Life Experiences in Social Medicine*. He died in 2004.

Count Gibson left Tufts in 1969 to become chair of the Department of Family, Community, and Preventive Medicine at Stanford. He remained committed to providing health care for minority activists engaged in struggle. When the group of American Indians occupied Alcatraz Island in San Francisco Bay, Gibson was one of the few white physicians welcomed onto the island to treat the protesters. He championed the farm workers' rights movement led by César Chavez, assisting the National Farm Workers' Union, and was an advocate for the rights of the mentally and physically disabled. After he retired from Stanford in 1999, Gibson and his wife moved to Connecticut, where he died in 2002. In 1990 the Columbia Point Health Center was renamed the Geiger-Gibson Health Center, and in 2004 the George Washington University School of Public Health established the Geiger-Gibson Program in Community Health Policy.

H. Jack Geiger moved from Tufts to Stony Brook in the early 1970s, where he headed the SUNY Department of Community Medicine. In 1978 he joined the faculty of the CUNY Medical School in Harlem. For

more than two decades he directed a program at CUNY committed to
training minority physicians for primary care service in underserved areas.
Geiger remained active politically, continuing to work with Physicians for
Social Responsibility. He was also a founding member and president of
both Physicians for Human Rights, an organization that investigated human rights abuses throughout the world, and the Committee for Health
in Southern Africa. A prolific writer on health care issues and systems,
Geiger worked in the field as well. His activism took him to international
hot spots, including Bosnia, Iraq, and the West Bank. He taught for a year
as visiting professor of community medicine at the University of Natal
Medical School in South Africa. Of his many awards and honors, that of
the Institute of Medicine of the National Academy of Sciences lauds
Geiger for "creating a model of the contemporary community health center to serve the poor and disadvantaged and for contributions to the advancement of minority health." Along with his colleagues John Hatch and
L. C. Dorsey, Geiger is writing a book on the founding and development
of the Mound Bayou community health center.

Phyllis Cunningham and Josephine Disparti followed similar career
paths. They received master's in public health degrees from the University
of North Carolina in the late 1960s and moved to New York, where they
taught together at the CCNY School of Nursing. Each received an Ed.D.
degree from Columbia Teachers College. After CCNY terminated its nursing education program, Disparti became director of assessment and evaluation for the National League of Nursing. Both remained politically
involved after their return to New York in the early 1970s, but not with
MCHR. After leaving his position as executive director of MCHR, Johnny
Parham was a vice president with the United Negro College Fund before
becoming the first executive director of the Thurgood Marshall Fund,
which awards merit scholarships to students who attend historically black
public colleges and universities. He retired in 1999.

Three founders of the Student Health Organizations have followed
different career paths. Bill Bronston returned to California in 1975, and
has held several positions in the California Department of Health, including medical director of the State Department of Rehabilitation. Active in
the disability rights movement, he created Tower of Youth, an organization
that encourages young people, including those at risk and with disabilities,
to develop their talents in the creative arts, including film and television.
Bronston has led delegations to Cuba and is a spokesperson for universal
health care. Mick McGarvey was a commissioned officer with the U.S.

Public Health Service before becoming senior vice president for Managed Care of Blue Cross Blue Shield of New Jersey. Fitzhugh Mullan joined the Public Health Service in 1972. From 1977 through 1981 he directed the National Health Service Corps, and in 1991 was appointed assistant surgeon general. He joined the staff of the journal *Health Affairs* as an editor, and has written widely on health care issues. In addition to *White Coat, Clenched Fist,* Mullan has written a history of the Public Health Service, *Plagues and Politics;* a collective biography of selected primary health care physicians, *Big Doctoring in America;* and a memoir, *Vital Signs: A Young Doctor's Struggle with Cancer.* He is currently Murdock Head Professor of Medicine and Health Policy at the George Washington University School of Public Health, professor of pediatrics at the GW Medical School, and a member of the medical staff of a community health center in Washington that serves a predominantly Hispanic population.

Another of the Young Turks, Larry Brilliant, has had a remarkable career in international medicine. Brilliant moved to India in the 1970s, where he played a major role in the World Health Organization's campaign to eradicate smallpox. In 1978 he was the cofounder and chair of Seva, an international nonprofit health foundation, whose projects have restored sight to more than two million blind people living in underdeveloped countries. Returning to the United States, he was professor of International Health and Epidemiology at the University of Michigan for many years. Among his many honors is the International Health Hero Award from the University of California at Berkeley. In 2006, Brilliant was appointed executive director of Google.org, the philanthropic arm that disperses 1 percent of Google's profits.

Antiwar activist Susan Schnall worked as an administrator at several New York hospitals in community outreach programs, with special interest in the rights of the disabled. After nine years as associate executive director at Bellevue Hospital, she retired in 2006, and currently teaches at the School of Continuing and Professional Studies at New York University. Schnall has been active in the work of the Agent Orange Responsibility and Relief Organization, a group formed to put pressure on both the chemical companies that produced Agent Orange and the U.S. government to clean up those areas of Vietnam that still contain dioxin, and to compensate Vietnamese victims of Agent Orange.

Among the most visible MCHR alumni are Alvin Poussaint and Sidney Wolfe. After leaving Mississippi, Poussaint accepted a position at Tufts Medical School as director of a psychiatry program in a low-income housing project. In 1969 he joined the Harvard Medical School faculty as professor of psychiatry, and he has also served as director of the Media Center for Children at the Judge Baker Children's Center in Boston. Poussaint's first two books, *Why Blacks Kill Blacks* and *Raising Black Children*, which he coauthored with James P. Comer, won critical acclaim, as did *Lay My Burden Down: Suicide and the Mental Health Crisis Among African Americans*, with Amy Alexander as coauthor. His regular contributions to *Ebony* magazine, along with his high visibility in the national media, have gained him a large audience, and he was widely recognized as a leading authority on race relations and the pathology of racism. He has served as a consultant to government agencies and private corporations, and was a script consultant for many television programs, most notably *The Cosby Show*. With Bill Cosby he wrote *Come on People: On the Path from Victims to Victors*. When Harvard honored him at a dinner in 2005 for his many contributions, Poussaint used his time on the podium to talk about his work with the Medical Committee for Human Rights in Mississippi. In the audience that night was his high school classmate, Bob Moses.

Sid Wolfe ran for national chairperson of MCHR in 1970 and lost the election to Eli Messinger. The next year Wolfe met Ralph Nader, who had just started his advocacy group, Public Citizen, and proposed that he and Nader begin a health research project, the first specialty group within Public Citizen. Since that time, as director of the Health Research Group (HRG), Wolfe has used Public Citizen's visibility to call attention to dangerous drugs, persuading the Food and Drug Administration to withdraw sixteen medicines it had previously approved. Among the Health Research Group's many publications is the bestselling book *Worst Pills, Best Pills*, an almanac of the effectiveness of drugs. The HRG also puts out a monthly newsletter, *Health Affairs*. Wolfe's opposition to the practices of the pharmaceutical manufacturers, as well as his reports on dangerous medical devices, medical malpractice, and the performance of state medical boards, has made him a controversial figure. A 2005 *New York Times* profile noted that Wolfe "has fought companies rich and poor and has angered just about every constituency in the health care industry." Among his many awards and honors was the MacArthur Foundation Fellowship in 1990. For more than three decades Wolfe has been a visible—and effective— public advocate for health care consumers.[3]

Tom Bodenheimer continues to do research on health care issues. With Kevin Grumbach, he wrote *Understanding Health Policy*, now in its fifth edition, and *Improving Primary Care*. He has been a national correspondent

for the *New England Journal of Medicine.* In 1980, with several other physicians, Bodenheimer established Bay West Family Health Care, a private
practice in San Francisco that serves a predominantly poor and elderly population. By 2002 these doctors had found it increasingly difficult to meet
the needs of their patients while being squeezed by cuts in Medicare, Medicaid, and private health care plans. His article, "Primary Care—Will It
Survive?," published in 2006, argues that the combination of low pay (compared with medical specialists) and inequities in both government and
private insurance plans has been responsible for the large reduction in the
number of family physicians, with fewer and fewer medical students choosing to enter the field of primary care. Bodenheimer teaches family and community medicine at the University of California San Francisco.[4]

After leaving the Judson Mobile Unit Health Clinic in the early
1970s, June Finer worked part-time with Planned Parenthood in Brooklyn and later at an abortion clinic on the Upper East Side. In 1980 she
took a full-time position with the Lower East Side Service Center in its
drug treatment and rehabilitation program, remaining there until her retirement at the end of 1999. She now lives in New Paltz, New York.

In 1970 Walter Lear founded the Institute of Social Medicine and
Community Health and began assembling an archive, the U.S. Health
Activism History Collection, which includes the MCHR Papers. These materials are now housed in the University of Pennsylvania Rare Book and
Manuscript Collection. For the last four decades, Lear has been active in
local and national movements. In 1984 the mayor of Philadelphia appointed him to the Philadelphia Commission on Human Relations, the
first openly gay PCHR commissioner. Among his many honors, Lear was
the recipient of the 1994 Paul Cornely Award of the Physicians Forum
and the 2006 Helen Rodriguez-Trias Award for Social Justice, presented
by the American Public Health Association, which commended him for
sixty years of social justice activism. Lear is currently finishing a book on
the history of "left medicine" in the United States.

Quentin Young took over as director of the Medical Department at
Cook County Hospital in 1972, recruiting a staff of like-minded resident
physicians. Three years later these doctors went out on strike over working
conditions, and Young was fired, only to be reinstated by a federal judge.
Young left Cook County in 1981, resuming his private practice in Hyde
Park and establishing the Health and Medicine Policy Research Group,
an advocacy organization whose social action agenda resembles that of
MCHR. Young hosted a weekly, hour-long program, *Public Affairs,* on

Chicago Public Radio for nearly two decades, and he served as president of the American Public Health Association in 1997. For more than half a century, Young has been an advocate for a universal national health system in the United States. He was a founder of the Physicians for a National Health Program (PNHP), a group of some ten thousand doctors that lobbies for a comprehensive universal single-payer national health insurance program. In 2008, the eighty-five-year-old physician was dividing his time between seeing his patients and serving as the national coordinator for PNHP.

Mississippi holds a special place in the history of the Medical Committee. In the late 1960s James Anderson, Aaron Shirley, and Bob Smith—dedicated to improving the quality of health care for the state's African American citizens—had to contend with an uncooperative and at times hostile political establishment. Inspired by the Tufts-Delta comprehensive community health center in Mound Bayou, Shirley and Anderson made plans to open a center to serve the people of Jackson and surrounding Hinds County. Opposition quickly arose from white politicians and the state medical society. Since the proposed center was not sponsored by a university (like Tufts at Mound Bayou), the governor had the power to veto the grant, and he did just that. Shirley and Anderson got help from Donald Rumsfeld, the young director of the OEO in the Nixon administration. In Jackson on other business, Rumsfeld had dinner with Shirley at a black-owned restaurant, and ten days later he overturned the governor's veto and reinstated the grant. The Jackson-Hinds Comprehensive Health Center was in business.[5]

Like its counterpart in Mound Bayou, the center in Jackson dealt with environmental problems such as unsanitary privies and wells in the patients' homes. It also initiated programs to provide mental health services, housing for senior citizens, and a comprehensive health clinic in an inner-city school with a counseling program to prevent drug use and teenage pregnancies. Patients at the health center were urged to register and vote. Shirley and Anderson also worked with those who hoped to start centers in their own communities. By 1979 Jackson-Hinds, now the largest health center in the state, had become "a national showplace," with federal bureaucrats and health care planners making the pilgrimage to Jackson to observe and learn.

Unfortunately, the "mother" institution at Mound Bayou had fallen on hard times. Jack Geiger, John Hatch, and L. C. Dorsey had left by 1971. Black middle-class leaders in Mound Bayou persuaded the OEO to turn the center's operation and ownership over to a local board, and for the next fifteen years the health center was beset by a range of problems, including lack of funding, political cronyism, and mismanagement. Federal authorities eventually demanded a new governing board, and in 1987 Dorsey came back to serve as executive director. During her eight-year tenure she did much to put the center back on its feet, establishing satellite operations in surrounding counties, initiating home health services in two counties, and restoring fiscal soundness to the operation of what is now called the Delta Health Center.[6]

In 1993 Shirley was one of two dozen Americans selected for a MacArthur Foundation "genius" grant of $350,000, giving him time to put in motion his dream of converting a large, bankrupt shopping mall in the middle of Jackson into a "state-of-the-art ambulatory health care facility providing quality health care for the urban poor." Needing allies with assets and influence to pull off such an ambitious undertaking, Shirley turned to the University of Mississippi Medical Center for help.[7]

The Jackson Medical Mall, which opened in 1995, covers fifty-three acres, all under one roof. It houses programs run by the state health department and by the Medical School, which moved its outpatient clinics and specialty services to the mall. The University's Pediatrics Department and the Department of Medicine are in charge of primary care. In all, there are more than fifty separate health care offices in the mall, including Jackson State University's School of Allied Health. The medical facility is also home to the Jackson Heart Study, a ten-year examination of cardiovascular disease among African Americans, funded by the National Institutes of Health. In addition to providing examinations and treatment for 6,300 Jackson-area residents, the Heart Study has an educational component at Tougaloo College and Jackson State University, providing new opportunities for minority students to pursue careers in public health and research. The Mall also contains Jackson City government offices, shops, and restaurants, and serves as a community center with a busy calendar of events. This remarkable community health care endeavor has attracted widespread interest, with health care administrators studying the feasibility of replicating this model nationwide. To honor the Jackson Medical Mall's founder, in 2005 the University of Mississippi Medical Center established an endowed chair in Aaron Shirley's name.[8]

Bob Smith expanded his private practice, establishing the Mississippi

Family Health Center in 1970, the first minority multispecialty clinic in the state, providing medical care to all patients, regardless of their ability to pay. Over the years, additional physicians and staff have led to increased services at the center, which has been a training facility in family practice for more than two hundred African American medical students and other health professionals, many of them from Mississippi. Smith was instrumental in developing cooperative relationships between Tougaloo College and the medical schools at Brown and Tufts, and served as an adjunct professor at both institutions. After winning the right to practice at local hospitals in the mid-1960s, Smith became a charter staff member of Hinds General Hospital when it opened in 1967. Elected chief of family medicine in 1974, he then became the first African American to serve as chief of staff at Hinds. Of the many awards and honors he has received, none seems more appropriate than a tribute from the city of Jackson: the downtown thoroughfare where four decades earlier the young physician had been harassed and arrested by local police is now Robert Smith Parkway.

As founding director of what is now the Mississippi Primary Health Care Association, the local component of the National Neighborhood Health Center organization, Smith maintained his involvement in the movement he helped bring into being. He was instrumental in establishing several health centers, including the Aaron Henry Health Center in Clarksdale. His operation in Jackson, now called Central Mississippi Health Services, became a federally funded comprehensive health center in 2002. It operates three sites, including the George and Ruth Owens Wellness Center at Tougaloo College, fulfilling one of Bob Smith's longtime dreams. The Jackson-Hinds Center has moved to a new modern building, and now has expanded to five sites, three of them in rural areas. In all, by 2005 there were twenty-two health center organizations in Mississippi, operating 141 delivery sites, and serving more than 280,000 patients. And where there were fewer than 50 black doctors practicing in the state back in the 1960s, that number has increased to around 350 in 2008. Given the racial and economic problems that still plague the Magnolia State, that is no small achievement.[9]

Acknowledgments

When I decided to write this book I knew very little about the Medical Committee for Human Rights. There were no monographs or even memoirs that discussed MCHR in detail. A couple of small collections of the organization's papers at several libraries would prove to be of limited assistance. Then Jack Geiger told me about a physician named Walter Lear, who had for years been gathering files from several organizations he categorized as the "Health Left" in American medicine, including MCHR. When I first met Dr. Lear at his home in Philadelphia he took me up to the third floor and opened the door to dozens of boxes of Medical Committee papers. (I immediately thought of the oft-repeated story of the historian who discovers a trove of documents in somebody's attic!) For the next twelve months I worked in Walter Lear's "attic," examining papers that were cataloged only by year. And when I had questions about certain people or developments, all I had to do was to go down a flight of stairs and ask the authority on the subject. To invoke the old cliché, Dr. Lear is truly the person "without whom this book could not have been written."

And I would have also been at a loss without the cooperation of the many Medical Committee activists who shared their stories with me. Particularly helpful were the late Desmond Callan, H. Jack Geiger, Phyllis Cunningham, Fitzhugh Mullan, Josephine Disparti, Alvin Poussaint, and Robert Smith.

Three colleagues read and made extensive comments on the manuscript. Susan Reverby, a distinguished scholar of the history of social medicine (and a former activist in MCHR), was an immense help to a civil rights historian working in new territory. Steven Lawson and Jim Patterson, two friends of many years, helped shape this book. Their wise counsel, encouragement, and critical comments were invaluable. My debt to them is enormous.

Over the years other scholars have had a direct impact on my work, none more so than Robert H. Ferrell. As an undergraduate at Indiana University, I took my first college history course from Bob Ferrell during the second semester of my senior year. He then persuaded me to do whatever it took to get into the graduate history program at IU. And he taught me how to write. Bill Chafe, Nancy Hewitt, Charles Payne, Connie Curry, Barbara Steinson, Anne Firor Scott, Patricia Sullivan, Tim Tyson, David Gellman, John Schlotterbeck, and Neil McMillen have enriched my life, academically and personally, as have younger scholars like Emilye Crosby, Jim Giesen, Hasan Jeffries, Danielle McGuire, Tiyi Morris, and Todd Moye. Thanks also to Carol Mann, Matt Herron, Charmian Redding, and Bill Wingell.

Other friends and family members have been supportive in a number of ways. These include Bob Bottoms, Neal Abraham, Donna and Bill Stark, Mary Giles, Ernie Limbo, Charles Eagles, Bill Ferris, Susan Glisson, Seetha Srinivasan, Claire and Larry Morse, Julie and George Hutchinson, and Dave and Marie Dittmer.

It was a pleasure to work with "the good editors" at Bloomsbury Press: Pete Beatty, Jenny Miyasaki, Katie Henderson, Paula Cooper, and Nancy Inglis. Editor and publisher Peter Ginna became interested in this project early on and has been a constant source of sound advice and encouragement. I consider myself fortunate indeed to have worked with such a talented and congenial crew. I am also grateful to the National Endowment for the Humanities and to the National Humanities Center for year-long fellowships.

Ellen Dittmer and I have been partners for more years than either of us cares to admit. She has always had a way with words. At first reluctant to do what she knew needed to be done, she then jumped in with enthusiasm, slashing away at my sentences, giving shape to my thoughts, and taking what I once thought was a decent manuscript and making it much, much better. This book is dedicated to our grandchildren, who are coming of age in a world much different from ours. They embody our hopes for a better America, with equality and good health care for all.

Notes

Dr. Walter Lear compiled the largest collection of materials on the Medical Committee for Human Rights, and placed it unprocessed at the Institute of Social Medicine and Community Health in Philadelphia, where I examined it. Unless otherwise noted, all citations in the book are from Walter Lear's collection. While an effort has been made to standardize the format of the citations for consistency, the citations may not be identical to the headings on the actual documents. (The papers have now been processed, and are available at the Rare Book and Manuscript Library at the University of Pennsylvania.) Biographical information on Walter Lear comes from my interviews with him on July 11–12, 17, and 28, 2000, and on January 18, 2001. All interviews were conducted in Philadelphia, Pennsylvania.

I had numerous conversations with Dr. Robert Smith from 2000 to 2007, all of which occurred in Jackson, Mississippi. Unless otherwise noted, biographical information on Dr. Smith comes from these interviews.

PREFACE

1. Martin Luther King, remarks at the second annual convention of the Medical Committee for Human Rights, Chicago, March 26, 1966.

PROLOGUE

1. Interview with Robert Smith, all interviews conducted between 2000 and 2007, Jackson, Miss.
2. Robert Smith interview.
3. John Dittmer, *Local People: The Struggle for Civil Rights in Mississippi* (Urbana: University of Illinois Press, 1994), 37, 45–46.
4. Ibid., 42–45.
5. Ibid., 32–33, 70. See also Vanessa N. Gamble, *A Place for Ourselves: The Black Hospital Movement, 1920–1944* (New York: Oxford University Press, 1995).

6. Robert Smith interview; Thomas J. Ward Jr., *Black Physicians in the Jim Crow South* (Fayetteville: University of Arkansas Press, 2003), 39–40; David Barton Smith, *Health Care Divided: Race and Healing a Nation* (Ann Arbor: University of Michigan Press, 1999), 15.

7. Smith, *Health Care Divided*, 39.

8. Robert Smith interview.

9. Interview with Aaron Shirley, Feb. 20, 2001, Jackson, Miss.; Gilbert Mason, with James Patterson Smith, *Beaches, Blood, and Ballots: A Black Doctor's Civil Rights Struggle* (Jackson: University Press of Mississippi, 2000), 37–38.

10. The AMA resolution is quoted in "Racism Rules the AMA Policies," *Journal of the National Medical Association* (Jan. 1949): 34–35. Interview with A. B. Britton, July 11, 2001, Jackson, Miss.; "General Practitioner of the Year," *Journal of the National Medical Association* (Nov. 1966): 488. The senior African American physician in Jackson was William E. Miller, who received his M.D. from the University of Illinois in 1930 and a master of public health degree from Harvard a year later.

11. James C. Cobb, *The Most Southern Place on Earth* (New York: Oxford University Press, 1992), 262–63.

12. Douglas Connor, with John F. Marzalek, *A Black Physician's Story: Bringing Hope in Mississippi* (Jackson: University Press of Mississippi, 1985), 78; Aaron Shirley interview.

13. *Time*, Aug. 23, 1968, 46–47.

14. Robert Smith interview.

15. Dittmer, *Local People*, chaps. 4 and 5.

16. Interview with Walter Lear, July 2000–Jan. 2001, Philadelphia, Pa.

17. Statement by Walter J. Lear, May 4, 1948; Association of Internes and Medical Students Committee Against Discrimination, *Discrimination in Medicine: A Report*, Dec. 1950, reprinted by the Institute of Social Medicine and Community Health.

18. Smith, *Health Care Divided*, 17, 33, 34. For more information on the National Medical Association, see W. Michael Byrd and Linda A. Clayton, *An American Health Dilemma*, (New York: Routledge Press, 2 vols.: vol. 1, 2000; vol. 2, 2002).

19. Smith, *Health Care Divided*, 48.

20. Interview with John L. S. Holloman, Nov. 14, 2000, New York; *Health Care Is a Human Right: A Collection of Biographies of the Medical Committee for Human Rights, 1964–1997* (New York: privately printed, 1997), 47; *New York Times*, March 2, 2002.

21. Dittmer, *Local People*, 157–69; Robert Smith interview.

22. *MCCR Newsletter*, n.d.; Walter Lear interview; *New York Times*, June 19, 1963. Holloman's mention of Birmingham referred to the SCLC's campaign there in the spring of 1963, made famous by the photographs of police with dogs attacking black children.

23. MCCR, press release, June 21, 1963.

24. *Medical Tribune*, July 5, 1963; *Proceedings of the Annual Meeting of the American Medical Association*, June 17–23, 1963, 286–88; *New York Times*, June 21, 1963.

25. *New York Times*, June 21, 1963; Robert Smith interview.

CHAPTER 1: THE GOOD DOCTORS

1. David Barton Smith, *Health Care Divided: Race and Healing a Nation* (Ann Arbor: University of Michigan Press, 1999), 47. See also P. Preston Reynolds, "Hospitals and Civil Rights, 1945–1963: The Case of *Simkins v. Moses H. Cone Memorial Hospital*," *Annals of Internal Medicine* (June 1, 1997), 898–906.

2. *MCCR Newsletter*, Aug. 1963.

3. Ibid.; Walter Lear to Adam Clayton Powell, June 26, 1963.

4. Minutes of the June 20, 1963, MCCR meeting; Minutes of the Steering Committee, MCCR, June 26, 1963; MCCR, *The Appeal to the AMA: Progress Report, July 12, 1963.*

5. John L. Holloman and Walter Lear to Edward R. Annis, July 31, 1963.

6. *New York Times,* July 2, 3, 1963; *MCCR Newsletter*, July 1963.

7. *New York Times*, Aug. 14, June 21, 1963.

8. Interview with Walter Lear, July 2000–Jan. 2001, Philadelphia, Pa.; *MCCR Newsletter*, Aug. 1963.

9. Walter Lear interview.

10. Interview with Leo and Trudy Orris, Sept. 13, 2000, New York; Debra Schultz, *Going South: Jewish Women in the Civil Rights Movement* (New York: NYU Press, 2001), 1, 2, 15.

11. Orris interview; Schultz, *Going South*, 80–81, 131–32.

12. Interview with Robert Smith, all interviews conducted between 2000 and 2007, Jackson, Miss.

13. Ibid.; interview with A. B. Britton, July 11, 2001, Jackson, Miss.

14. Walter Lear to Margaret B. Dolan, Aug. 9, 1963; Lear to Sheldon Rahn, Aug. 14, 1963.

15. Minutes of the Steering Committee, MCCR, June 26, 1963; Walter Lear interview.

16. Lear to Joseph Grogan, June 14, 1965; Lear to Occidental Restaurant, Feb. 19, 1965.

17. Interview with Aaron Shirley, Feb. 20, 2001, Jackson, Miss.

18. Interview with James Anderson, July 12, 2001, Jackson, Miss.

19. John Dittmer, *Local People: The Struggle for Civil Rights in Mississippi* (Urbana: University of Illinois Press, 1994), 215.

20. Ibid., 213.

21. Ibid., 208–11.

22. John Dittmer, "The Politics of the Mississippi Movement," in Charles Eagles, ed., *The Civil Rights Movement in America* (Jackson: University Press of Mississippi, 1986), 80–81.

23. Robert Smith interview.

24. Carol Rogoff to Tom Levin, June 18, 1964, Medical Committee for Human Rights collection, Schomburg Center for Research in Black Culture, New York Public Library (hereafter cited as Schomburg Center).

25. Ibid. *New York Times*, Sept. 10, 1995; Tom Levin to Charles Evers, June 23, 1964, MCHR collection, Schomburg Center; SNCC, "Mississippi Summer Program," ibid., n.d.; James Forman to Tom Levin, June 28, 1964, ibid.

26. Interview with Tom Levin, Sept. 14, 2000, New York.

27. Schultz, *Going South,* 5.

28. Levin to Evers, June 23, 1964; interview with Desmond Callan, Jan. 16, 2001, Hillsdale, N.Y.; Tom Levin interview. That the Medical Committee for Human Rights had a number of members who had been or still were affiliated with the Communist Party is indisputable. I found no evidence that the party attempted to infiltrate MCHR in an effort to take it over, or to dictate its policies. Given that even in the twenty-first century past association with the Communist Party carries a stigma in many circles, I have decided not to "name names" of party members unless given permission. On a couple of occasions a person being interviewed told me to turn off the tape recorder, then said that he or she had been a party member in the 1960s, and asked that I not make this information public. I shall respect their privacy.

29. Tom Levin to Aaron Henry, June 24, 1964, telegram, MCHR collection, Schomburg Center.

30. Interview with Martin Gittelman, Sept. 14, 2000, New York; Committee for Emergency Aid in Mississippi, press release, June 25, 1964.

31. John L. Holloman to Benjamin Wainfield, July 1, 1964; "Report by Leslie Falk, Jackson, Miss., Field Medical Administrator from July 12 to July 25, 1964."

32. Falk, "Report"; Robert Smith interview.

33. Robert Smith interview; Minutes of the Medical Committee for Human Rights (Mississippi Project), July 6, 1964; Tom Levin and Jerome Tobis to A. B. Britton, telegram, July 7, 1964, MCHR collection, Schomburg Center. Levin to Art Thomas, July 16, 1964, ibid.; *New York Times,* July 18, 1964.

CHAPTER 2: FREEDOM SUMMER IN MISSISSIPPI

1. Leslie A. Falk, "Health Care for All: A Life in Social Medicine," unpublished manuscript in my possession, 18, 24, 27, 106, 124, 166, 188, 203; interview with Leslie Falk, May 25, 2001, Sherburne, Vermont; "Fighting for the Underdog," *Hopkins Medical News* (Spring/Summer 2001): 37.

2. Leslie Falk, "Program for Mississippi Project"; Falk, "Some People Seen." In 1980 an emotionally disturbed Dennis Sweeney shot and killed Allard Lowenstein, who had been Sweeney's mentor before he went to Mississippi.

3. Interview with Robert Smith, all interviews conducted between 2000 and 2007, Jackson, Miss.; Leslie Falk interview; MCHR, *Security Handbook*, attachment 5. A majority of the volunteers were from the New York–New England area. But word of the Medical Committee's program received national press attention, and health care professionals from across the country came to Mississippi during the summer.

4. Minutes of the Executive Committee Meeting, MCHR, July 20, 1964.

5. Interview with Tom Levin, Sept. 14, 2000, New York; interview with H. Jack Geiger, Sept. 13, 2000, New York.

6. Joseph H. Brenner and Robert Coles to "Dear Doctors," June 24, 1964; Robert Coles to Tom Levin, June 24, 1964; David Miller to Tom Levin, n.d.; Elliott Hurwitt to Dr. Hamilton, Aug. 19, 1964, all in MCHR Collection, Schomburg Center.

7. Hurwitt to Hamilton, MCHR Collection, Schomburg Center; *Preliminary Report on Medical Situation in Batesville*, no author listed, July 13, 1964; Falk, "Program for Mississippi Project."

8. Robert Smith interview. Hubbard's public support of Lyndon Johnson led to his isolation in Mississippi—Barry Goldwater carried the state with 85 percent of the vote—and by the late 1960s Hubbard had moved back to New York.

9. *Report of Dr. Martin Gittelman, Canton, July 30, 1964*; Count Gibson, *Report of the Medical Coordinator for August 23–30, 1964.*

10. Alfred Kogan, M.D., *Report on Meeting with Dr. Archie Gray, Aug. 3, 1964*; Tom Levin interview; Robert Smith interview.

11. Memorandum to MCHR by Virginia Wells, July 17–24, 1964.

12. *Report of Visit to Kings Daughters Hospital,* Martha Wright, July 7, 1964; *Field Report, Leon Radler, M.D., Canton, August 3–8, 1964.*

13. Hyman Gold, M.D., "Physicians in Mississippi," *Physicians Forum* 2 (Spring–Summer 1965): 17–18.

14. Jerome Tobis to "Dear Doctor," July 25, 1964; Robert Smith interview; interview with Aaron Shirley, Feb. 20, 2001, Jackson, Miss.; John Hatch to Thomas Ricketts, n.d., John Hatch Papers, Wilson Library, University of North Carolina at Chapel Hill.

15. H. Jack Geiger interview; Robert Smith interview.

16. Minutes of the Executive Committee Meeting, MCHR, July 20, 1964.

17. Robert Smith interview.

18. Jasper F. Williams to Mrs. Johnson, Aug. 6, 1964; "Resolution from the Illinois Delegation"; Quentin Young to Montague Cobb, Aug. 13, 1964, Quentin Young Papers, State Historical Society of Wisconsin.

19. For more on the freedom schools and the summer project, see John Dittmer, *Local People: The Struggle for Civil Rights in Mississippi* (Urbana: University of Illinois Press, 1994). chaps. 11, 12.

20. MCHR, *Security Handbook*; Anonymous, "On Coming to Meridian"; Memorandum to All COFO Personnel from the Medical Committee on [sic] Human Rights, n.d.; David Levine, "Vicksburg Report."

21. Sally Belfrage, *Freedom Summer* (New York: Viking Press, 1965), 99.

22. Edward Belsky and Mary Holman, "Clarksdale Area," Aug. 2–9, 1964; H. J. Browne, "Clarksdale Medical Team," Aug. 2–8, 1964; Aaron Henry, undated report, MCHR collection, Schomburg Center; Belfrage, *Freedom Summer*, 99.

23. Interview with June Finer, Jan. 17, 2001, New Paltz, N.Y.; interview with Peter Orris, June 19, 2007, Chicago.

24. Memorandum to All COFO Personnel; Tom Levin interview; Lee Hoffman, *Report on Activities in Clarksdale*, Aug. 16–28, 1964.

25. Hoffman, *Report on Activities in Clarksdale.*

26. Ibid.; Arthur F. Dunn, *Report from Holly Springs*, Aug. 22, 1964; "Mary V. Wiles, R.N., Aug. 8–20, 1964."

27. Richard Brenner, report, Aug. 6, 1964; interview with Martin Gittelman, Sept. 14, 2000, New York; June Finer interview.

28. Coles quoted in John Dittmer, *Local People*, 327; interview with Desmond Callan, Jan. 16, 2001, Hillsdale, N.Y.; Tom Levin, Edward Sachar, Lee Hoffman, reports, Aug. 15, 1964. Years later "battle fatigue" was given the medical name post-traumatic stress disorder (PTSD), a condition that affected thousands of GI veterans of Vietnam and the Gulf wars.

29. Tom Levin to Elliott Hurwitt et al., July 28, 1964, MCHR collection, Schomburg Center; L. Redler, M.D., "Greenwood: 8/1–8/2, 1964."

30. Emanuel Schreiber, "The Idea of a Retreat Center for COFO," Sept. 10, 1964.

31. Martin Gittelman interview; Gittelman also held counseling sessions for students who would attempt to desegregate white public schools in the fall.

32. Robert Smith interview.

33. Schreiber, "The Idea"; Count Gibson, *Report of Medical Coordinator for August 23–30.*

34. Martin Gittelman interview; interview with Alvin Poussaint, May 24, 2001, Boston; *Special Report: Medical Committee for Human Rights,* n.d.

35. Dittmer, *Local People,* 251; Dr. Joel Bates, report, July 13–19, 1964.

36. June Finer, "Shooting of Silas McGhee," Aug. 17, 1964; Dittmer, *Local People,* 276–79.

37. "Medical Committee Asks Censure of Mississippi Physician," press release, MCHR, Aug. 18, 1964; Elliott Hurwitt to Norman A. Welch, Aug. 18, 1964; James R. Cavett Jr. to Hurwitt, Jan. 6, 1965.

38. Dittmer, *Local People,* 247, 283.

39. Charles Goodrich, untitled report, MCHR collection, Schomburg Center.

40. David Spain, "Mississippi Eyewitness: The Three Civil Rights Workers—How They Were Murdered," *Ramparts,* special issue (1964): 43, 46.

41. Jerry Mitchell, "Spy Agency Took Aim at NY Pathologist," *Clarion-Ledger,* April 6, 2000; Aaron O. Wells, "The Doctor," *Nation,* Dec. 28, 1964, 515–16; Spain, "Mississippi Eyewitness," 47; Seth Cagin and Philip Dray, *We Are Not Afraid: The Story of Goodman, Schwerner and Chaney and the Civil Rights Campaign in Mississippi* (New York: Macmillan, 1988), 406–7.

42. Spain, "Mississippi Eyewitness"; Dittmer, *Local People,* 283.

43. Mitchell, "Spy Agency"; Jerry Mitchell, "44 Days That Changed Mississippi," *Clarion-Ledger,* April 6, 2000; Cagin and Dray, *We Are Not Afraid,* 407; Joel G. Brunson to Louis Lasagna, June 25. Late in 1967 an all-white Mississippi jury convicted seven men, including Neshoba County deputy sheriff Cecil Price and Klan leader Sam Bowers, of the federal crime of "violating the civil rights" of Chaney, Schwerner, and Goodman. All of the defendants were released from prison by the mid-1970s. In 2005, Mitchell's investigative reporting helped lead to the trial and conviction of Edgar Ray Killen, who orchestrated the Klan killings. Killen was the beneficiary of a mistrial in 1967 when a single juror voted for his acquittal.

44. "Special Report," MCHR, Oct. 21, 1964; Dittmer, *Local People,* 302.

CHAPTER 3: THE MEDICAL ARM
OF THE CIVIL RIGHTS MOVEMENT

1. *Special Report: Medical Committee for Human Rights,* n.d.

2. Ibid.

3. Minutes of Meeting, Sept. 12, 1964, New York City; "By-laws of Medical Committee for Human Rights, Inc.," 1; Elliott Hurwitt to Aaron Wells, Sept. 14, 1964; Claire Hurwitt, open letter, Sept. 12, 1964. Elliott Hurwitt would rejoin the Medical Committee, but not in a leadership role.

4. Memo Re: Medical Committee for Human Rights: Mississippi Project. To: Medical Committee Personnel. From: Jesse Morris, n.d.

5. Ibid.; interview with Desmond Callan, Jan. 16, 2001, Hillsdale, N.Y.

6. Interviews with H. Jack Geiger, Sept. 13, 2000, March 28, 2001, New York. Unless otherwise noted, all biographical material in this chapter comes from these interviews. Geiger has written an autobiographical essay, "A Life in Social Medicine," in Ellen L. Bassuk, *The Doctor-Activist: Physicians Fighting for Social Change* (New York: Plenum Press, 1996), 11–27.

7. Claire Bradley to Aaron Wells, Oct. 21, 1964.

8. See John Dittmer, *Local People: The Struggle for Civil Rights in Mississippi* (Urbana: University of Illinois Press, 1994), chap. 12.

9. Ibid., 330.

10. Ibid., 318; Alfred Kogan and Tom Levin to "Dear Fellow Mississippi Volunteers," Oct. 16, 1964.

11. "Special Report," Oct. 21, 1964; Claire Bradley to Aaron Wells, Sept. 21, 1964.

12. Al Moldovan to "Dear Colleague," Sept. 21, 1964; Moldovan, "Treasurer's Report— 1964–1965," 3; Claire Bradley to "Dear Doctors," Sept. 9, 1964.

13. Art Thomas to Aaron Wells, Sept. 18, 1964.

14. Interviews with Phyllis Cunningham, Nov. 16, 2000, March 31, 2001, New York. Unless otherwise indicated, all biographical material in this chapter comes from these interviews.

15. Phyllis Cunningham to Claire Bradley, Sept. 12, 1964; "Phyllis Cunningham, Discussion in Jackson, Mississippi, December 12, 1964."

16. Cunningham to Bradley, Oct. 12, 1964.

17. Ibid.

18. Phyllis Cunningham to Constance Friess, Nov. 15, 2004.

19. Interviews with Josephine Disparti, March 29, 2001, March 23, 2007, New York. Unless otherwise noted, all biographical material comes from these interviews.

20. Dittmer, *Local People,* 191–93. After John Doar of the Justice Department intervened, the charges against Turnbow were dropped for lack of evidence.

21. M. Phyllis Cunningham, Helene Richardson Sanders, and Patricia Weatherly, "We Went to Mississippi: MCHR's Rural Health Project," draft copy, 1–2; Josephine Disparti interviews; interview with Josephine Disparti and Phyllis Cunningham, July 26, 2001, New York.

22. Josephine Disparti interview, March 29, 2001; Constance Friess, "Mississippi Medical Problems as of October 24 to November 1—Summary," 1964.

23. H. Jack Geiger interview, Sept. 13, 2000; Ian Smith to Aaron Wells, Oct. 9, 1964; *New York Times,* Oct. 7, 1964.

24. Phyllis Cunningham to Claire Bradley, Oct. 12, 1964.

25. Friess, "Mississippi Medical"; *Report by Josephine Disparti, November 13, 1964*; *Report by Josephine Disparti, November 23, 1964.*

26. Josephine Disparti and Phyllis Cunningham interviews, July 26, 2001, New York; Claire Bradley to Donald Cornaly, Sept. 23, 1964; Cunningham quoted in Ronda Kotelchuck and Howard Levy, "MCHR: An Organization in Search of an Identity," *Health/PAC Bulletin,* no. 63 (March/April 1975): 6.

27. MCHR Executive Committee Minutes, Dec. 14, 1964; Des Callan, *Report on the Greenville–Jackson Meeting,* Dec. 11–13, 1964; interview with Tom Levin, Sept. 14, 2000.

28. Sidney Greenberg to Bob Smith, Feb. 22, 1964; Smith to Greenberg, March 13, 1965.

29. Desmond Callan interview.

30. Ibid.; Parry Teasdale, "Dr. Desmond Callan, 76, Dies," *Independent,* July 26, 2002.

31. Desmond Callan interview.

32. Callan, *Report on the Greenville–Jackson Meeting.*

33. Ibid.

34. Ibid.

35. Ibid.; MCHR Executive Committee Minutes, Dec. 15, 1964.

36. H. Jack Geiger interviews.

37. Ibid.

38. *Boston Globe,* July 30, 2002; H. Jack Geiger interviews.

39. H. Jack Geiger, "The First Community Health Centers: A Model of Enduring Value," *Journal of Ambulatory Care Management* 28 (2005): 295.

40. Callan, *Report on the Greenville–Jackson Meeting.*

41. MCHR Executive Committee Minutes, Dec. 15, 1964.

CHAPTER 4: SELMA AND JACKSON

1. Desmond Callan, untitled manuscript in his private papers, n.d.; Desmond Callan, "A Mississippi Health Program: A Modest Proposal," Jan. 5, 1965.

2. Callan, "A Modest Proposal."

3. Interview with Desmond Callan, Jan. 16, 2001, Hillsdale, N.Y.

4. Ibid.; Minutes of the Executive Committee Meeting, MCHR, Feb. 15, 1965; Johnny Parham, *Report of the Executive Director,* March 22, 1965.

5. Minutes of the Executive Committee Meeting, MCHR, Feb. 15, 1965; Hosea Williams and Lafayette Surney to Aaron Wells, March 5, 1965.

6. Interview with Alfred Moldovan, November 15, 2000, New York.

7. Ibid.; *New York Times,* March 8, 1965.

8. No author, *Report on Activities of the Medical Committee in Selma, Alabama, March 1965,* n.d.

9. Reed and Lewis quoted in John Lewis, with Michael D'Orso, *Walking with the Wind: A Memoir of the Movement* (New York: Simon & Schuster, 1998), 328, 327.

10. Al Moldovan interview; *New York Times,* March 8, 1965; C. H. Wright, M.D., "The Siege of Selma"; Tom Levin to Johnny Parham, March 12, 1965.

11. David Garrow, *Bearing the Cross: Martin Luther King, Jr., and the Southern Christian Leadership Conference* (New York: Morrow, 1986), 400–401.

12. Ibid., 402; Al Moldovan interview.

13. H. Jack Geiger, Richard Hauskenecht, Alfred Moldovan, Leon Redler, and Belinda Straight, letter to *Medical Tribune,* April 19, 1965; interview with H. Jack Geiger,

Sept. 13, 2000. The Alabama official was bluffing. His office did not intervene later when the out-of-state physicians provided first aid to demonstrators beaten by police in Montgomery.

14. Garrow, *Bearing the Cross,* 396, 405–6; Lewis, *Walking with the Wind,* 355; Clayborne Carson, *In Struggle: SNCC and the Black Awakening of the 1960s* (Cambridge: Harvard University Press, 1981), 160.

15. Levin to Parham, March 15, 1965; E. Richard Weinerman, M.D., *Report from Alabama, March 16–19, 1965.*

16. Weinerman, *Report from Alabama*; Johnson, quoted in Lewis, *Walking with the Wind,* 339; Garrow, *Bearing the Cross,* 409.

17. Weinerman, *Report from Alabama*; MCHR *"Newsletter,"* March 1965.

18. Garrow, *Bearing the Cross,* 420; interview with David French, February 12, 2002, Washington, D.C.; Lewis, *Walking with the Wind,* 343; MCHR Chicago Chapter, "Crisis in Selma," April 24, 1965.

19. Interview with Tom Levin, Sept. 14, 2000; Aaron O. Wells, "The National Chairman's Report," *Health News,* Aug. 1965, 2; Mary Holman to "Dear Jim," March 24, 1965, MCHR collection, Boston Public Library.

20. Interview with Josephine Disparti March 29, 2001, New York; interview with Alvin Poussaint, May 21, 2003, Boston; interview with June Finer, March 29, 2001, New Paltz, N.Y.

21. Alvin Poussaint interview; Chicago Chapter, "Crisis in Selma."

22. H. Jack Geiger interview; Tom Levin interview; minutes of the executive board, MCHR, March 22, 1965.

23. Tom Levin interview; Cobb quoted in *Medical Tribune* 6, no. 102 (1965), clipping; *Journal of the National Medical Association* (March 1966): 130.

24. Wells, quoted in *MCHR Newsletter,* May 1965; Leonidas Berry to Aaron Wells, May 3, 1965.

25. Aaron Wells to Montague Cobb, March 16, 1965; Wells to Leonidas Berry, June 2, 1965; Berry to Wells, July 1, 1965; "NMA Votes to Recruit White Physicians," *Medical Tribune* 6, no. 102 (1965), clipping; H. Jack Geiger interview; David French to Aaron Wells, Dec. 9, 1964; interview with Robert Smith.

26. Interview with Johnny Parham, March 30, 2002, New York; *MCHR Newsletter,* March 1965.

27. Johnny Parham, "Report of the Executive Director," March 22, 1965, copy in Parham's personal papers.

28. Ibid.; Johnny Parham interview.

29. "By-Laws of the Medical Committee for Human Rights, Inc."; "Resolution on Chapter Structure and Membership Adopted at First Annual Conference," MCHR, Washington, D.C., April 23–25, 1965; "Fund-Raising Resolution Passed at MCHR Annual Conference," Washington, D.C., April 23–25, 1965.

30. Minutes of the Executive Board, MCHR, April 19, 1965.

31. *MCHR Newsletter,* May 1965; "National Executive Board" (list of members); "MCHR National Executive Committee (as of Governing Council Meeting, June 20, 1965)."

32. *MCHR Newsletter,* May 1965; Alvin Poussaint interview. See also the biographical

essay on Poussaint in George R. Metcalf, *Up from Within: Today's New Black Leaders* (New York: McGraw-Hill, 1971), 234–60.

33. Alvin Poussaint interview; Josephine Disparti interview.

34. Alvin Poussaint interview.

35. Interview with Robert Smith, all interviews conducted between 2000 and 2007, Jackson, Miss.; H. Jack Geiger interview; Sinonia Spinka to Dr. Robert Smith, Jan. 4, 1965, personal collection of Robert Smith; Aaron O. Wells to John Doar, April 7, 1965.

36. John Dittmer, *Local People: The Struggle for Civil Rights in Mississippi* (Urbana: University of Illinois Press, 1994), 344.

37. Ibid., 344–46.

38. "Statement by Phyllis Cunningham, R.N., Employed by Medical Committee for Human Rights and the Student Nonviolent Coordinating Committee," n.d.; "Rights Drive Nurse Tells of Miss. Jail Horrors," *Pittsburgh Post-Gazette,* July 1, 1961, clipping.

39. Josephine Disparti interview; interview with June Finer, May 23, 2007, New Paltz, N.Y.

40. June Finer interview; Dittmer, *Local People,* 345; *New York Times,* July 1, 9, 1965; Alvin Poussaint to Johnny Parham, July 13, 1965.

41. "List of Brutalities in the Jackson Freedom Democratic Party Arrests Beginning June 14, 1965," MCHR, press release, June 19, 1965.

42. Ibid.; John McKee Pratt, "Mississippi Fair, 1965," *Health Rights,* Aug. 1965, 4–5; Dittmer, *Local People,* 345.

43. "List of Brutalities"; Memorandum to National Office, MCHR, from Fredric Solomon Re: Congressional Briefing, June 30, 1965; "Statement on Police Brutality in the South," MCHR, press release, n.d.; *New York Herald Tribune,* June 23, 1965, clipping; June Finer, report, May 1965–July 1965, 6.

44. Dittmer, *Local People,* 346.

45. Alvin Poussaint, *Report on Southern Projects,* Jan. 16, 1966; Johnny Parham to Chapter Presidents, telegram, June 10, 1965; Parham, "Day Letter to All Chapters," June 23, 1965.

46. Minutes of the National Governing Council Meeting, MCHR, June 20, 1965.

CHAPTER 5: SUMMER, 1965

1. Aaron Wells, "The National Chairman's Report," *Health Rights* (Aug. 1965) 2; "Chapter and Field Reports," MCHR, Sept. 1965, 1–6.

2. "Chapter and Field Reports," 6–7; Minutes of the Steering Committee— 8-17-65; Philip Stewart to Edward Barsky, Sept. 8, 1965.

3. Interview with Samuel Siegel, March 28, 2001, New York.

4. David Barton Smith, *Health Care Divided: Race and the Healing of a Nation* (Ann Arbor: University of Michigan Press, 1999), 51; interview with Quentin Young, Oct. 12, 2001, Chicago; Arthur Falls to Johnny Parham, June 4, 1965; "Chapter and Field Reports," 1.

5. "Chapter and Field Reports," 5–6; *MCHR Newsletter,* Jan. 1965.

6. "Chapter and Field Reports," 1–4; Walter Lear to H. Jack Geiger, Sept. 20, 1965; Los Angeles Physicians for Social Responsibility "Newsletter," Sept. 6, 1965; Minutes of the Steering Committee Meeting, MCHR Los Angeles Chapter, Dec. 15, 1965.

7. Adam Fairclough, *Race and Democracy: The Civil Rights Struggle in Louisiana, 1915–1972* (Athens: University of Georgia Press, 1995), 345, 355.

8. Ibid., 356–58; Wagner Bridger and Marvin Belsky to "Dear Colleagues," March 17, 1965.

9. June Finer, report, May 1965–July 1965; interview with June Finer, May 23, 2007, New Paltz, N.Y., "Chapter and Field Reports," 9.

10. *New York Times*, July 9, 1965; statement by Leneva Tiedeman, July 9, 1965; statement by Frank Lossy, July 9, 1965; Lance Hill, *The Deacons for Defense: Armed Resistance and the Civil Rights Movement* (Chapel Hill: University of North Carolina Press, 2004), 140–44; Fairclough, *Race and Democracy*, 368–69. Crowe survived the shooting. Charges against Austin were later dropped when he agreed to leave Bogalusa. Hill, *Deacons for Defense*, 253.

11. *New York Times*, July 11, 1965; Johnny Parham, telegram, July 11, 1965; Hilda Braverman to Johnny Parham, July 11, 1965; C. H. Wright, "Report to MCHR," Bogalusa, LA, July 17–24, 1965.

12. Wright, "Report to MCHR."

13. Ibid.; Hilda Braverman to Johnny Parham, July 28, 1965, Aug. 16, 1965; Braverman, MCHR, Memorandum to CORE Projects, Re: Visit of MCHR Personnel, n.d.; Philip R. Stewart and Binnie Chiles, "Baton Rouge and New Orleans Reports," n.d.

14. Braverman to Parham, Aug. 16, 1965; "Chapter and Field Reports," 9; Leneva Tiedeman to Johnny Parham, Sept. 3, 1965.

15. Maria C. Phaneuf to June Finer, Aug. 2, 1965; June Finer, report.

16. Robert V. Jacobson, report, July 17, 1965–Aug. 1, 1965.

17. June Finer interview, Nov. 14, 2001.

18. Willis Butler, M.D., report, on Interview with Dr. P. B. Moss, 9-30-65; Willis Butler, M.D., report on interview with Dr. Walter Greene, 10-6-65; Willis Butler, "Summary of Three Week Tour of Duty as a Volunteer," Sept. 12, 1965.

19. Memorandum to Johnny Parham Jr. by Alvin F. Poussaint, n.d.,; June Finer and Willis Butler to Parham, Oct. 5, 1965.

20. Zanvel Klein, report, Sept. 9, 1965; R. Greenberg, M.D., report, Sept. 12, 1965.

21. Thomas Waddell, M.D., "Summary of 16 Day Tour," Nov. 6, 1965; Abe Chaplin and George Sigel, "MCHR activities: Selma, Ala., Jackson, Miss., Baton Rouge, La.," Aug. 30, 1965.

22. Waddell, "16 Day Tour"; Leneva Tiedeman to Johnny Parham, Nov. 12, 1965; Phyllis Cunningham to Alvin Poussaint, Oct. 10, 1966; *Medical Committee for Human Rights, Selma, Alabama*, pamphlet, n.d.

23. Alvin Poussaint, *Report on Southern Projects*, July 1, 1965–Dec. 1, 1965.

24. John Dittmer, *Local People: The Struggle for Civil Rights in Mississippi* (Urbana: University of Illinois Press), chap. 15.

25. William Bronston, "A New Generation: The Student Medical Conference," *Health Rights*, Aug. 1965, 8; MCHR, "Orientation Program for Health Profession Students Prior to Mississippi Summer, June 27–July 3, 1965."

26. *Pittsburgh Press,* July 4, 1965, clipping; Richard Weinerman to Johnny Parham Jr., June 10, 1965; Parham to Weinerman, July 14, 1965. Leon Kass went on to become chair of the President's Council of Bioethics during the first term of President George W. Bush. He became an outspoken opponent of embryonic stem cell research and cloning.

27. Alvin Poussaint, "Medical Committee for Human Rights, 1966," Annual Report, 8; interview with Fitzhugh Mullan, Feb. 14, 2002, Bethesda, Md.; Poussaint, *Report on Visit to Southern District Assignment Areas,* July 17 and 18, 1965; Poussaint, "Notes Taken During Meeting with MCHR Student Volunteers—July 24, 1965."

28. Ibid.; Conger quoted in Fitzhugh Mullan, *Big Doctoring in America: Profiles in Primary Care* (Berkeley: University of California Press, 2002), 62.

29. Fitzhugh Mullan interview; Fitzhugh Mullan, *White Coat, Clenched Fist: The Political Education of an American Physician* (New York: Macmillan, 1976, and Ann Arbor: University of Michigan Press, paperback ed., 2006), 5, 11.

30. Fitzhugh Mullan interview; Mullan, diary entry, July 17, in Quentin Young Papers, State Historical Society of Wisconsin (hereafter cited as Young Papers); Mullan, *White Coat,* 4.

31. Mullan, August 1, diary entry, in Young Papers.

32. Stokely Carmichael and Ekwueme Michael Thelwell, *Ready for Revolution: The Life and Struggles of Stokely Carmichael (Kwame Ture)* (New York: Scribner, 2003), 377; Mullan, *White Coat,* 16.

33. Mullan, *White Coat,* 17; Fitzhugh Mullan interview.

34. Mullan, *White Coat,* 18.

35. Fitzhugh Mullan interview; Mullan to Alvin Poussaint, Sept. 28, 1965, in Young Papers; Chicago MCHR, Winter Bulletin, 1965–66, in ibid.

36. Dittmer, *Local People,* 368–69.

37. Al Moldovan to Tom Levin, April 10, 1965; Minutes of the Executive Committee Meeting, MCHR, June 7, 1965; Tom Levin, Robert Smith, and Helen Bass Williams to Mike Holloman, July 2, 1965.

38. Johnny Parham to Tom Levin, July 7, 1965; Levin to Parham, July 10, 1965.

39. H. Jack Geiger to Warren McKenna, May 10, 1965, Medical Committee for Human Rights Collection, Schomburg Center for Research in Black Culture, New York Public Library.

40. Robert Smith to James Hendrick, July 22, 1965; interview with Robert Smith, all interviews conducted between 2000 and 2007, Jackson, Miss.; interview with Aaron Shirley, Feb. 20, 2001; and interview with James Anderson, July 12, 2001.

41. *New York Times,* obituary, July 23, 2000.

42. Ibid.; Josephine Martin and Robert Schwartz to Tom Levin, July 15, 1965; Schwartz and Martin to Johnny Parham, Oct. 30, 1965; interview with Unita Blackwell and Robert Schwartz, July 25, 2001, New York; Josephine Martin, "Front Line Psychiatry for Civil Rights Workers," n.d., Josephine Martin Collection, University of Southern Mississippi Library. For an autobiography that deals with their life together, see Robert J. Schwartz, *Can You Make a Difference? A Memoir of a Life for Change* (New York: Lantern Books, 2002).

43. Dittmer, *Local People,* 381–82.

CHAPTER 6: THE LAST MARCH

1. Alvin F. Poussaint, "Report on Southern Projects, July 1, 1965 to Dec. 31, 1965"; personal data sheet, Pat Weatherly; Johnny Parham to Helene Richardson, June 24, 1965; Jeannette Badger, "In Retrospect," n.d.; "Report of the Executive Director," July 19, 1965.

2. Interview with Josephine Disparti, March 29, 2001, New York; Disparti to Johnny Parham, July 8, Aug. 13, 1965; Helene Richardson to "Betty," July 19, 1965, in Quentin Young Papers, State Historical Society of Wisconsin.

3. Interview with Phyllis Cunningham, Nov. 16, 2000; Memorandum Concerning Future Plans for the Southern Program of MCHR by Cunningham, n.d., Young Papers; Alvin Poussaint to Johnny Parham, June 20, 1965.

4. Helene Richardson and Patricia Weatherly, "Holmes County Clinic: An Experiment in Rural Health Care," *Health Rights* (Spring 1966), 11, 19–21.

5. Interviews with H. Jack Geiger, Sept. 13, 2000, March 28, 2001, New York.

6. Alvin F. Poussaint to F. Peter Libassi, Civil Rights Division, HEW, March 3, 1966; Des Callan to Al Moldovan, Dec. 5, 1965; no author, "Complaint for Hospitals," n.d. For more on Title VI enforcement outside of Mississippi, see Preston P. Reynolds, "The Federal Government's Use of Title VI and Medicare to Racially Integrate Hospitals in the United States, 1963 through 1967," in *American Journal of Public Health* (1997): 1850–58.

7. No author, "Complaint: Scott County Hospital," n.d.; *Title VI . . . One Year Later: A Survey of Desegregation of Health and Welfare Services in the South*, U.S. Commission on Civil Rights (Washington, D.C.: Government Printing Office, 1966), 5.

8. Rowland Evans and Robert Novak, "Title VI of Civil Rights Will Be in a Minor Key," n.d., clipping; Phyllis Cunningham to Mary Holman, June 8, 1965; David Barton Smith, *Health Care Divided: Race and Healing a Nation* (Ann Arbor: University of Michigan Press, 1999), 125.

9. Alvin Poussaint to Robert Kastenmeier, Dec. 8, 1965; Johnny Parham to "Chapter Chairmen," Sept. 16, 1965.

10. *New York Times*, Dec. 17, 1965; *Washington Post,* Dec. 17, 1965.

11. John W. Gardner to Robert Kennedy, Feb. 1, 1966; Robert Kennedy to Alvin Poussaint, Feb. 15, 1966; National Medical Association, press release, August 9, 1966; Smith, *Health Care Divided*, 161–63.

12. Surgeon General William H. Stewart to "Dear Hospital Administrator," March 4, 1966; Public Health Service, press release, March 7, 1966; no author, "Hospital Compliance: Selected States as of May 7, 1966"; *New York Times*, June 13, 16, 1966.

13. Smith, *Health Care Divided*, 132, 133; interview with Paul Plotz, Feb. 14, 2002, Bethesda, Md.

14. Paul Plotz interview; Des Callan to Johnny Parham, May 16, 1966, Medical Committee for Human Rights Collection, Schomburg Center for Research in Black Culture, New York Public Library; Peter Libassi to Alvin Poussaint, March 4, 1966; Memorandum to SNCC Staff by Phyllis Cunningham, April 25, 1966.

15. Paul Plotz interview.

16. Ibid.; *Detroit Free Press*, Oct. 30, 1966, clipping.

17. *New York Times,* June 9, 1966; Paul Plotz interview; Lynn M. Pohl, "The Permeable Color Line: Medical Interaction and Hospital 'Desegregation' in a Mississippi Community," 1977, paper in my possession, 29.

18. Pohl, "Permeable Color Line," 29; Harold M. Graning to Johnny Parham, March 1, 1966; interview with Robert Smith, all interviews conducted between 2000 and 2007, Jackson, Miss.

19. *New York Times,* Sept. 29, 30, 1966; Smith, *Health Care Divided,* 165; *New York Times,* Oct. 22, 1966.

20. Pohl, "Permeable Color Line," 26; Frank E. G. Weil to Alvin Poussaint, Sept. 24, 1966, personal papers of Alvin Poussaint.

21. Mary Holman, "Summary of Lobby Activity for MCHR," April 1966, personal papers of Mary Holman; Medicare form, ibid.

22. Evelyn Dupont, *Office Operations: A Report,* n.d.; interview with Johnny Parham, March 30, 2002, New York.

23. Johnny Parham interview; Smith obituary, *New York Times,* April 5, 2001.

24. Esther Smith to Dizzy Gillespie, July 16, 1965; Edward Barsky, "Fund Raising Report," June 7, 1965; Minutes of the Executive Committee Meeting, MCHR, Aug. 2, 1965.

25. Johnny Parham interview; interview with Alfred Moldovan, Nov. 15, 2000; Memorandum to Johnny Parham and others by Mrs. Cecile Marshall, March 7, 1966; Minutes of the Governing Council, MCHR, March 24, 1966.

26. Mike Holloman to Johnny Parham, Dec. 4, 1965.

27. Mike Holloman, telegram, Feb. 4, 1966; Alfred Moldovan, *Interim Treasurer's Report,* Confidential, March 1, 1966, 21.

28. Alfred Moldovan interview; Esther Smith to Mike Holloman, Feb. 25, 1966; Tuni Berman to Holloman, Feb. 25, 1966.

29. Johnny Parham to Mike Holloman, March 16, 1966.

30. Interview with Desmond Callan, Jan. 16, 2001, Hillsdale, N.Y.; Minutes of the Governing Council, MCHR, March 24, 1966.

31. Minutes of the Governing Council, MCHR, March 24, 1966; Desmond Callan and Johnny Parham interviews.

32. Summary Minutes of the National Governing Council, MCHR, March 24 and 26, 1966.

33. Ibid.

34. Phyllis Cunningham interview.

35. Alfred Moldovan interview.

36. Paul Plotz and Desmond Callan interviews; interview with David French and Sidney Wolfe, Feb. 13, 2002, Washington, D.C.

37. Minutes of the Governing Council, MCHR, March 27, 1966; Minutes of the Executive Committee, MCHR, July 19, 1966; Phyllis Cunningham interview; Samuel Bachrack to Johnny Parham, April 4, 1966; interview with June Finer, Nov. 4, 2000, New Paltz, N.Y.

38. Minutes of the Governing Council, MCHR, March 27, 1966; Mary Holman to Johnny Parham, March 23, 1966.

39. John Dittmer, *Local People: The Struggle for Civil Rights in Mississippi* (Urbana: University of Illinois Press), 389; interview with Alvin Poussaint, May 24, 2001, Boston.

40. Dittmer, *Local People*, 392–93.

41. Alvin Poussaint and Phyllis Cunningham interviews.

42. Robert Smith interview.

43. Ibid.; Alvin Poussaint interview.

44. Dittmer, *Local People*, 395–98.

45. Ibid., 397.

46. Ibid., 398; Alvin Poussaint interview.

47. Alvin Poussaint interview; Dittmer, *Local People,* 399–400.

48. Robert Smith and Alvin Poussaint interviews.

49. Robert Smith interview; Dittmer, *Local People*, 400–1.

50. Dittmer, *Local People*, 401.

51. Robert Smith and Phyllis Cunningham interviews.

52. Alvin Poussaint interview; Poussaint, "The Stresses of the White Female Worker in the Civil Rights Movement," *American Journal of Psychiatry* 123, no. 4 (October 1966), 401–7. Phyllis Cunningham immediately took exception to the stereotype of the white woman activist in Poussaint's essay, and told him so. Mary Holman tried to diffuse the issue with a poem she wrote and sent to Poussaint, titled "Doggerel for a Black Psychiatrist," which poked fun at Poussaint as well as the subjects of his essay. Poussaint wrote back that the poem was "witty and extremely well done," and went on to claim that "the paper is overall sympathetic to the plight of the white female worker," a conclusion that escaped many readers. Phyllis Cunningham interview; Mary Holman to Al Poussaint, April 28, 1966, Mary Holman's personal papers; Poussaint to Holman, May 6, 1966, ibid.

53. Dittmer, *Local People*, 402; Alvin Poussaint, "Speech to Be Delivered at Meredith March Rally."

54. Rosalie Ross to Phyllis Cunningham, n.d.

CHAPTER 7: THE WAR AT HOME

1. "MCHR Summer Program (1966) in the South for MCHR Volunteers," n.d.; Alvin Poussaint, "Brief Report on the Southern Program," Aug. 17, 1966.

2. Interview with Walter Lear, July 11, 2001, Philadelphia; interview with Quentin Young, Oct. 12, 2001, Chicago; *MCHR Newsletter 2,* July 13, 1966, *MCHR Newsletter 3,* July 29, 1966; Rosalie Ross to Phyllis Cunningham, Aug. 29, 1966; Mark Newman, *Divine Agitators: The Delta Ministry and Civil Rights in Mississippi* (Athens: University of Georgia Press, 2004), 112.

3. Phyllis Cunningham to Cecile Boatwright, July 8, 1966; Cunningham to Elaine Bernstein, Oct. 15, 1966; Cunningham to Patricia Weatherly, Oct. 17, 1966.

4. Interview with Phyllis Cunningham, March 31, 2001, New York; Cunningham to Elaine Bernstein, Oct. 15, 1966, Alvin Poussaint personal papers; Patricia Weatherly and Cunningham to Edward Netingam, Nov. 26, 1966, personal collection of Desmond Callan.

5. Phyllis Cunningham, interview; Charles M. Payne, *I've Got the Light of Freedom: The Organizing Tradition and the Mississippi Freedom Struggle* (Berkeley: University of California Press, 1995), 383–84.

6. David French to "Dear Sir," Oct. 22, 1966.

7. Minutes of the National Governing Council, MCHR, San Francisco, Calif., Oct. 29–30, 1966; Memorandum to MCHR Chapter Leaders by Quentin Young, Sept. 22, 1966, Quentin Young Papers, State Historical Society of Wisconsin.

8. Minutes of the National Governing Council, MCHR, Young Papers; "Result of National Billing as of August 31, 1966."

9. Henry S. Kahn to "Dear Fellow Officer," Oct. 4, 1966, Young Papers.

10. "Structure Committee," n.d., Young Papers; Minutes of the National Governing Council MCHR.

11. Ibid.

12. Interview with William Bronston, March 27, 2002, Carmichael, Calif.; James T. Patterson, *Grand Expectations: The United States, 1945–1974* (New York: Oxford University Press, 1996), 595–96.

13. "Medical Group Urges Vietnam War Cessation and Negotiations," MCHR, press release, May 25, 1967; Martin Luther King to Quentin Young, May 1, 1967; Council of Health Organizations, press release, Dec. 27, 1971. The 1967 resolution on Vietnam cost the MCHR members, including Paul Cornely, its most prestigious African American sponsor.

14. Patterson, *Grand Expectations*, 599, 616; E. L. Davis to Curtis Tarr, n.d.

15. Patterson, *Grand Expectations,* 599, 616; MCHR, "MCHR Program for Draft Exams," Feb. 9, 1969.

16. MCHR, "Suggestions to Physicians Preparing Reports for Selective Service Registrants," May 1968; MCHR, "MCHR List of Medical Disabilities," n.d..

17. Messinger quoted in undated *New York Times* clipping; *New York Times*, Nov. 16, 1970; "Draft-Defying Doctors," *Time*, Nov. 16, 1970, 67; Murray Abowitz and Arlene Farwell to "Dear Colleague," Nov. 5, 1969; anonymous interview.

18. *Newsweek*, Aug. 3, 1970, 42–43; *Time*, Aug. 3, 1970.

19. Murray Abowitz, "Rough Draft," Los Angeles MCHR/PSR, n.d., ca. March 1970.

20. Abowitz, ibid.; MCHR, "MCHR List of Medical Disabilities." The category "IV-F" meant "not qualified for any service."

21. Patterson, *Grand Expectations,* 617; Abowitz, "MCHR List"; *New York Times*, n.d., clipping; *Newsweek*, Aug. 3, 1970, 43.

22. Abowitz, "MCHR List"; *Newsweek*, Aug. 3, 1970, 43; *New York Times*, n.d., clipping.

23. Elinor Langer, "The Court-Martial of Captain Levy: Medical Ethics v. Military Law," *Science* 156 (June 1967): 1346–47.

24. Ibid., 1346–68; Walter Goodman, "Choose Your War; Or, the Case of the Selective C.O.," *New York Times Magazine,* March 23, 1969, 35, 128.

25. *Newsweek*, June 2, 1967, 15–16; Goodman, "Choose Your War," 128.

26. Langer, "Court-Martial," 1349–50; *Nation*, May 29, 1967, 676–7; *New York Times,* April 19, 1969.

27. *Health Rights News*, October 1967, 12; Medical Committee to End the War in Vietnam, "Newsletter," Spring 1968, 3; MCHR, "Resolution by the Governing Council . . . on Health and Military Services," May 10, 1967; T. G. G. Wilson, letter to *New York Times,* Aug. 10, 1967.

28. Minutes of the National Executive Committee, MCHR, May 10, 1970; Henry S. Kahn, Memo on Organizing Project for Army's Medical Field School, April 29, 1970; Kahn, "Project Report: Military Education Project," July 21, 1971.

29. *San Antonio Express-News*, Aug. 1, 1971, clipping.

30. Interview with Susan Schnall, May 22, 2007, New York; *San Antonio Express-News*, Aug. 1, 1971, clipping. Schnall tells the story of the demonstration and her arrest in David Zeiger's documentary film about antiwar activity among military personnel, *Sir! No Sir!*

31. Henry Kahn to "Brothers and Sisters," Aug. 13, 1971; Jane Fonda, *My Life So Far* (New York: Random House, 2005), 272–73; Amily Hamanoff to Pat Murchie, Oct. 1, 1971.

32. Kahn, "Brothers and Sisters"; Amily Hamanoff to Pat Murchie, Oct. 1, 1971; Susan Schnall interview.

33. *Indianapolis Star,* Nov. 3, 1969; Chicago MCHR "Newsletter," Nov. 24, 1969; "Statement of the Beaver 55," n.d.

34. *Health Rights News*, March–April 1971, 10; interview with Quentin Young, Sept. 29, 2006.

35. *Health Rights News*, March–April 1971, 10.

36. Jane Kennedy, "Letters from Prison," *Health Rights News*, Jan. 1971, 14.

37. Bannon quoted in *Health Rights News*, March–April 1971, 1, and *Health Rights News,* May–June 1971, 11; Leonard R. McConnell, chairman, Parole Board, to Eli Messinger, March 24, 1971; Gilbert S. Omenn to Senator Vance Hartke, Jan. 30, 1971; Jane Kennedy, "Note to My Friends," Feb. 3, 1971; *Detroit Free Press*, July 24, 1971, clipping.

38. Eli Messinger to Gus Harrison, director of Michigan Department of Corrections, Feb. 13, 1971; Gilbert Omenn to Senator Birch Bayh, Jan. 30, 1971; Tom Fitzpatrick, "Prison News—The Sad and the Glad," *Chicago Sun-Times*, n.d., clipping; Jack Murchie, "Jane's Friends See Parole Board," *Health Rights News*, March–April 1971, 10; Barbara Yippee, *Health Liberation News,* n.d., clipping; Quentin Young interview (Oct. 12, 2001). Jane Kennedy's exposure of conditions in prisons foreshadowed the development of the MCHR task forces on prison health reform in the early 1970s.

39. Eli Messinger to "Dear Friend," draft letter, n.d.; Minutes of the Governing Council, MCHR, Jan. 10–12, 1969, 6.

40. Steven Fox, "Medical Aid for Vietnam," *Health Rights* (Spring 1966), 6–7, 18; Paul Lowinger, draft of MCHR press release, n.d.; *Health Rights News*, June 1972, 10.

CHAPTER 8: THE MEDICAL ARM OF THE NEW LEFT

1. Ronda Kotelchuck and Howard Levy, "MCHR: An Organization in Search of an Identity," *Health/PAC Bulletin*, no. 63 (March/April 1975), 5.

2. David Garrow, *Bearing the Cross: Martin Luther King, Jr., and the Southern Christian Leadership Council* (New York: William Morrow, 1986), 557–58; Nick Kotz, *Judgment Days: Lyndon Baines Johnson, Martin Luther King, Jr., and the Laws That Changed America* (Boston: Houghton Mifflin, 2005), 373–74; William Chafe, *The Unfinished Journey: America Since World War II* (New York: Oxford University Press, 4th ed., 1999), 365.

3. Garrow, *Bearing the Cross*, 579, 583.

4. Martin Luther King, "Open Letter to Members of the Health Professions," March 22, 1968; "Convention Resolutions," *Health Rights News*, May 1968, 3; Mary Holman to Johnny Parham, Dec. 27, 1967.

5. Arthur Frank, Jesse Roth, Sidney Wolfe, and Henry Metzger, "Medical Problems of Civil Disorders," *New England Journal of Medicine*, Jan. 30, 1969, 247–48.

6. Ben W. Gilbert and the staff of the *Washington Post, Ten Blocks from the White House: Anatomy of the Washington Riots of 1968* (New York: Praeger, 1968), 14–33.

7. "Emergency Medical Plan Put to an Early Test," *Medical World News*, May 17, 1968, 67; Washington MCHR to "Dear Friend," April 12, 1968, Quentin Young Papers, State Historical Society of Wisconsin.

8. Frank et al., "Medical Problems," 249; interview with Paul Plotz, Feb. 14, 2002, Bethesda, Md.

9. Frank et al., "Medical Problems," 251–53; "Emergency Medical Plan," 67.

10. Frank et al., "Medical Problems," 248.

11. Gilbert, *Ten Blocks*, 197, 199; Florence Ridlon, *A Black Physician's Struggle for Civil Rights: Edward C. Mazique, M.D.* (Albuquerque: University of New Mexico Press, 2005), 258–59.

12. Ridlon, *Black Physician's Struggle*, 268; Quentin Young to Lionel Swan, March 29, 1968, Young Papers.

13. Ridlon, *Black Physician's Struggle*, 272–73; Mary Holman to John Dittmer, Aug. 21, 2001; Arthur Frank to Quentin Young, June 4, 1968, Young Papers.

14. Ridlon, *Black Physician's Struggle*, 268–70.

15. McGrory quoted in Gerald D. McKnight, *The Last Crusade: Martin Luther King, Jr., the FBI, and the Poor People's Campaign* (Boulder, Colo.: Westview Press, 1998), 114–15; Charles Fager, *Uncertain Resurrection: The Poor People's Campaign* (Fayetteville, N.C.: Kimo Press, 1982), 95.

16. "Medicine in the Mud for Poor People's March," *Science News* 83, June 8, 1968, 545; Harvey Webb Jr., "Dentistry at Resurrection City," Young Papers, n.d., clipping.

17. Ridlon, *Black Physician's Struggle*, 262, 279.

18. Franks quoted in "Medicine in the Mud," 545; Edward C. Mazique, "Health Services and the Poor People's Campaign," *Journal of the National Medical Association* 60 (July 1968), 332–33.

19. Ridlon, *Black Physician's Struggle*, 277; Gilbert, *Ten Blocks*, 201–2.

20. Ridlon, *Black Physician's Struggle*, 271.

21. James Simon Kunen, *The Strawberry Statement—Notes of a College Revolutionary* (New York: Random House, 1968), 14–15, 17; Mark Kurlansky, *1968: The Year That Rocked the World* (New York: Random House, 2004), 195–96. See also Roger Kahn, *The Battle for Morningside Heights: Why Students Rebel* (New York: William Morrow, 1970).

22. *New York Times*, April 24–27, 1968; Kunen, *Strawberry Statement*, 20–29; Kurlansky, *1968*, 198–202.

23. "Statement of June Finer, M.D.," n.d.; Kahn, *The Battle*, 129–32.

24. "Statement of June Finer, M.D."

25. Kahn, *The Battle*, 193, 199.

26. Ibid., 199, 205.

27. Interview with June Finer, May 23, 2007, New Paltz, N.Y.; "Statement of June Finer, M.D."; Kahn, *The Battle*, 129–30.

28. Marvin Harris, "Big Bust on Morningside Heights," *Nation*, June 10, 1969, 757; "Statement of June Finer, M.D."

29. *New York Times*, April 30, May 1, 1968.

30. Lewis Chester, Godfrey Hodgson, and Bruce Page, *An American Melodrama: The Presidential Campaign of 1968* (New York: Viking Press, 1969), 516–19, 521; James T. Patterson, *Grand Expectations: The United States, 1945–1974* (New York: Oxford University Press, 1996), 694. Frank Kush's *Battleground Chicago: The Police and the 1968 Democratic National Convention* (Westport, Conn.: Praeger, 2004) is more sympathetic to the Chicago police.

31. Interview with Quentin Young, Oct. 12, 2001, Chicago.

32. Ibid.; "MCHR Treats Over 1,000 in Chicago," *Health Rights News*, November 1968, 3.

33. Chester et al., *American Melodrama*, 522–23; Patterson, *Grand Expectations*, 695.

34. Quentin Young interview; "MCHR Treats Over 1,000," 3.

35. Author unknown, "Notes on a Conversation with Ruth Migdal, 16 Oct 1968," Young Papers; "MCHR Treats Over 1,000"; Jane Kennedy, "Violence in Chicago," *American Journal of Nursing* (October 1968): 2169–70.

36. Chester et al., *American Melodrama*, 582–83.

37. *New York Times,* Aug. 29, 1968.

38. Ibid.; Thomas S. Harper, M.D., " 'Affront' in Chicago," *Medical Tribune*, Sept. 19, 1968, clipping in Young Papers, Kennedy "Violence in Chicago," 2169.

39. Patterson, *Grand Expectations*, 696.

40. Godfrey Hodgson, *America in Our Time: From World War II to Nixon, What Happened and Why* (New York: Vintage Books, 1976), 372–73; Kurlansky, *1968*, 381.

41. *New York Times*, Sept. 7, 1968; Chester et al., *American Melodrama*, 600–1.

42. Chester et al., *American Melodrama*, 600–1.

43. *The Strategy of Contusion,* MCHR, press release, Sept. 10, 1968; Chester, *American Melodrama*, 603–4.

44. "Medical Records Subpoenaed," *Chicago MCHR Newsletter*, Sept. 21, 1968, 1–4.

45. Quentin Young interview; Robert Cohen, *When the Left Was Young: Student Radicals and America's First Mass Student Movement, 1929–1941* (New York: Oxford University Press, 1993), 292.

46. Quentin Young interview.

47. Ibid.; Quentin David Young, curriculum vitae, Young Papers; Quentin Young to Abner Mikva, Oct. 10, 1968, ibid.

48. "Special Supplement," *Health Rights News*, November 1968, 8. *Health Rights News* published Young's HUAC testimony in its entirety.

49. Ibid., 9–12.

50. Ibid., 19, 36, 29, 26. Young's taking the First Amendment had been a shrewd political move. Nonetheless, he did not want to be thought a Communist, which was the clear implication behind the questions he refused to answer. Before his second day of testimony he told reporters that he was not a member of the Communist

Party, and then on the witness stand said that what he told the reporters outside the committee room was true. In a sense, Young was having it both ways, refusing on principle to talk about his affiliations before the committee, while stating in public that the accusation that he was a member of the party was false.

51. Philip Shapiro's papers are housed in the Department of Special Collections in the Green Library at Stanford University.

52. Hodgson, *America in Our Time*, 302–3; interview with Richard Fine, March 28, 2002, San Francisco.

53. Paul Chaat Smith and Robert Allen Warrior, *Like a Hurricane: The Indian Movement from Alcatraz to Wounded Knee* (New York: The New Press, 1997), 1–5, 24, 61–62.

54. *Health Rights News*, April 1970; *San Francisco Examiner*, July 22, 1970, clipping; Richard Fine interview.

55. Richard Fine interview; Smith and Warrior, *Like a Hurricane*, 31, 34, 66, 108.

56. Alvin M. Josephy Jr., *Red Power: The American Indians' Fight for Freedom* (New York: American Heritage Press, 1971), 15, 144–56.

57. Smith and Warrior, *Like a Hurricane*, 200–217.

58. Ibid., 225, 233; Mary Crow Dog and Richard Erdoes, *Lakota Woman* (New York: Grove Weidenfeld, 1990), 147; Signe Waller, *Love and Revolution: A Political Memoir* (New York: Rowman and Littlefield, 2002), 497; Barbara Yippee, *Report from Wounded Knee*, March 30, 1973.

59. *Health Rights News*, Aug./Sept. 1973; excerpt from Waller diary in Waller, *Love and Revolution*, 495–98.

60. "Wounded Knee: Dear Fellow MCHR Member," n.d.

CHAPTER 9: THE YOUNG TURKS

1. Fitzhugh Mullan, *White Coat, Clenched Fist: The Political Education of an American Physician* (New York: Macmillan, 1976; Ann Arbor: University of Michigan Press, paperback ed., 2006), 153; *Washington Post, New York Times, San Francisco Chronicle*, June 17, 1968.

2. "Statement to the American Medical Association by the Medical Committee for Human Rights"; "Statement to the AMA," Bay Area Poor People's Campaign, June 16, 1968, Quentin Young Papers, State Historical Society of Wisconsin; *Washington Post*, June 17, 1968.

3. *San Francisco Chronicle*, June 16, 1968.

4. "AMA Is Challenged to Fulfill Promise on Negroes," *Medical World News*, Feb. 23, 1968, 39; *New York Times*, June 19, 1968.

5. *Medical World News*, July 19, 1968, 31–32; *New York Times*, June 18, 1968; *Philadelphia Evening Bulletin*, Dec. 3, 1968, clipping

6. *New York Times*, June 19, 1968; AMA, press release, July 11, 2008, American Medical Association Web site.

7. Walter Lear to Eli Messinger, April 1, 1970.

8. MCHR, "Financial Activity from Jan. 1, 1969 to December 31, 1969"; MCHR, "Numbers of Dues-Paying Members Based on Receipts in National Office," Feb. 14, 1969; "MCHR Financial Statement for 1970."

9. Alan Venable to Pat Lievow, Oct. 20, 1970; Larry Brilliant, statement, n.d., ca. 1970.

10. Minutes of the Governing Council, MCHR, Sept. 29–Oct. 1, 1967; Michael R. McGarvey, Fitzhugh Mullan, and Steven S. Sharfstein, "A Study in Medical Action—Student Health Organizations," *New England Journal of Medicine,* July 1968, 74–75. The best scholarly account of SHO is Naomi Rogers, "'Caution: The AMA May Be Damaging to Your Health': The Student Health Organizations (SHO) and American Medicine, 1965–1970," *Radical History Review* 80 (Spring 2001): 5–34.

11. McGarvey et al., "A Study"; interview with William Bronston, March 27, 2002, Carmichael, Calif.

12. McGarvey et al., "A Study," 75; interview with Michael McGarvey, March 30, 2001, New York.

13. William Bronston interview.

14. Michael McGarvey interview.

15. McGarvey, "A Study," 76; Michael McGarvey and William Bronston interviews.

16. McGarvey, "A Study," 76; McGarvey interview; "SHO: The Memory Lingers," *Health Rights News,* September 1971.

17. Tom Levin to Quentin Young, June 28, 1967, Young Papers; William Bronston interview; interview with Fitzhugh Mullan, Feb. 14, 2001, Bethesda, MD; *Report from the Seminar on Student Activities,* n.d., Young Papers.

18. Quentin Young to Bill Bronston and Mick McGarvey, April 26, 1967, Young Papers; Joseph Stokes Jr. to Young, May 31, 1967, ibid.; Young to Stokes, June 10, 1967, ibid.; Rogers, "Caution," 12.

19. "SHO Business: A New Role?" *Medical World News,* May 9, 1969; Pamela Osbourne, Suzan Simons, et al., *Taylor Homes Area Site Report,* n.d.; Gerald Kirk, *West Side Area Coordinator Report on 1968 Student Health Project,* n.d., 1; McGarvey, "A Study," 77.

20. "SHO Business"; Rogers, "Caution," 16.

21. Committee for Black Admissions, press release, Sept. 6, 1968; "Integration Battlefront," *Journal of the National Medical Association* (Jan. 1969): 82; Lyndon Johnson, "Address to the National Medical Association," *Journal of the National Medical Association* (Nov. 1968): 450–53.

22. Michael McGarvey interview; Sidney N. Repplier to Ned Van Dyke, July 6, 1970.

23. "Integration Battlefront," *Journal of the National Medical Association* (Sept. 1969): 377; Edmund C. Casey, "Manpower and Health Care Delivery," *Journal of the National Medical Association* (Sept. 1972): 450.

24. "SHO Business."

25. McGarvey, "A Study," 78; Larry Brilliant, "SHO Meets in Detroit," *Health Rights News,* May 1968; Fitzhugh Mullan interview. SHO members' fears of government infiltration were not unwarranted, given the record of the FBI in the 1960s and 1970s.

26. "SHO Meets in Detroit"; Michael McGarvey, Fitzhugh Mullan, and William Bronston interviews.

27. "SHO Meets in Detroit"; Rogers, "Caution," 16; Fitzhugh Mullan interview.

28. Mullan, *White Coat,* 70, 92, 91, 97; no author, "Brief History of the Lincoln Collective," n.d., ca. 1973.

29. Mullan, *White Coat*, 98; *New York Times*, Aug. 27, Dec. 21, 1970.
30. *New York Times*, Nov. 18, 1970; Mullan, *White Coat*, 102–3. See also Susan Reverby and Marsha Love, "The Emancipation of Lincoln: A Study in Institutional Organizing," *Health/PAC Bulletin*, no. 4(Jan. 1972): 1–16.
31. *New York Times*, July 15, 16, 1970; Mullan, *White Coat*, 142–44.
32. *New York Times*, Nov. 29, 1970; Mullan, *White Coat*, 166–68.
33. *New York Times*, ibid.
34. Ibid.; Mullan, *White Coat*, 169–71.
35. *New York Times*, Nov. 19, 1970, Jan. 24, July 16, 1971.
36. Mullan, *White Coat*, 176; Victor Sidel to Eli Messinger, Dec. 4, 1970; Messinger to Sidel, Dec. 30, 1970.
37. Mullan, *White Coat*, 207; interview with Susan Schnall, May 22, 2007, New York.
38. Mullan, *White Coat*, 206; "Brief History."
39. Mullan, *White Coat*, 209.
40. *Health Rights News*, April 1970, Jan. 1971.
41. Ibid., April 1970.
42. Ibid.; Dean Latimer, "What Is the Sound of One Clap Dripping?" *Realist*, Jan./Feb. 1971, 6–7; *Manhattan Tribune*, Oct. 17, 1970, clipping in June Finer's personal papers.
43. James T. Patterson, *Grand Expectations: The United States, 1945–1974* (New York: Oxford University Press, 1996), 659–60; William Chafe, *The Unfinished Journey: America Since World War II* (New York: Oxford University Press, 1986), 413.
44. Minutes of the National Executive Committee, MCHR, postscript, Dec. 7, 1969; Bruce A. Dixon, "I Remember Fred," *Black Commentator*, December 7, 2004.
45. *Health Rights News*, Feb. 1970; Minutes of the Executive Board, Philadelphia MCHR, March 2, 1970; Ann Garland, "My Opinion (Color It Black)," undated statement.
46. *Health Rights News*, Feb. 1970; Interview with Quentin Young, Sept. 29, 2006, Chicago.
47. Tom Bodenheimer, "Free Clinics: Strategy for Survival," *Health Rights News*, March 1972.

CHAPTER 10: HEALTH CARE IS A HUMAN RIGHT

1. *New York Times*, Dec. 10, 1967; H. Jack Geiger interview, Sept. 13, 2000, New York; Bonnie Lefkowitz, "The Health Center Story: Forty Years of Commitment," *Journal of Ambulatory Care Management* 28 (2005), 296. See also Lefkowitz, *Community Health Centers: A Movement and the People Who Made It Happen* (New Brunswick: Rutgers University Press, 2007).
2. Interview with John Hatch, March 13, 2002, Durham, N.C.; Lefkowitz, "Health Center Story," 295.
3. H. Jack Geiger, undated statement in author's possession.
4. John Hatch interview; interview with Josephine Disparti, March 29, 2001, New York.
5. Ibid.; Lefkowitz, "Health Center Story," 297.
6. John W. Hatch, "Community Development in a Rural Comprehensive Community Health Program," 1970, 2–5, in Delta Health Center Records #4613, Manuscripts Department, Wilson Library, University of North Carolina at Chapel Hill.

7. Interview with Robert Smith, all inteviews conducted between 2000 and 2007, Jackson, Miss; H. Jack Geiger interviews; interview with Aaron Shirley, Feb. 20, 2001, Jackson, Miss.; Mark Newman, *Divine Agitators: The Delta Ministry and Civil Rights in Mississippi* (Athens: University of Georgia Press, 2004), 176; Richard Hall, "A Stir of Hope in Mound Bayou," reprint of a 1969 *Life* article, Delta Health Center Records; Fitzhugh Mullan, "The National Health Service Corps and Health Personnel Innovations: Beyond Poorhouse Medicine," in Victor Sidel and Ruth Sidel, eds., *Reforming Medicine: Lessons of the Last Quarter Century* (New York: Pantheon, 1984), 183–88.

8. Hatch, "Community Development," 20.

9. Paul Starr, *The Social Transformation of American Medicine* (New York: Basic Books, 1982), 371; John Dittmer, *Local People: The Struggle for Civil Rights in Mississippi* (Urbana: University of Illinois Press, 1994), 383–86.

10. John Hatch interview; Newman, *Divine Agitators*, 176.

11. Lefkowitz, *Community Health Centers*, 38–39; Dittmer, *Local People*, 383.

12. John Hatch interview; H. Jack Geiger, "A Health Center in Mississippi," in Lawrence Cory et al., eds., *Medicine in a Changing Society* (St. Louis: C. V. Mosby Company, 1972), 158.

13. Geiger, "Health Center," 163.

14. Interview with L. C. Dorsey, July 9, 2002, Jackson, Miss.; "Dorsey Selected as New Director of Health Center," *Delta Democrat-Times*, Delta Health Center Records, clipping; Dorsey, "Dirt Dauber Nests, Socks Nailed over Doorways, Prayer and OTC's: Space Age Medicine in the Poor Community," 10–12, manuscript in my possession; Bruce Morgan, "Up from Mississippi," *Tufts Medicine* (Spring 2003): 17, 25.

15. Lefkowitz, "Health Center Story," 297; Starr, *Social Transformation*, 371.

16. Report of H. Jack Geiger and Count Gibson, "Action in the North," Oct. 16, 1965; H. Jack Geiger interview; Executive Committee Notes, MCHR, Dec. 13, 1965; Minutes of the National Governing Council, MCHR, Oct. 16–17, 1965.

17. H. Jack Geiger interview; interview with Desmond Callan, Jan. 16, 2001, Hillsdale, N.Y.

18. Lefkowitz, *Community Health Centers*, 27, 42–44, 54; Geiger, "The First Community Health Centers," 315.

19. Starr, *Social Transformation*, 261–66; *Time*, May 11, 1970, 60–61.

20. Starr, *Social Transformation*, 275–80; *Time*, May 11, 1970, 60–61.

21. W. Michael Byrd and Linda A. Clayton, *An American Health Care Dilemma*, vol. 2 (New York: Routledge Press, 2002), vol. 2, 240; Starr, *Social Transformation*, 283.

22. Starr, *Social Transformation*, 286–89.

23. Ibid., 384–85.

24. Ibid.

25. Walter Reuther, "The Health Care Crisis: Where Do We Go from Here?" *American Journal of Public Health* (Jan. 1969): 14–15.

26. *New York Times*, June 21, Dec. 10, 1967.

27. Ibid., July 2, 1967; *Wall Street Journal*, Feb. 7, 1968.

28. Pat Murchie to James Taylor, Dec. 1971; Luke Wilson to Quentin Young, Dec. 28, 1971; interview with Quentin Young, March 12, 2002, Chicago; MCHR, "Proposal for a 1971–72 National Program."

29. Minutes of the Executive Committee Meeting, MCHR, May 13–16, 1971.

30. Starr, *Social Transformation*, 381; Byrd and Clayton, *An American Health Care Dilemma,* vol. 2, 395.

31. Starr, *Social Transformation*, 396.

32. Starr, *Social Transformation*, 395–97; Byrd and Clayton, *An American Health Care Dilemma,* vol. 2, 306; Tom Bodenheimer, "A Radical Alternative to National Health Insurance," n.d.; Tom Bodenheimer, Steve Cummings, and Elizabeth Harding, eds., *Billions for Band-Aids: An Analysis of the U.S. Health Care System and of Proposals for Its Reform* (San Francisco: MCHR, 1972), 102.

33. Bodenheimer et al., *Band-Aids,* 107–8; Starr, *Social Transformation*, 394.

34. MCHR, "Awake Americans," leaflet; Laura Green to "Dear Friend," June 1971.

35. Bodenheimer et al., *Band-Aids,* 107–8; MCHR, "Preliminary Position Paper on National Health Care, September, 1971"; Quentin Young quoted in Gregg W. Downey, "Medical rights committee plans 'crusade for medical justice,'" *Modern Hospital* (June 1971), MCHR reprint.

36. Bodenheimer et al., *Band-Aids,* table of contents; interview with Thomas Bodenheimer, March 29, 2002, San Francisco.

37. Thomas Bodenheimer interview; "Resolution on MCHR National Health Proposal," MCHR National Convention, April 18, 1971.

38. Thomas Bodenheimer interview; Bodenheimer quoted in Gregg W. Downey, typewritten transcription of an interview, copy in Quentin Young Papers, State Historical Society of Wisconsin; Downey, "Medical rights committee"; MCHR, "A Proposal for a National Health Care Plan."

39. Bill Bruzzone to Thomas Bodenheimer, July 21, 1971; Lefkowitz, *Community Health Centers,* 27; Thomas Bodenheimer and Quentin Young (March 12, 2000) interviews.

40. Howard Levy and Ronda Kotelchuck, "MCHR: An Organization in Search of an Identity," *Health/PAC Bulletin*, no. 63 (March/April 1975): 18–21; *Congressional Record*, Dec. 17, 1971, vol. 117; Shirley Chisholm to "Dear Friend," Nov. 10, 1971.

41. MCHR Occupational Health Project, *Health Hazards in the Workplace* (Chicago: MCHR, 1972).

42. Greg Downey, "Occupational Health Issue May Be Rallying Point for Doctors and Unions," *Modern Hospital* (Feb. 1973): 39–40.

43. Ibid.; Howard Levy and Ronda Kotelchuck, "MCHR," 20.

44. MCHR, *Report of the NEC Meeting,* Sept. 2–4, 1972; *Occupational Health Project Report,* June 1972, 11, and June 1973, 5.

45. Walter Lear to Roxanne Jones, Oct. 13, 1970; "Statement of the Medical Committee for Human Rights on Lead Poisoning in Children," Sept. 17, 1970; "Sickle Cell Anemia Program," *MCHR Organizational Newsletter,* Aug. 19, 1971.

46. Tom Wicker, *A Time to Die* (New York: Quadrangle Press, 1975), 314; "Proposal for a National Prison Health Program within the Medical Committee for Human Rights," n.d.

47. "Abortion," *Health Rights News*, Aug. 1973; "Abortion Law Reform Urged by Physicians Group," MCHR, press release, May 10, 1967; Malika McCray, "Radical Health Activism: The Boston Chapter of the Medical Committee for Human

Rights, 1964–1981" (master's thesis, Tufts University, 2007), 92–93; interview with Quentin Young, Oct. 12, 2001, Chicago.

48. Interview with William Bronston, May 27, 2002, Carmichael, Calif.; interview with Susan Schnall, May 22, 2007, New York; "Council of Health Organizations Statement on Drug Abuse," n.d.; Memorandum to the National Executive Committee Re: Patients' Rights Grant, by Susan Schnall and Jackie Kelly, n.d.; "Resolutions—From Gay Caucus," April 27–30, 1972; interview with Walter Lear, Oct. 21, 2000, Philadelphia.

CHAPTER 11: YEARS OF DECLINE

1. "Statement of the Women's Caucus—MCHR National Convention," 1971; Kotelchuck and Levy, "MCHR: An Organization in Search of an Identity," *Health/PAC Bulletin*, no. 63 (March/April 1975): 17; *Guardian*, July 14, 1971; interview with Susan Schnall, May 22, 2007, New York.
2. Kotelchuck and Levy, ibid.; Pat Murchie to Julian White, Feb. 15, 1972.
3. "Health Radicals: Crusade to Shift Medical Power to the People," *Science*, Aug. 6, 1971, 506; Quentin Young to "Dear MCHR Activist," Nov. 29, 1972; Frank Goldsmith, *Organizational Report,* Aug. 19, 1971; *MCHR Organizational Newsletter,* Oct. 29–31, 1971.
4. Patricia Murchie to MCHR New York Chapter, Sept. 25, 1971; Quentin Young to MCHR New York Chapter, Oct. 15, 1971; Helena van Raan to Frank Goldsmith, Dec. 8, 1971; Kotelchuck and Levy, "MCHR," 24.
5. MCHR New York Chapter to Quentin Young, May 25, 1972; Ann Garland and Gwen Smith to "National Executive Committee, New York Chapter and all MCHR Chapters," June 1, 1972; Kotelchuck and Levy, "MCHR," 24; interview with Eli Messinger, March 25, 2001, New York.
6. *Health Rights News*, Dec. 1972.
7. Kotelchuck and Levy, "MCHR," 25; "Proposed Budget—June 1, 1972 to May 31, 1973," n.d.; Minutes of the NEC meeting, June 9–10, 1973, Medical Committee for Human Rights (hereafter cited as Minutes, NEC). *Health Rights News,* December 1972; Minutes, NEC, Oct. 21–23, 1973.
8. Kotelchuck and Levy, "MCHR," 23; Quentin Young to Ronda Kotelchuck and Howard Levy, April 2, 1975; interview with Peter Orris, June 19, 2007, Chicago.
9. *Health Rights News*, April 1973; Minutes, NEC, June 9–10, 1973.
10. Minutes, NEC, June 9–10, 1973; *Report of the MCHR Regional Meeting in Boston,* Oct. 6–7, 1973.
11. Minutes, NEC, Oct. 21–23, 1973; Susan Schnall and Peter Orris interviews.
12. "MCHR: A Power to Reckon Without," *Medical World News*, May 10, 1973, 19; *Health Rights News*, Sept. 1972, clipping.
13. "What Is the Revolutionary Union?" n.d.; Activist Caucus to "Dear Health-PAC," n.d., ca. 1975.
14. "Dear Health-PAC."
15. Susan Schnall interview.
16. "Dear Health-PAC"; *American Medical,* May 19, 1975, 1; Young to Kotelchuck and Levy, April 2, 1975; Proposed Agenda, MCHR 12th Annual Convention,

Freeport, Illinois, n.d.; Activist Caucus, "Summary of the May 9–11, 1975, National MCHR Convention" (hereafter cited as "Summary").

17. Jim Ferlo, "MCHR Pre-NEC Meeting," Oct. 12, 1975.

18. "Summary"; MCHR Pittsburgh Chapter, "Statement on the Crisis of MCHR's National Leadership and National Office," Oct. 17, 1975; Susan Schnall, Marty Schiffer, Peter Schnall, Paul Geffner, and Joe Pissarevsky, "Position Paper on 1976 MCHR Convention," n.d.

19. "Draft Criticism of the Role of the Revolutionary Communist Party (RCP) and the Forces Aligned with It in the Medical Committee for Human Rights," submitted by several Boston members of the Activist Caucus, May 4, 1976; "Statement from Durham-Chapel Hill MCHR: Decision to Withdraw from National MCHR," n.d., ca. July 1977.

20. National Committee to Overturn the Bakke Decision, "Fight Racism, Overturn the Bakke Decision," n.d.

21. Ibid.; Jim Ryan and Ed Bernstein to "Dear Friends," April 9, 1978.

22. Peter Moyer, untitled campaign statement, 1978; MCHR New York Chapter Steering Committee to "Dear Friends," May 20, 1978; "Call to a Conference on the Bakke Case," n.d.

23. Steering Committee to "Dear Friends," May 20, 1978; *Revolution*, Jan. 1978, clipping.

24. *MCHR Interchapter Newsletter*, n.d.; James T. Patterson, *Restless Giant: The United States from Watergate to Bush v. Gore* (New York: Oxford University Press, 2005), 31.

25. *Guardian*, Oct. 11, 1978; "Norman Bethune Caucus Expelled," *MCHR News*, Fall 1979, clipping.

26. *Report from MCHR National Meeting*, Oct. 19, 1980; Peter Marshall to "Dear Friend," Jan. 8, 1981.

CODA

1. Fitzhugh Mullan, *White Coat, Clenched Fist: The Education of an American Physician* (New York: Macmillan, 1976; Ann Arbor: University of Michigan Press, 2006, paperback ed.), 20–22; Signe Waller, *Love and Revolution: A Political Memoir* (New York: Rowman and Littlefield, 2002), 25–26.

2. Waller, *Love and Revolution*, 26–27; Mike Dooley, "Jim Waller, M.D.," *MCHR News*, Spring 1980, 17.

3. Waller, *Love and Revolution*, 30, 61–66, 76–77; Jean Sharpe and Yonni Chapman to Walter Lear, Nov. 22, 1976. The material that follows comes from Signe Waller's memoir, *Love and Revolution*, 27–31, 85, 196–99, 224–27.

4. *Health Rights News*, Spring 1980, 17. In a civil suit filed in 1985, a jury found the defendants liable for the wrongful death of Mike Nathan, and awarded $351,500 to his widow, Marty, and their daughter. She shared the settlement with the other victims, and started the Greensboro Justice Fund, of which she is executive director. Waller, *Love and Revolution*, 461; Greensboro Truth and Reconciliation Commission, Public Hearing #3, testimony of Dr. Martha Nathan, Sept. 30, 2005, http://www.greensborotrc.org/.

5. "Grand Opening and Dedication, the Desmond Callan Community Health Center, November 3, 2006," program notes, copy in my possession.
6. *New York Times*, Dec. 25, 2008.
7. Interview with Thomas Bodenheimer, March 29, 2002, San Francisco.

AFTERWORD: THE MCHR LEGACY

1. The biographical material that follows comes from my interviews, from obituaries, Internet sources, and from *Health Care Is a Human Right: A Collection of Biographies of the Medical Committee for Human Rights (MCHR)*, privately printed in 1997.
2. "Grand Opening and Dedication, the Desmond Callan Community Health Center, November 3, 2006," program notes, copy in my possession.
3. *New York Times*, Feb. 15, 2005.
4. Thomas Bodenheimer, "Primary Care—Will It Survive?" *New England Journal of Medicine* 355 (Aug. 31, 2006): 861–64.
5. Interview with Robert Smith, all interviews conducted between 2000 and 2007, Jackson, Miss.; interview with James Anderson, July 12, 2001, Jackson, Miss.; Bonnie Lefkowitz, *Community Health Centers: A Movement and the People Who Made It Happen* (New Brunswick: Rutgers University Press, 2007), 40–41; interview with Aaron Shirley, Sept. 11, 2007, Jackson, Miss.
6. Lefkowitz, *Community Health Centers*, 43–45; interview with H. Jack Geiger, March 28, 2001, New York.
7. Lefkowitz, *Community Health Centers*, 43–45; Aaron Shirley interview.
8. Lefkowitz, *Community Health Centers*, 43–45; Jackson Medical Mall Foundation, "Mall Growth and Development," www.jacksonmedicalmall.org/history.html.
9. Robert Smith interview; Mississippi Primary Health Care Association, Health Center Fact Sheet, Jan. 12, 2007; Lefkowitz, *Community Health Centers*, 46.

Index